GASTROENTEROLOGY AND HEPATOLOGY

The Comprehensive Visual Reference

GASTROENTEROLOGY AND HEPATOLOGY

The Comprehensive Visual Reference

series editor
Mark Feldman, MD

Southland Professor and Vice Chairman
Department of Internal Medicine
University of Texas Southwestern
    Medical Center at Dallas

Chief, Medical Service
Veterans Affairs Medical Center
Dallas, Texas

volume 7
Small Intestine

volume editor
Lawrence R. Schiller, MD, FACP, FACG

Clinical Associate Professor
Department of Internal Medicine
University of Texas Southwestern Medical Center
Baylor University Medical Center
Dallas, Texas

With 19 contributors

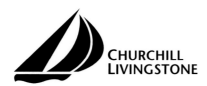

**CHURCHILL
LIVINGSTONE**

Developed by Current Medicine, Inc.
Philadelphia

Current Medicine, Inc.

400 Market Street
Suite 700
Philadelphia, PA 19106

Managing Editor	*Lori J. Bainbridge*
Development Editors	*Ira D. Smiley and Raymond Lukens*
Editorial Assistant	*Scott Thomas Hurd*
Art Director	*Paul Fennessy*
Design and Layout	*Robert LeBrun*
Illustration Director	*Ann Saydlowski*
Illustrators	*Liz Carrozza, Beth Starkey, Larry Ward, Lisa Weischedel, and Debra Wertz*
Typesetting	*John Tomcavage*
Production	*Lori Holland*
Indexer	*Maria Coughlin*

Small intestine / Lawrence R. Schiller, volume editor.
p. cm. — (Gastroenterology and hepatology: v. 7)
Includes bibliographical references and index.
ISBN 0-443-07865-3
1. Intestine, Small—Diseases—Atlases. I. Schiller, Lawrence R., 1951- . II. Series.
[DNLM: 1. Intestine, Small—atlases. 2. Intestinal Diseases—atlases. 1996 A-754 /
WI 17 G257 1997 v. 7]
RC860.S63 1997
616.3'4—dc21
DNLM/DLC
for Library of Congress
97-5655
CIP

Library of Congress Cataloging-in-Publication Data
ISBN 0-443-07865-3

Printed in Singapore by Imago Productions (FE) Pte Ltd.

10 9 8 7 6 5 4 3 2 1

DISTRIBUTED WORLDWIDE BY CHURCHILL LIVINGSTONE, INC.

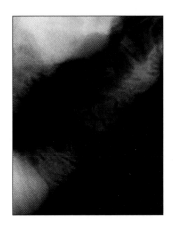

Series Preface

In recent years dramatic developments in the practice of gastro-enterology have unfolded, and the specialty has become, more than ever, a visual discipline. Advances in endoscopy, radiology, or a combination of the two, such as endoscopic retrograde cholangiopancreatography and endoscopic ultrasonography, have occurred in the past 2 decades. Because of advanced imaging technology, a gastroenterologist, like a dermatologist, is often able to directly view the pathology of a patient's organs. Moreover, practicing gastroenterologists and hepatologists can frequently diagnose disease from biopsy samples examined microscopically, often aided by an increasing number of special staining techniques. As a result of these advances, gastroenterology has grown as rapidly as any subspecialty of internal medicine.

Gastroenterology and Hepatology: The Comprehensive Visual Reference is an ambitious 8-volume collection of images that pictorially displays the gastrointestinal tract, liver, biliary tree, and pancreas in health and disease, both in children and adults. The series is comprised of 89 chapters containing nearly 4000 images accompanied by legends. The images in this collection include not only traditional photographs but also charts, tables, drawings, algorithms, and diagrams, making this collection much more than an atlas in the conventional sense. Chapters are authored by experts selected by one of the eight volume editors, who carefully reviewed each chapter within their volume.

Disorders of the gastrointestinal tract, liver, biliary tree, and pancreas are common in children and adults. *Helicobacter pylori* gastritis is the most frequent bacterial infection of humans and is a risk factor for peptic ulcer disease and gastric malignancies. Colorectal carcinoma is the second leading cause of cancer mortality in the United States, with nearly 60,000 deaths in 1990. Pancreatic cancer resulted in an additional 25,000 deaths. Liver disease is also an important cause of morbidity and mortality, with more that 25,000 deaths from cirrhosis alone in 1990. Gallstone disease is also common in our society, with increasing reliance on laparoscopic cholecystectomy in symptomatic individuals. Inflamma-tory bowel diseases (ulcerative colitis, Crohn's disease) are also widespread in all segments of the population; their causes still elude us.

The past few decades have also witnessed striking advances in the therapy of gastrointestinal disorders. Examples include "cure" of peptic ulcer disease by eradicating *H. pylori* with antimicrobial agents, healing of erosive esophagitis with proton pump inhibitor drugs, remission of chronic viral hepatitis B or C with interferon-α2b, and hepatic transplantation for patients with fulminant hepatic failure or end-stage liver disease. Therapeutic endoscopic techniques have proliferated that ameliorate the need for surgical procedures. Endoscopic advances include placement of peroral endo-scopic gastrostomy tubes for nutritional support, insertion of stents in the bile duct or esophagus to relieve malignant obstruction, and the use of injection therapy, thermal coagulation, or laser therapy to treat bleeding ulcers and other lesions, including tumors. *Gastroenterology and Hepatology: The Comprehensive Visual Reference* will cover these advances and many others in the field of gastroenterology.

I wish to thank a number of people for their contributions to this series. The dedication and expertise of the other volume editors—Willis Maddrey, Rick Boland, Paul Hyman, Nick LaRusso, Roy Orlando, Larry Schiller, and Phil Toskes—was critical and most appreciated. The nearly 100 contributing authors were both creative and generous with their time and teaching materials. And special thanks to Abe Krieger, President of Current Medicine, for recruiting me for this unique project, and to his talented associates at Current Medicine.

The images contained in this 8-volume collection are available in print as well as in slide format, and the series is soon being formatted for CD-ROM use. All of us who have participated in this ambitious project hope that each of the 8 volumes, as well as the entire collection, will be useful to physicians and health professionals throughout the world involved in the diagnosis and treatment of patients of all ages who suffer from gastrointestinal disorders.

Mark Feldman, MD

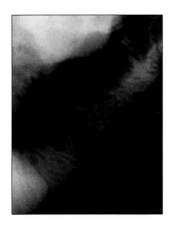

Volume Preface

The small intestine is small in diameter. As the longest segment of the gastrointestinal tract, and with the greatest absorptive surface area of any organ in the body, the small intestine is the indispensable point of entry for all nourishment that sustains life. As the biggest interface with our environment, it has a vital, and as yet incompletely understood, role in the immune system and host defenses.

Diseases of the small intestine can have devastating effects on the body. They may be difficult to evaluate and manage, often present only when advanced, and can produce widespread manifestations. A proper appreciation of these disorders is rooted in knowledge of the normal structure and function of the small intestine and the alterations caused by disease. Indeed, such knowledge is the basis for most of the diagnostic tests and therapies for small-bowel problems.

In this volume the authors describe the elegant physiology that allows the intestine to do its vital work and the disturbances that accompany dysfunction. The evaluation and management of many important diseases are presented in depth. Driven by the figures and tables provided, each author has included detailed legends that enlightens the reader and enriches one's understanding of disorders of the small intestine. Although not a replacement for a comprehensive text-book, this collection will make familiar concepts more accessible and the esoteric more familiar. Careful study of the figures, tables, and legends will enhance anyone's insight about this area of gastroenterology.

An effort of this magnitude requires the attention of many individuals. The authors of each chapter spent countless hours finding photographs and figures, designing new illustrations, and writing succinct legends for this volume. What seems quite smooth took many rewrites to get right. I appreciate their dedication to this task and their compliance with my requests. The staff and managers at Current Medicine provided expert advice on layout and design and are responsible for the clean, legible style of this volume. Finally, I would like to thank the series editor, Mark Feldman, for his counsel and suggestions throughout the production process. He read every word, looked at every figure and table, and helped to make this volume first-rate.

Although every effort was made to make this volume comprehensive and topical, I have no doubt that some readers will feel that we have missed illustrating one or more subjects of interest. I urge these readers to contact me with their suggestions so that future editions can correct these deficiencies.

Lawrence R. Schiller, MD

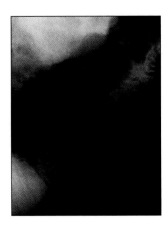

Contributors

Ralph A. Giannella, MD
Mark Brown Professor of Medicine
Department of Internal Medicine
University of Cincinnati
Cincinnati, Ohio

William Hutson, MD
Assistant Professor
Department of Medicine
University of Pittsburgh School of Medicine
University of Pittsburgh Medical Center
Pittsburgh, Pennsylvania

Samuel Klein, MD
Professor
Department of Internal Medicine
Washington University School of Medicine
Barnes-Jewish Hospital
St. Louis, Missouri

Edward L. Lee, MD
Professor
Department of Pathology
Department of Veterans Affairs North Texas
    Health Care System
University of Texas Southwestern Medical Center
Dallas, Texas

Gordon D. Luk, MD
Chief, Gastroenterology
Department of Veterans Affairs Medical Center
Dallas, Texas

Eamonn M.M. Quigley, MD, FRCP
Associate Professor
Department of Internal Medicine
University of Nebraska
University Hospital
Omaha, Nebraska

Francisco C. Ramirez, MD
Assistant Professor of Clinical Medicine
Department of Medicine
University of Arizona
Associate Chair of Medicine for Gastroenterology
Carl T. Hayden VA Medical Center
Phoenix, Arizona

James C. Reynolds, MD
Professor of Medicine
Chief, Division of Gastroenterology and Hepatology
Allegheny University of the Health Sciences
Philadelphia, Pennsylvania

Arvey I. Rogers, MD
Professor
Department of Medicine
University of Miami
Veterans Affairs Medical Center
University of Miami Hospital and Clinics
Jackson Memorial Hospital
Miami, Florida

Charles M. Rosen, MD
Instructor of Clinical Medicine
Department of Medicine
University of Miami
Mount Sinai Medical Center
Miami, Florida

David B. Sachar, MD, FACP
The Dr. Burrill B. Crohn Professor of Medicine
Mount Sinai School of Medicine of the
    City University of New York
Director of the Dr. Henry D. Janowitz Division
    of Gastroenterology
The Mount Sinai Hospital
New York, New York

Ellen J. Scherl, MD
Assistant Attending
Department of Medicine
Mount Sinai Medical School
Mount Sinai Hospital
New York, New York

Lawrence R. Schiller, MD, FACP
Clinical Associate Professor
Department of Internal Medicine
University of Texas Southwestern Medical Center
Baylor University Medical Center
Dallas, Texas

Joseph H. Sellin, MD
Professor
Department of Internal Medicine/Gastroenterology
University of Texas, Houston
The Digestive Disease Center of Houston
Houston, Texas

Herbert J. Smith, MD
Professor of Radiology
Department of Veterans Affairs
    North Texas Health Care System
University of Texas Southwestern Medical School
Dallas, Texas

Atsushi Sugitani, MD
Clinical Fellow
Department of Transplant Surgery
University of Pittsburgh Medical Center
Pittsburgh, Pennsylvania

Robert W. Summers, MD
Professor of Internal Medicine
Department of Internal Medicine
University of Iowa College of Medicine
University of Iowa Hospitals and Clinics
Iowa City, Iowa

Javier Tabasco-Minguillan, MD
Assistant Professor of Medicine
Division of Transplantation Medicine
University of Pittsburgh Medical Center
Pittsburgh, Pennsylvania

Henrik Westergaard, MD
Associate Professor
Department of Internal Medicine
University of Texas Southwestern
    Medical Center
Parkland Hospital
Dallas, Texas

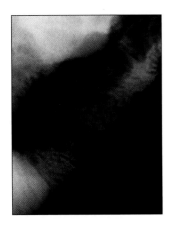

Contents

Chapter 1

Functional Anatomy, Fluid, and
  Electrolyte Absorption

JOSEPH H. SELLIN

Functional Anatomy 1.2
General Principles of Mucosal Transport 1.5
Heterogeneity of Transport Function 1.10
Regulation of Mucosal Transport 1.11
Intracellular Regulation 1.13
Abnormal Regulation Producing Disease: Cholera .1.14

Chapter 2

Nutrient Digestion and Absorption

HENRIK WESTERGAARD

Diet Composition 2.2
Cephalic Phase 2.2
Gastric Phase 2.4
Lipid Digestion and Absorption 2.8
Carbohydrate Digestion and Absorption 2.11
Protein Digestion and Absorption 2.12
Micronutrient Absorption 2.15

Chapter 3

Small-Bowel Motility

ROBERT W. SUMMERS

Anatomy 3.2
The Small Intestinal Nervous System 3.7
Intrinsic Innervation 3.9
Fluid Flow and Motility in the Intestine 3.11

Chapter 4

Secretory Diarrhea

LAWRENCE R. SCHILLER

General Features of Secretory Diarrheas 4.2
Differential Diagnosis of Secretory Diarrhea 4.4
Specific Syndromes of Secretory Diarrhea 4.5
VIPoma 4.15
Other Tumors Producing Circulating Secretagogues 4.16
Nonspecific Treatment 4.22

Chapter 5
Nutrient Malabsorption
SAMUEL KLEIN

Classification 5.2
Premucosal Disease 5.2
Mucosal Disease 5.6
Postmucosal Disease 5.15
Evaluation of Suspected Malabsorption 5.15
Nutritional Therapy Complications 5.19

Chapter 6
Gastric and Small Intestinal Motility Disorders
EAMONN M.M. QUIGLEY

Evaluation of Gastric and Small Intestinal Motility—Current Status 6.2
Clinical Disorders 6.7
Management 6.16

Chapter 7
Crohn's Disease of the Small Intestine
ELLEN J. SCHERL AND DAVID B. SACHAR

Anatomic Pathology 7.2
Clinical Pathologic Correlation: Disease Patterns 7.7
Clinical Pathophysiology Related to Small-Bowel Disease 7.9
(Clinical) Natural History 7.10
Diagnosis 7.11
Differential Diagnosis: Problems of Identity 7.11
Epidemiology and Risk Factors 7.14
Etiology 7.14
Therapy 7.15
Surgical Treatment and Postoperative Recurrence 7.19

Chapter 8
Neoplastic Diseases
GORDON D. LUK, HERBERT J. SMITH, AND EDWARD L. LEE

Epidemiology, Pathogenesis, and Presentation .8.2
Adenomas and Adenocarcinomas 8.4
Carcinoid Tumors 8.7
Lymphoma 8.8
Stromal Tumors 8.9
Other Tumors and Masses 8.11

Chapter 9

Small-Bowel Bleeding

FRANCISCO C. RAMIREZ

Clinical Presentation and Evaluation of Small-Bowel Hemorrhage 9.1
Causes of Small-Bowel Hemorrhage 9.2
Management of Small-Bowel Hemorrhage 9.2

Chapter 10

Mesenteric Vascular Insufficiency

ARVEY I. ROGERS AND CHARLES M. ROSEN

Pathophysiology 10.1
Clinical Aspects 10.2
Presentation and Treatment 10.2
Anatomy 10.2
Physiology and Pathophysiology 10.5
Classification and Etiology 10.6
Clinical Syndromes 10.8

Chapter 11

Small-Bowel Transplantation

JAVIER TABASCO-MINGUILLAN, WILLIAM HUTSON, ATSUSHI SUGITANI,
    AND JAMES C. REYNOLDS

Indications and Contraindications 11.2
Operative Procedure 11.5
Complications 11.6
Follow-up and Future Directions 11.14

Chapter 12

Infections of the Intestine

RALPH A. GIANNELLA

General Aspects of Infectious Diarrhea 12.2
Pathogenesis of Infectious Diarrhea 12.3
Cholera 12.5
Escherichia coli 12.6
Salmonella 12.9
Shigella 12.10
Campylobacter 12.11
Yersinia enterocolitica 12.12
Clostridium difficile 12.12
Food Poisoning 12.14
Traveler's Diarrhea 12.14
Sexually Transmitted Enteric Infections 12.15
Giardiasis 12.16
Entamoeba histolytica 12.17
Cryptosporidium 12.17
Microsporidia 12.18
Cytomegalovirus 12.18

Index I.1

Chapter 1

Functional Anatomy, Fluid, and Electrolyte Absorption

JOSEPH H. SELLIN

The intestine performs two seemingly contradictory tasks. It serves as a barrier to the hostile luminal environment, but at the same time, transports fluid, electrolytes, nutrients, and macromolecules across the barrier. Several characteristics of the intestine allow it to perform both these goals. The small intestine is a polarized epithelium with cellular and paracellular pathways across the epithelium; specific apical and basolateral cell membrane domains; characteristic electrochemical gradients across cell membrane. Significant heterogeneity exists along the small intestine, axial heterogeneity from duodenum to ileum, and vertical heterogeneity along the crypt: villus axis. This heterogeneity produces regional differences in transport function, which allows the intestine to absorb nutrients, fluid, and electrolytes in an efficient process. Mucosal transport is tightly regulated by neural, paracrine, endocrine, and immune systems, resulting in functional flexibility to meet the needs of the body.

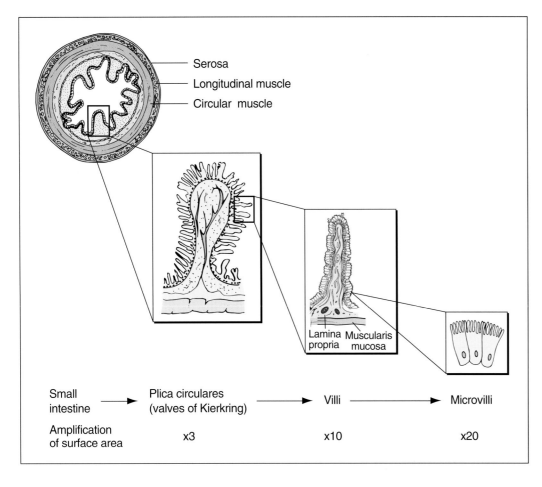

FIGURE 1-1.

Functional design of the small intestine: amplification of surface area. The anatomy of the small intestine is designed to amplify the surface area, thereby expanding the interface of luminal contents with enterocytes. The microvillus membrane has a surface area 600-fold larger than a simple cylinder with the diameter of the small intestine.

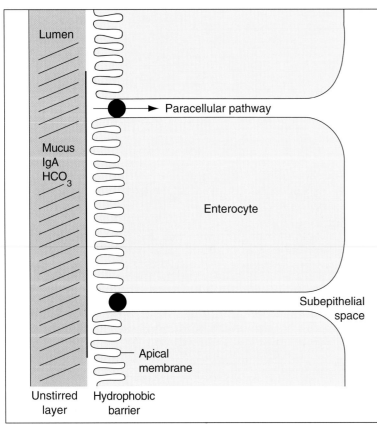

FIGURE 1-2.

Barrier function. The intestine is designed to provide a barrier separating the hostile, variable environment of the intestinal lumen from the carefully controlled subepithelial space. There are several components to the barrier. Secreted mucus, immunoglobulin A, and bicarbonate provide a unique microenvironment that protects the enterocytes. Mucus forms a viscous hydrated gel and binds bacteria. Secreted immunoglobulin A binds bacterial antigens. Bicarbonate neutralizes luminal acid. The unstirred layer is a theoretical diffusion barrier separating the bulk of the intestinal lumen from the area adjacent to the epithelium. The physiologic significance of the unstirred layer at the villus tip is uncertain, but it probably creates a functional diffusion barrier lower on the villus and into the crypt lumen. The apical membrane of the epithelial cells is the most obvious barrier. The lipid bilayer of the plasma membrane is a very high hurdle to the permeation of the hydrophilic solutes, but allows diffusion of hydrophobic molecules (*eg*, lipids). Intrinsic membrane proteins are necessary for entry of hydrophilic solutes into the cell. The paracellular pathway provides a low electrical resistance shunt around cells and blocks the movement of macromolecules around cells.

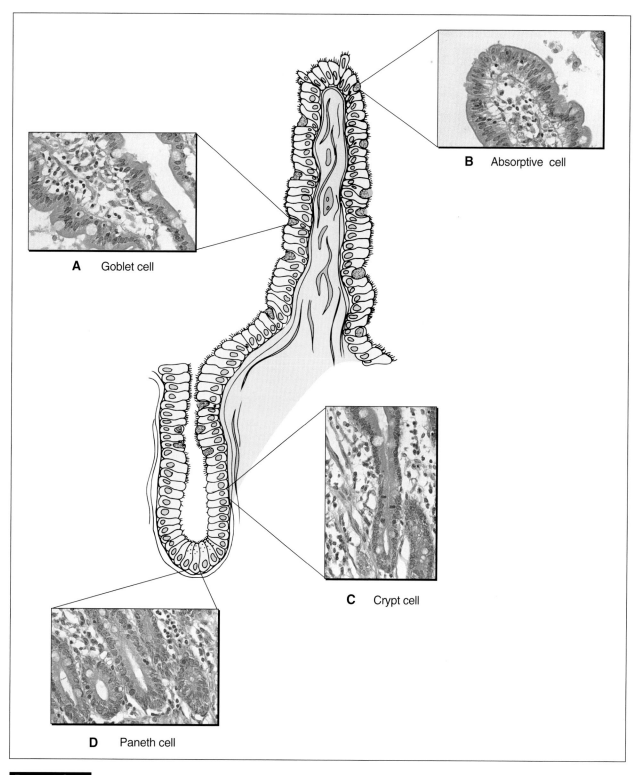

A Goblet cell

B Absorptive cell

C Crypt cell

D Paneth cell

FIGURE 1-3.

Cell types in the small intestine. Several histologically distinct cell types exist in the small intestine. There are major classifications. **A**, Goblet cells demonstrate an apical pole distended by clear mucin granules, suggesting the shape of a wine goblet. Mucus secretion most likely serves a protective role against noxious stimuli. Goblet cells are denser in the proximal compared to distal intestine, and sparser on the villus tip, with poorly developed terminal web and microvilli. **B**, Absorptive cells with well-developed microvilli, a prominent terminal web, a clear area immediately below the microvilli, enriched in cytoskeletal elements. **C**, Crypt cells are smaller, with fewer, less-developed microvilli and narrow apices.

D, Paneth cells are found in the base of the crypt. They characteristically demonstrated basophilic cytoplasm and eosinophilic secretory granules. Paneth cells are more common in the ileum than in the jejunum. The function of Paneth cells is obscure, but it probably is involved in the intestinal barrier function.

Other distinct types of cells are found in the intestine. M cells are characteristically found over Peyer's patches. They rapidly transport luminal macromolecules and some microorganisms by transcytosis. M cells represent a leak in the barrier function, but probably are also important for processing and presenting antigen to mucosal immune system. Other cell types include endocrine, caveolated, and cup cells.

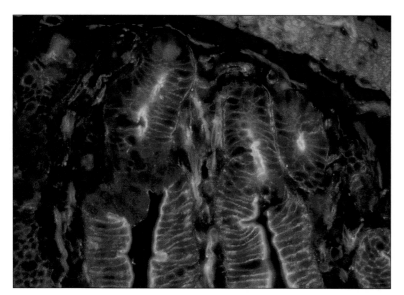

FIGURE 1-4.

Cell polarity. Apical and basolateral membranes differ structurally, in lipid composition, and in the distribution of membrane proteins. Most obviously, the apical membrane has a well-developed microvillus system that amplifies the apical surface approximately 20-fold. The basolateral membrane has no specific structural components other than those associated with junctional complexes (*see* Figure 1-6).

The apical membrane is distinct in its high content of glycosphingolipids compared with the basolateral membrane and nonpolarized cells. The ratio of glycosphingolipid:phospholipid:cholesterol is approximately 1.2:1.0:1.0 compared with the basolateral ratios of 0.4:1.0:0.5. Polarized cells accurately direct proteins to the apical or basolateral membrane. This sorting defines cell function and is necessary for vectoral transport. Proteins for nutrient absorption find their way to the apical membrane; the sodium pump must locate to the basolateral membrane. The specific mechanisms for this sorting are not fully understood.

In this photomicrograph of a small intestine from a mouse, the apical membrane is immunolabeled with phalloidin, localizing actin in red, and the basolateral protein-β catenin is labeled in green, demonstrating specific membrane domains.

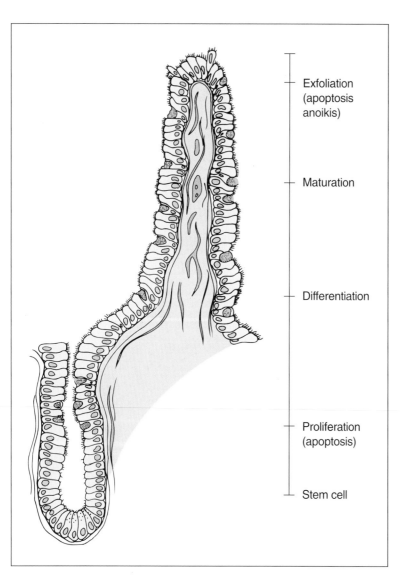

Exfoliation (apoptosis anoikis)

Maturation

Differentiation

Proliferation (apoptosis)

Stem cell

FIGURE 1-5.

Crypt dynamics. The epithelial cells of the small intestine turn over in a rapid, continuous, and coordinated process. Although not specifically identified or characterized, anchored stem cells give rise to proliferative cells of the crypt. As the cells migrate from the crypt to the villus, cells stop dividing and become more differentiated. Exfoliation occurs as mature cells are shed into the intestinal lumen. Epithelial integrity is maintained as adjacent cells appear to extend cell processes underneath the extruded cell to link with each other, thus forming new junctional complexes. Apoptosis, or programmed cell death, is integral to maintaining the cellular balance in the crypt:villus unit. Apoptosis may also serve to remove genetically abnormal cells early in the course of differentiation. In the small intestine, apoptosis has been demonstrated in the area adjacent to the presumptive stem cell. In contrast, in the colon, apoptosis occurs somewhat more distant from the stem cells, at the surface, perhaps permitting some abnormal cells to escape from apoptotic control. The mechanisms involved in exfoliation have not been clearly defined. Cells may go through the apoptotic process and then exfoliate. Alternatively, cells may lose contact with the basement membrane as a primary event and then die, a process termed *anoikis*.

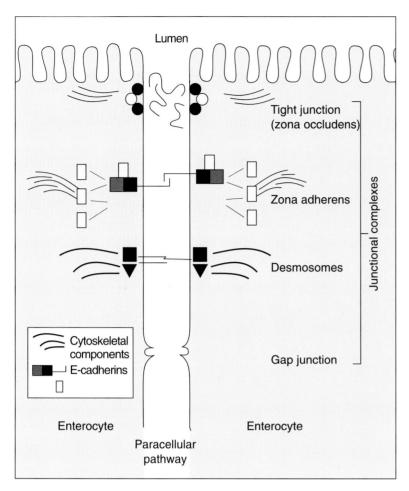

Lumen

Tight junction
(zona occludens)

Zona adherens

Junctional complexes

Desmosomes

Gap junction

Cytoskeletal
components

E-cadherins

Enterocyte

Enterocyte

Paracellular
pathway

FIGURE 1-6.

Paracellular pathway. The characteristics of the paracellular pathway are defined by specific junctional complexes that span the intercellular space. There are four types of complexes: (1) the zona occludens, or tight junction; (2) the zona adherens, or intermediate junction; (3) the desmosomes; and (4) gap junctions. Specific proteins localized to each complex link adjacent cells and the cytoskeleton. Original models of the paracellular pathway as a static barrier are being replaced by a more dynamic model in which the junctional complexes are involved in signaling and regulation, most likely through protein phosphorylation or dephosphorylation.

The tight junction is the most apical complex and is believed to control permeability across the paracellular pathway through a series of strands and grooves. Molecular definition of the specific components of the tight junction (*eg*, Z0-1, Z0-2, occludin, cingulin) may permit a clearer understanding of how the tight junction functions as a barrier for ions and macromolecules. The zona adherens is critical for cell-to-cell adhesion. Transmembrane glycoproteins (*E-cadherins*) function as cell-to-cell adhesion molecules across the zona adherens and complex with a family of proteins termed *catenins*. E-cadherin and catenins are critical for defining cell polarity. Alterations in cadherin-catenin distribution and function have been implicated in carcinogenesis. Desmosomes serve an auxiliary role in cell-to-cell adhesion. Gap junctions are important in cell-to-cell communication.

GENERAL PRINCIPLES OF MUCOSAL TRANSPORT

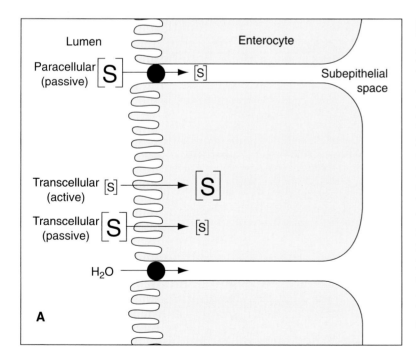

Lumen

Enterocyte

Paracellular
(passive)

Subepithelial
space

Transcellular
(active)

Transcellular
(passive)

H_2O

A

FIGURE 1-7.

A, Active and passive transport. Luminal contents face two possible pathways across the epithelium, either around the enterocytes (paracellular) or through the cells (transcellular). Paracellular transport is always passive; transcellular transport may be either passive or active. Whether movement of a particular solute is active or passive depends on chemical and electrical gradients. Chemical gradients describe the differences in concentration between two compartments (*ie*, lumen and cell). Electrical gradients refer to the potential difference across membranes. An ion such as sodium or chloride will respond to both electrical and chemical gradients whereas for uncharged particles, only a chemical gradient is relevant. Because electrical and chemical gradients for a particular ion may be either in similar or opposite directions, the sum of these forces can be calculated as an electrochemical gradient. Passive transport proceeds in the direction of the electrochemical gradient for a specific solute or ion whereas active transport involves movement against a gradient and requires the expenditure of energy. Water transport is always passive in response to osmotic forces due to the shift of solute from lumen to subepithelial space, or vice versa.

(*continued on next page*)

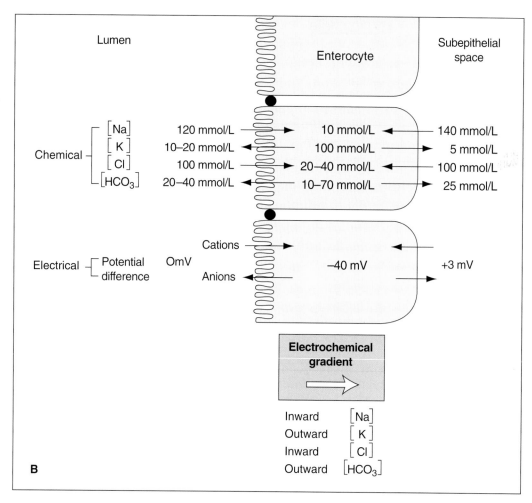

FIGURE 1-7. (CONTINUED)

B, Electrochemical driving forces across the intestinal epithelium. Electrical and chemical gradients across the apical and basolateral membranes of enterocytes determine how particular ions move into and out of cells. A favorable ("downhill") electrochemical gradient allows an ion to move passively, as in sodium's entry into the cell. An unfavorable ("uphill") electrochemical gradient necessitates the expenditure of energy (*ie*, sodium's exit from the cell). Compared with sodium, the conditions for potassium are reversed. Because of the variabilities in the methods for measurement of intracellular concentrations of anions, these tend to be less accurate than for cations.

Ion transport may be classified as electrogenic or electroneutral. Electrogenic transport implies a net transfer of charge across the epithelium; the charge may be either positive (Na) or negative (Cl). For example, electrogenic Na absorption may occur via either an Na channel or by nutrient-coupled absorption. Cl secretion is electrogenic (discussed later in this chapter). Electroneutral absorption implies either similarly directed movement of both a cation and anion (symport) or the oppositely directed movement of similarly charged ions (antiport). Sodium-hydrogen exchange is an example of electroneutral transport.

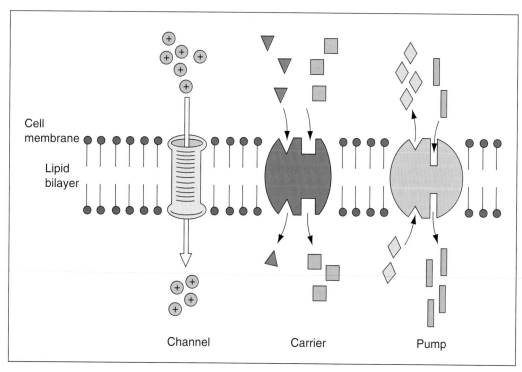

however, require specific transmembrane proteins for movement into or out of cells. There are three major types of such proteins. *Ion-specific channels* are protein pores that permit rapid passive diffusion of particular ions down an electrochemical gradient. Specific examples include the sodium channel that mediates salt absorption in the rectum and cystic fibrosis transmembrane conductance regulator (CFTR), a chloride channel involved in secretion that is defective in cystic fibrosis. *Carriers* are integral membrane proteins that carry either specific solutes or multiple ions across a membrane at a much slower rate than channels; like channels, carriers transport down an electrochemical gradient. Carriers often take advantage of the electrochemical gradient for a specific ion or solute, most frequently sodium, to transport another solute "uphill" against its gradient; this has been termed *secondary active transport*. *Pumps* are carriers that move a solute or ion against an electrochemical gradient directly linked to the expenditure of energy. The omnipresent ouabain-sensitive Na-K ATPase (Na pump) is the most familiar example.

FIGURE 1-8.

How solutes cross membranes: channels, carriers, and pumps. Nonpolar molecules may diffuse across the lipid bilayer of cell membranes. Ions, electrolytes, and charged or polar solutes,

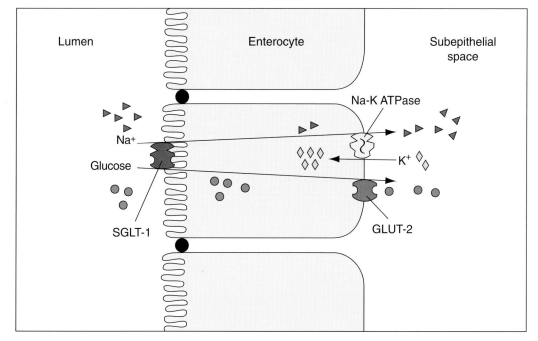

FIGURE 1-9.

Nutrient-coupled absorption of sodium. Sugars and amino acids harness the favorable electrochemical gradient for sodium entry across the apical membrane of enterocytes to drive nutrient absorption. A specific carrier (SGLT-1) with binding sites for both sodium and glucose transports both solutes into the enterocytes. Sodium is extruded across the basolateral membrane by the sodium pump (Na-K ATPase), thereby maintaining the driving force for sodium entry across the apical membrane. Glucose accumulates within the enterocyte and exits through a sodium-independent transporter (GLUT-2) that facilitates diffusion across the basolateral membrane. Similar systems for amino acid absorption are operative in the small intestine. This mechanism is present throughout the small intestine.

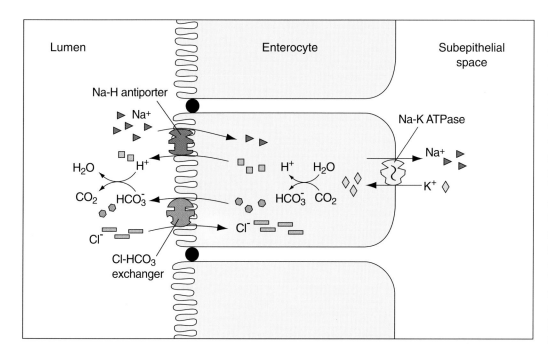

FIGURE 1-10.

Sodium-hydrogen exchange and sodium-chloride absorption. Sodium absorption in the small intestine may be nutrient-independent, but linked to chloride. Although in some species there may be a single apical carrier coupling sodium and chloride directly, in the mammalian intestine there are dual exchangers, an Na:H antiporter and a chloride:bicarbonate (HCO_3) exchanger. The electrochemical gradient for sodium across the apical membrane is critical for this. The net result of the synchronous operation of these two transporters is uptake of sodium chloride into the cell with addition of water and carbon dioxide to the lumen. The Na-H antiporter is located throughout the small intestine, but the Cl-HCO_3 exchanger is only located in the ileum. Neutral NaCl absorption is seen, therefore, only in the ileum. In the jejunum, Na-H exchange causes luminal acidification and mediates bicarbonate absorption (luminal disappearance).

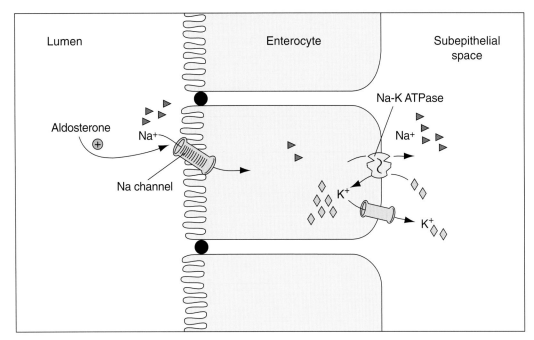

FIGURE 1-11.

Electrogenic sodium absorption: sodium channels. Sodium absorption independent of nutrients or anions typically occurs through ion-specific sodium channels in the apical membrane of enterocytes. Well-characterized amiloride-inhibitable sodium channels in the colon, responsive to mineralocorticoids are responsible for conserving colonic fluids. Less well-characterized channels in the ileum and cecum also absorb sodium. Sodium enters the cell via electrodiffusion through sodium channels and is then pumped across the basolateral membrane by the sodium pump. Electrogenic sodium absorption is responsible in part for maintenance of a lumen-negative potential difference across the gut mucosa. Potassium entering via the sodium pump is recycled out of the cell through K channels.

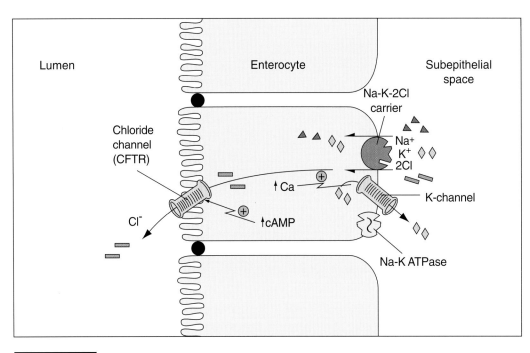

FIGURE 1-12.

Chloride secretion. Chloride is pivotal to fluid secretion in the intestine. The gut exhibits a low basal rate of chloride secretion, which can be augmented by a variety of mediators, including hormonal, neural, luminal, and inflammatory factors. The basic model of chlo-

ride secretion includes a specific basolateral entry step and apical exit step. The basolateral entry step is a single, electroneutral carrier that binds sodium, potassium, and chloride in a 1:1:2 ratio. This carrier can be inhibited by the loop diuretics, furosemide and bumetanide.

The favorable gradient for sodium entry allows potassium and chloride to accumulate within the cell. Sodium exits through the sodium pump. Chloride exits the cell through chloride channels on the apical membrane. There may be multiple chloride channels sensitive to various mediators, but one of the principal channels underlying the chloride secretion of secretory diarrheas is cystic fibrosis transmembrane conductance regulator (CFTR), the specific protein that is abnormal in cystic fibrosis. Postassium entering through the Na-K-2Cl carrier is recycled across the basolateral membrane through potassium channels. Both chloride and potassium channel regulation by second messengers like cAMP and intracellular CA^{++} modulate chloride secretion.

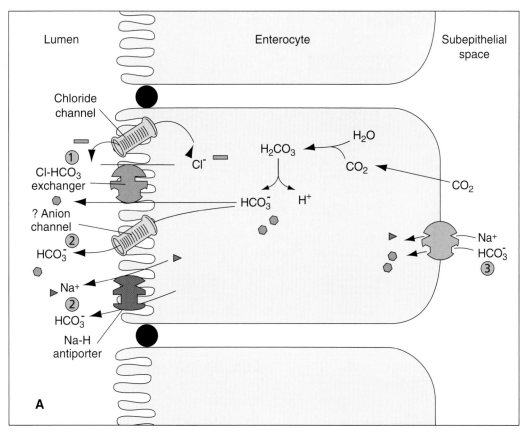

A

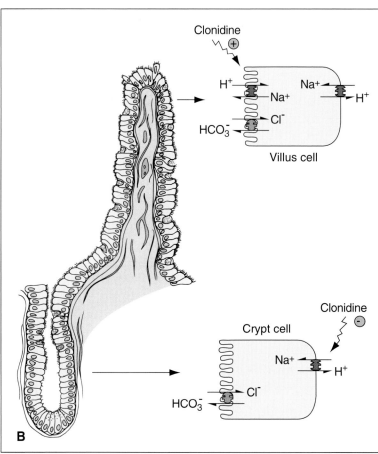

B

FIGURE 1-13.

A, Bicarbonate transport. The small intestine, particularly the ileum, secretes bicarbonate ions (HCO_3). There are multiple potential mechanisms for bicarbonate secretions: (1) HCO_3, arising either from intracellular metabolism and production or entering across the basolateral membrane, may be exchanged for chloride by the chloride-bicarbonate exchanger; chloride can be recycled via an apical chloride channel. (2) Bicarbonate may accumulate intracellularly above its electrochemical equilibrium and exit across the apical membrane through an anion channel, perhaps a chloride channel. This might be electrogenic unless balanced by absorption of an anion or secretion of a cation. (3) Na^-HCO_3 symport with varying ratios of ions may be involved in either basolateral entry or apical exit steps.

B, Alternatively, the differential expression of sodium-hydrogen and chloride-bicarbonate exchangers on the apical membrane of crypt and villus cells may account for an electroneutral component of bicarbonate secretion. Crypt cells express Na-H exchangers (NHEs) only on the basolateral membrane, creating a mechanism for electroneutral bicarbonate secretion. α-2 Adrenergic agonists, such as clonidine, have differential effects on NHEs along the crypt villus axis.

Bicarbonate absorption predominates in the jejunum and is mediated by an apical sodium-hydrogen exchanger, which results in acidification of the luminal fluid and disappearance of HCO_3 from the lumen. There may be additional mechanisms which involve HCO_3 specifically.

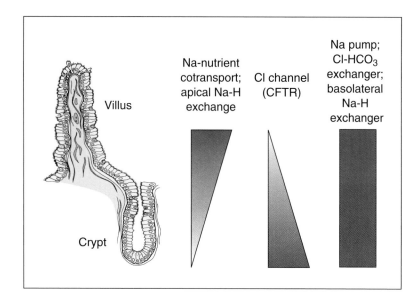

FIGURE 1-14.

Heterogeneity along the crypt villus axis. A clear evolution of expression of specific proteins is present along the crypt–villus axis that reflects (or determines) the functional capacity of cells along this axis. For example, there is an increased expression of sodium-nutrient cotransporters and apical sodium-hydrogen exchangers toward the villus tip. In contrast, cystic fibrosis transmembrane conductance regulator (CFTR), the cyclic AMP-sensitive chloride conductance, is expressed primarily in cells in the upper crypt and lower villus. This reflects the functional dichotomy between the villus (absorption) and the crypt (secretion). There are some transporters that appear to be expressed uniformly along the axis: the sodium pump, the apical chloride-bicarbonate exchanger, and the basolateral sodium-hydrogen exchanger.

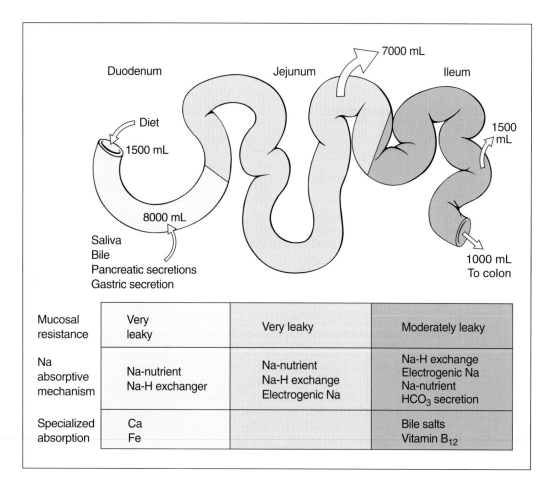

Mucosal resistance	Very leaky	Very leaky	Moderately leaky
Na absorptive mechanism	Na-nutrient Na-H exchanger	Na-nutrient Na-H exchange Electrogenic Na	Na-H exchange Electrogenic Na Na-nutrient HCO_3 secretion
Specialized absorption	Ca Fe		Bile salts Vitamin B_{12}

FIGURE 1-15.

Heterogeneity along the small intestine. Along the length of the small intestine, there are significant differences in transport function. In the upper small intestine, there is primarily an influx of fluid from oral intake, digestive secretions, and passive entry of water due to osmotic equilibration from ingestion of hypertonic foods. In the jejunum, especially during the postprandial period, fluid and electrolyte absorption occurs primarily through sodium-nutrient–coupled mechanisms. In the ileum chyme is depleted of nutrients, and sodium and water are absorbed predominantly by nutrient-independent mechanisms. If the proximal intestine is dysfunctional, the ileum compensates with more sodium-nutrient absorption. There are some regions of the intestine with specialized absorptive mechanisms for which other regions of the small intestine cannot fully compensate, such as Fe absorption in the duodenum and B_{12} absorption in the ileum.

REGULATION OF MUCOSAL TRANSPORT

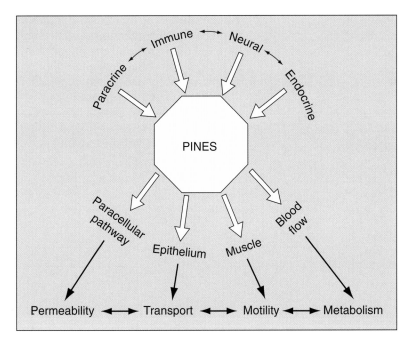

FIGURE 1-16.

Pines. The gut develops a coordinated response to environmental challenges that affects multiple elements of the epithelium beyond the enterocyte. Rather than focusing on the probably false dichotomy between motility-based or epithelial-secretory diarrheas, it is more advantageous to realize that the gut processes numerous inputs from the paracrine, immune, neural, and endocrine systems, and produces a response that may involve the epithelial cell, permeability, blood flow, and motility. In a world of lumpers and splitters, this may be an instance in which lumping is more appropriate. This regulatory system of the gut is termed *PINES*, an acronym for *p*aracrine-*i*mmuno-*n*euro-*e*ndocrine *s*ystem. An appreciation of the complex, multifaceted response that the gut exhibits during daily life is necessary for understanding the pathophysiology of diarrhea and other disorders, and employing appropriate therapies.

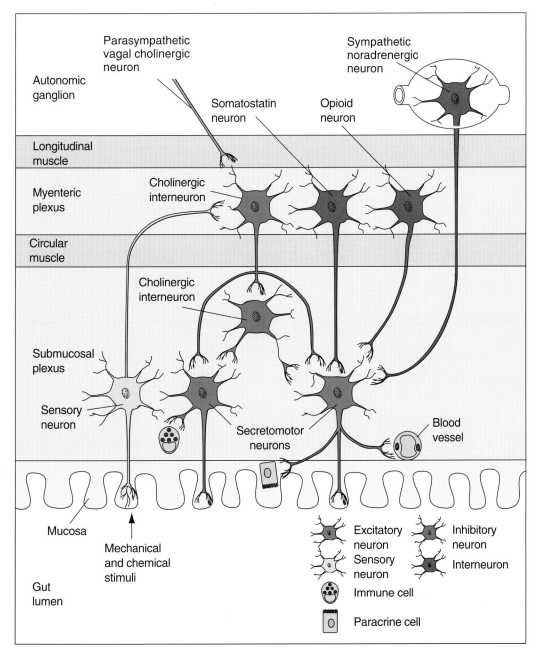

FIGURE 1-17.

Neural regulation of transport. Three divisions of the autonomic nervous system are involved in regulation of intestinal function: (1) parasympathetic, predominantly through cholinergic stimulation of secretion through vagal input; (2) adrenergic stimulation of absorption through prevertebral and sympathetic ganglia; and (3) the enteric nervous system (ENS), which integrates and coordinates the neural activity of the epithelia, vasculature, and smooth muscle. The enteric system consists of sensory neurons responsive to intraluminal stimuli, interneurons, and secretomotor neurons releasing vasoactive intestinal polypeptide and acetylcholine. Additional neural inputs and outputs modulate the function of secretory neurons and the interaction of the ENS with the smooth muscle and with immune and paracrine cells that may also influence mucosal transport.

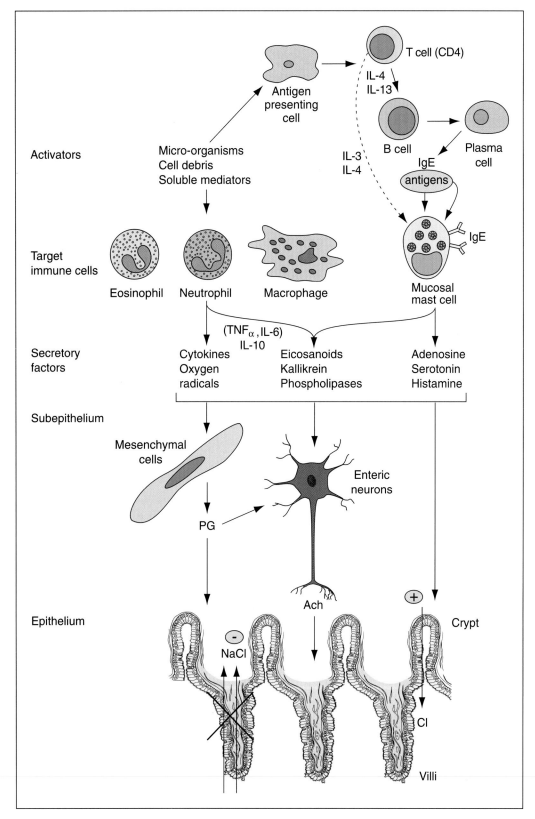

FIGURE 1-18.

Immune regulation of transport. Immune cells can be stimulated by multiple agonists originating either from the lumen (bacteria and bacterial products) and the interstitium (T cells). These intestinal immune cells release an array of secretory factors, which act either directly on the epithelium or indirectly by stimulating mesenchymal cells or enteric neurons to release prostaglandins or acetylcholine. (*Adapted from* Sellin [1]; with permission.)

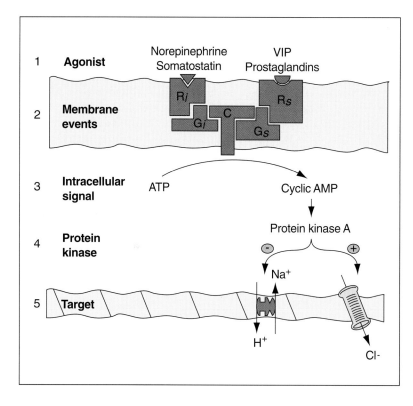

FIGURE 1-19.

Second messengers in five easy pieces, part I: cyclic nucleotides. Signaling of extracellular events and translation into appropriate cellular responses is accomplished through a complex system of second messengers. One major class of second messengers is cyclic nucleotides, including cyclic adenosine monophosphate (cAMP) and cyclic guanosine monophosphate (cGMP).

Five steps are involved in the transduction of an external signal into a change in cellular function: (1) binding of either a stimulatory or an inhibitory agonist to the appropriate receptor of the membrane-bound adenylate cyclase system. The extracellular agonist may be either a luminal secretagogue, most commonly a bacterial enterotoxin, or an endogenous factor, such as hormones or inflammatory mediators; (2) binding activates the corresponding tripartite cyclase system, including the receptor (R_i or R_s), a guanosine triphosphate (GTP)-dependent linking protein (G-protein [G_i or G_s]) and a catalytic enzyme unit (C); (3) an intracellular signal results from production of cAMP or cGMP from either adenosine triphosphate or guanosine triphosphate; (4) the increased intracellular cyclic nucleotide results in activation of specific protein kinases; (5) activated protein kinases phosphorylate target proteins, resulting in increased activity of chloride channels or inhibition of sodium-hydrogen exchangers. (*Adapted from* Sellin [1]; with permission.)

process can be modeled into five steps: (1) Neurotransmitters (*eg*, acetylcholine) or inflammatory mediators function as agonists that bind to specific membrane proteins which elicit an increase in intracellular calcium; (2) this results in activation of a G protein that stimulates phospholipase C (PLC), (3) which converts phosphoinositols (PI) to diacylglycerol and inositol triphosphate (DAG and IP_3); (4) elevated diacylglycerol in combination with phospholipids and intracellular calcium function as an intracellular signal, which activates protein kinase C, (5) which then acts on its specific target protein, modulating the activity of the sodium-hydrogen exchanger and chloride conductance.

Inositol triphosphate increases intracellular calcium by release from intracellular stores, targeting the calcium-binding protein calmodulin, which then sets in motion an alternative cascade of events leading to modulation of the target proteins: activation of Ca-calmodulin kinase.

Receptors linked directly to calcium channels (6) provide another pathway for increasing intracellular calcium (*eg*, a substance P receptor opens calcium channels, increasing intracellular calcium concentration). This leads to activation of specific protein kinases and modulation of target membrane transporters. (*Adapted from* Sellin [1]; with permission.)

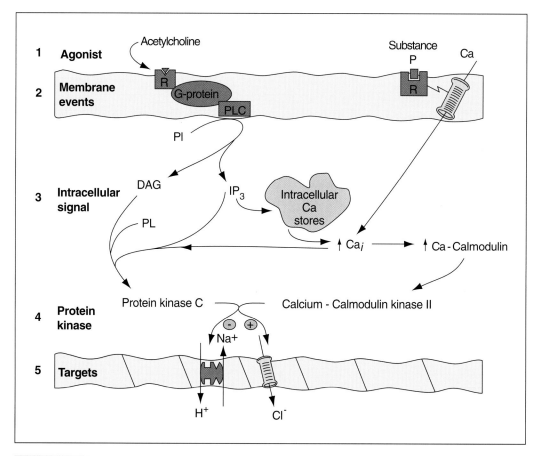

FIGURE 1-20.

Second messengers in five easy pieces, part II: calcium. The second major class of second messengers is intracellular calcium. As with cyclic nucleotides, the signal transduction

ABNORMAL REGULATION PRODUCING DISEASE: CHOLERA

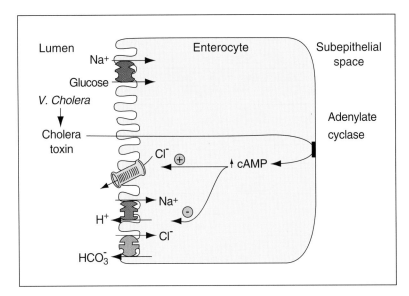

FIGURE 1-21.

Cholera: the simplified version. The intestinal response to cholera toxin has served as a paradigm of the evolving concepts of epithelial ion transport. The early models of toxin-intestinal interactions focused on the epithelial cell. Cholera toxin binds to the apical membrane, traverses the cytoplasm by unknown mechanisms, and targets adenylate cyclase, switching the catalytic unit to an unregulated "on" position by stimulating the G protein and causing a prolonged increase in intracellular cyclic adenosine monophosphate (cAMP), activating apical chloride channels, and inhibiting electroneutral sodium transport. The simultaneous inhibition of absorption and stimulation of secretion results in profound diarrhea. Na-nutrient cotransport is unaffected, providing the physiologic basis for oral rehydration therapy.

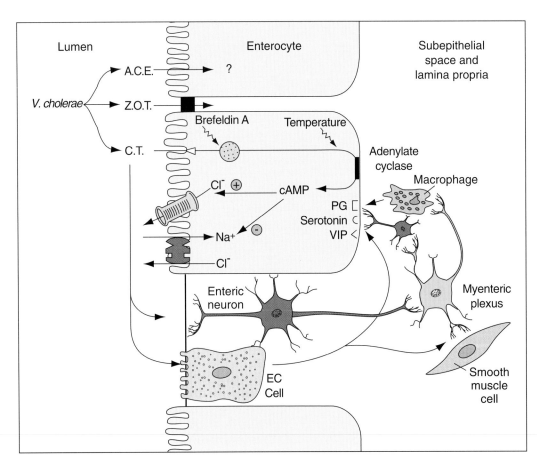

FIGURE 1-22.

Cholera: the revised version. The updated model of cholera extends beyond the enterocyte itself to include pines (the neuroimmunoendocrine system) and the intestinal smooth muscle. In addition to the classic cholera toxin (CT), two other toxins have been identified: zona occludens toxin (ZOT), which "loosens" the tight junctions, and accessory cholera toxin (ACE), the function of which is unknown. The intracellular processing of cholera toxin involves at least two discrete steps before reaching the basolateral adenylate cyclase; these steps are sensitive to either brefeldin A, an inhibitor of vesicular trafficking, or to temperature.

Cholera toxin targets both enteric neurons and endocrine cells (EC), stimulating the release of prostaglandins, serotonin, and vasoactive intestinal polypeptide, which amplify considerably the direct effects of the toxin on the enterocyte. Stimulation of the enteric nervous system by cholera toxin also significantly alters motor function. Thus, cholera toxin activates a full panoply of secretory stimuli that contribute to diarrhea.

REFERENCE

1. Sellin JH: Intestinal electrolyte absorption and secretion. In
    Gastrointestinal Disease: Pathophysiology, Diagnosis, Management, edn 5.
    Edited by Sleisenger MH, Fordtran JS. Philadelphia: W.B. Saunders;
    1993:954–976.

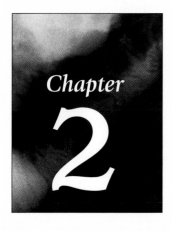

Chapter 2

Nutrient Digestion and Absorption

H E N R I K W E S T E R G A A R D

Nutrients are divided into macro- and micronutrients according to the amounts required daily. Lipids, carbohydrates, and proteins are macronutrients; their major role in the diet is to serve as energy sources to balance daily energy expenditures. Proteins, in addition, have nutritional value because they provide essential amino acids for protein synthesis, for which there is an absolute daily minimum requirement. Lipids also provide two essential fatty acids, but essential fatty acid deficiency is very rare when consuming a normal diet. Carbohydrates are nonessential and serve purely as a calorie source [1].

Vitamins, minerals, and trace elements are micronutrients. The intake and daily requirements of micronutrients range from micrograms to milligrams. A recommended daily allowance has been defined for micronutrients to ensure a sufficient daily intake to prevent development of specific micronutrient deficiency states [2].

Nutrient digestion involves a complex but highly integrated series of events that are governed by the autonomic nervous system and gastrointestinal hormones. The digestive processes can be divided into cephalic, gastric, and intestinal phases. The cephalic phase starts before food is ingested and is initiated by the thought, sight, taste, and smell of food, which stimulate salivary, gastric, and pancreatic secretions. The gastric phase involves the mechanical disruption of masticated food by gastric peristalsis (grinding) followed by limited enzymatic digestion in an acid environment. The emptying of partially digested food particles from the stomach in a sequential and regulated manner starts the intestinal phase of digestion. Gastric chyme in the duodenum releases cholecystokinin and secretin, which stimulate gallbladder emptying and pancreatic secretion of digestive enzymes and bicarbonate. Intraluminal digestion of macronutrients generates fatty acids, monoglycerides, oligosaccharides and disaccharides, and oligopeptides and amino acids. The lipolytic products are insoluble in water and require solubilization by bile acid micelles before absorption. The products of digested carbohydrate and protein are water soluble, but require further digestion by brush-border saccharidases and peptidases before absorption. Absorption of the digestive products proceeds rapidly in the proximal small intestine by passive and active transport processes. More than 95% of macronutrients are digested and absorbed before the intestinal chyme reaches the distal jejunum. The chyme then consists mainly of indigestible carbohydrate (fiber), bile acids, electrolytes, and water. Bile acids are absorbed in the ileum, and fiber is partially digested by bacterial enzymes in the colon to short-chain fatty acids, which are efficiently absorbed.

A well-balanced diet provides sufficient amounts of micronutrients to meet daily requirements [3]. Micronutrient absorption is relatively inefficient in contrast to macronutrient absorption. The absorption process of some micronutrients, such as vitamin B_{12} and calcium, has been well defined, but the precise details of the transport process for many other vitamins and trace elements still await characterization.

DIET COMPOSITION

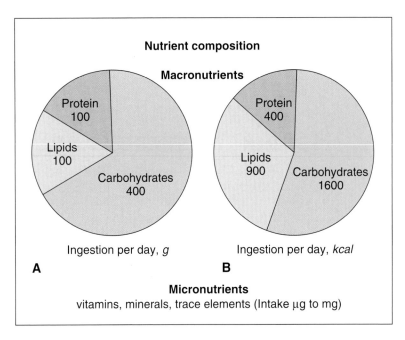

Nutrient composition

Macronutrients

Protein 100

Lipids 100

Carbohydrates 400

Ingestion per day, *g*

A

Protein 400

Lipids 900

Carbohydrates 1600

Ingestion per day, *kcal*

B

Micronutrients
vitamins, minerals, trace elements (Intake µg to mg)

Figure 2-1.

Nutrients in the diet are provided by various animal and vegetable products. The macronutrients—lipids, carbohydrates, and proteins—are complex molecules, and serve primarily as an energy source to balance energy expenditures to maintain a stable weight. In addition, lipids and proteins provide essential fatty acids and amino acids. The ingested amounts in grams (**panel A**) and kilocalories (**panel B**) per day are illustrated. The micronutrients, vitamins, minerals, and trace elements serve important roles in many metabolic processes; sufficient daily intake is essential to prevent development of states of deficiency. Nutritional guidelines have been developed to ensure adequate intake [2].

CEPHALIC PHASE

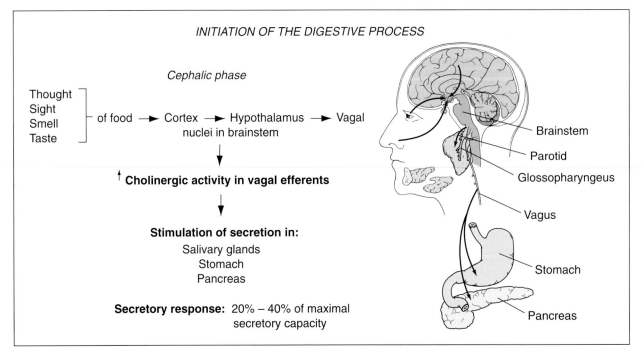

INITIATION OF THE DIGESTIVE PROCESS

Cephalic phase

Thought
Sight
Smell
Taste

of food → Cortex → Hypothalamus → Vagal
nuclei in brainstem

↑ **Cholinergic activity in vagal efferents**

Stimulation of secretion in:
Salivary glands
Stomach
Pancreas

Secretory response: 20% – 40% of maximal
secretory capacity

Brainstem

Parotid

Glossopharyngeus

Vagus

Stomach

Pancreas

Figure 2-2.

The digestive process is initiated by sensory signals elicited by the thought, sight, taste, and smell of food (cephalic phase). The signals are processed in the cortex and relayed through the hypothalamus to vagal and glossopharyngeal nuclei in the brain stem. This results in increased cholinergic activity in efferent nerves (vagus and glossopharyngeus), which supply salivary glands, stomach, and pancreas. The increase in cholinergic activity stimulates salivary, gastric, and pancreatic secretion. The secretory response is about 20% to 40% of maximal secretory capacity.

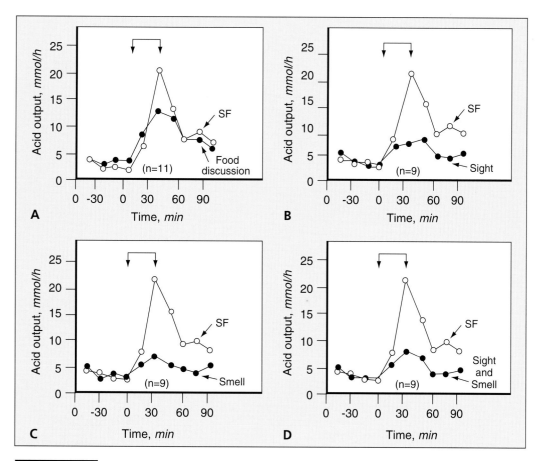

FIGURE 2-3.

A–D, The effect of discussion, sight, and smell of food on gastric acid output in mmol/hr as a function of time in normal human subjects. The acid output in response to sham feeding (SF) in the same subjects is also shown. SF consisted of being presented with an appetizing meal, chewing it thoroughly, and spitting it out without swallowing. The response to food discussions was 66% of the SF response, and the response to sight and smell was about 20% to 30% of the SF response (*From* Feldman and Richardson [4]; with permission).

TABLE 2-1. DIGESTION STARTS IN THE ORAL CAVITY

Mastication—Mechanical disruption of solid food

Increased salivary secretion—Moistening of food particles and mixing with salivary amylase, R-factors, and lingual lipase

Taste of food—Increased stimulation of gastric secretion

Swallowing of food bolus

TABLE 2-1

The oral cavity has important functions in the initial processing of solid food. Careful chewing breaks solid food into smaller pieces, which facilitates the swallowing process. The taste of food stimulates increased salivary secretion to moisten solid food and mix food with salivary amylase R-factors, and lingual lipase. [5]. The taste of food further stimulates gastric acid secretion through sensory impulses to vagal nuclei in the brain stem, which leads to increased efferent vagal activity (sham feeding response).

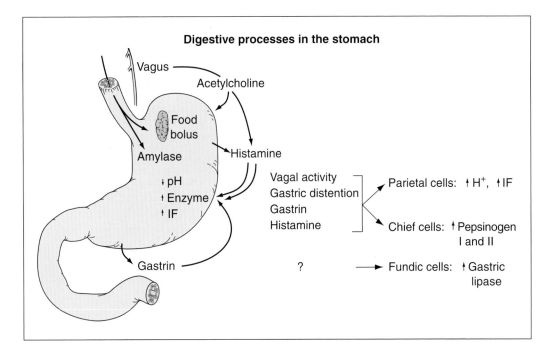

Digestive processes in the stomach

FIGURE 2-4.

The arrival of a swallowed food bolus in the stomach elicits a maximal secretory response in terms of acid and enzyme secretion. Acetylcholine from vagal efferents and intramural nerves stimulated by gastric distention histamine released from enterochromaffin-like cells, and gastrin from antral G cells stimulate acid and intrinsic factor (IF) secretion from parietal cells and pepsinogen I and II secretion from chief cells [6,7]. Gastric lipase is secreted from cells in the gastric fundus [8]. The regulatory mediators of lipase secretion have not been characterized. The three enzymes—pepsin, lipase, and amylase— attack proteins, lipids, and carbohydrates in the food bolus. The overall enzymatic breakdown of macronutrients in the stomach is about 20% to 30% of total digestion, and is primarily limited by the time food particles reside in the stomach.

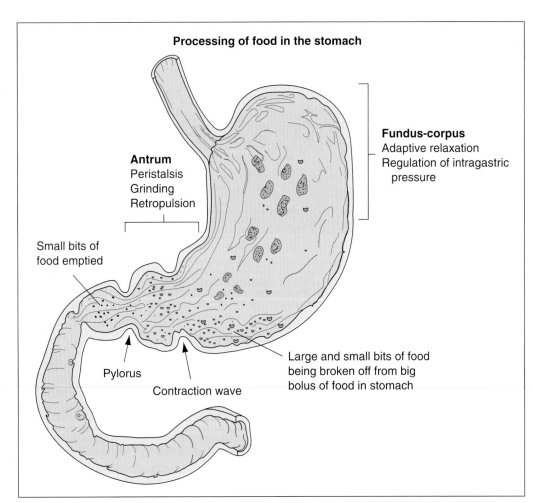

Processing of food in the stomach

Fundus-corpus
Adaptive relaxation
Regulation of intragastric pressure

Antrum
Peristalsis
Grinding
Retropulsion

Small bits of food emptied

Pylorus

Contraction wave

Large and small bits of food being broken off from big bolus of food in stomach

FIGURE 2-5.

The emptying of food from the stomach is regulated by neural and hormonal mechanisms. The arrival of food in the proximal stomach (fundus and corpus) causes an adaptive relaxation mediated by neuronal release of vasoactive intestinal polypeptide and nitric oxide. The relaxation accommodates the increasing gastric volume without an increase in the pressure gradient between the proximal and distal stomach. The presence of food in the stomach also induces increased antral peristaltic activity (grinding) with propulsion and retropulsion of food particles. The combined mechanical and enzymatic activity gradually decrease the size of food particles until they are sufficiently small (1–2 mm) to allow passage into the duodenum [9].

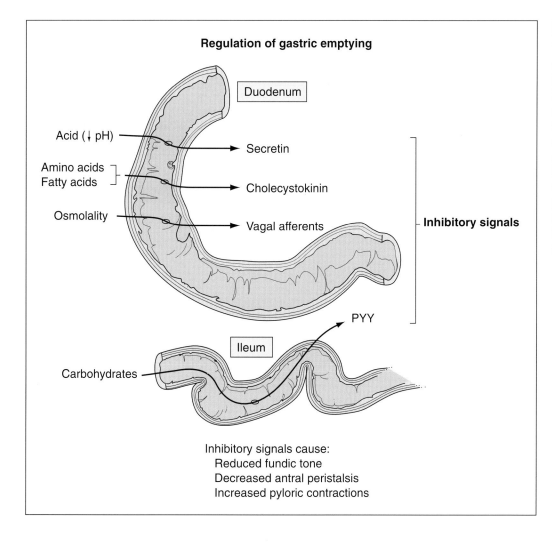

Regulation of gastric emptying

Duodenum

Acid (↓ pH) → Secretin

Amino acids
Fatty acids → Cholecystokinin

Osmolality → Vagal afferents

Inhibitory signals

PYY

Ileum

Carbohydrates

Inhibitory signals cause:
Reduced fundic tone
Decreased antral peristalsis
Increased pyloric contractions

FIGURE 2-6.

FIGURE 2-6.

The passage of acidic, hyperosmolar gastric chyme into the duodenum elicits several inhibitory signals that slow gastric emptying. Fatty acid and amino acids release cholecystokinin, and acid mediates secretin release from neuroendocrine cells in the duodenal and jejunal mucosa. Hyperosmolarity is sensed by osmoreceptors, and the inhibitory signals are transmitted through vagal afferents. Finally, carbohydrates release peptide YY (PYY) from the ileum. These signals inhibit gastric emptying by reducing fundic tone, decreasing antral peristalsis, and increasing pyloric contractions [10].

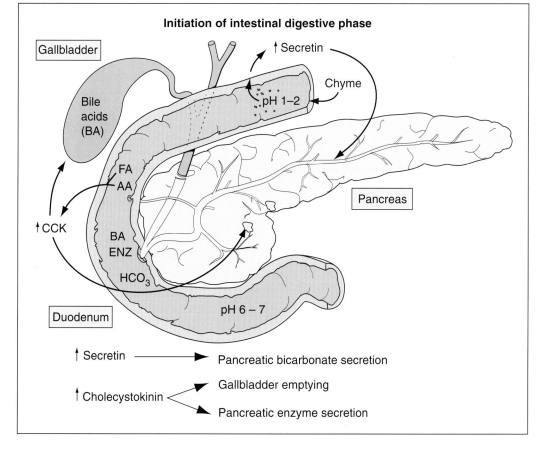

Initiation of intestinal digestive phase

Gallbladder

↑ Secretin

Chyme

Bile acids (BA)

pH 1–2

FA
AA

Pancreas

↑CCK

BA
ENZ

HCO₃

Duodenum

pH 6 – 7

↑ Secretin ⟶ Pancreatic bicarbonate secretion

↑ Cholecystokinin ⟵ Gallbladder emptying

Pancreatic enzyme secretion

FIGURE 2-7.

Cholecystokinin (CCK) and secretin are of major importance in the regulation of digestive function. Secretin released into the blood binds to secretin receptors on pancreatic ducts and stimulates bicarbonate (HCO_3) secretion. Secreted bicarbonate neutralizes gastric acid, and intraluminal pH increases from 1 to 2 in the duodenal bulb to 6 to 7 in the distal duodenum. Release of CCK causes gallbladder contraction directly and through activation of vagal efferents, and stimulates pancreatic enzyme secretion by binding to CCK receptors on pancreatic nerves and acini [11]. The arriving gastric chyme is thus bathed in gallbladder bile with a high bile-acid concentration, and pancreatic secretion with a high bicarbonate concentration and more than 20 different lytic enzymes. Therefore, the actions of CCK and secretin generate optimal conditions for continued macronutrient digestion in the proximal small intestine. AA—amino acids; BA—bile acids; ENZ—enzymes; FA—fatty acids.

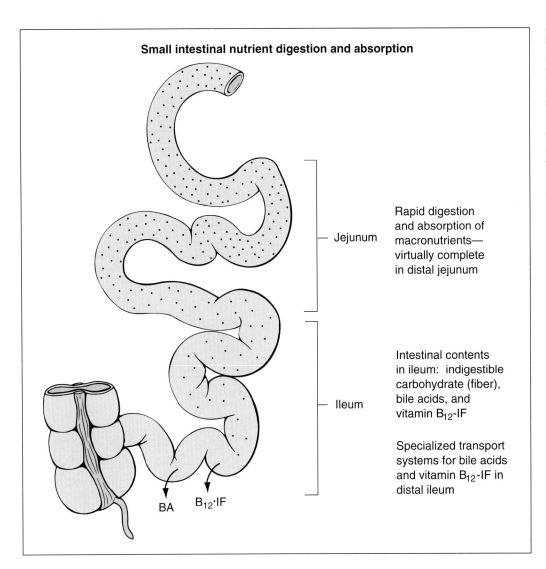

Small intestinal nutrient digestion and absorption

Jejunum — Rapid digestion and absorption of macronutrients— virtually complete in distal jejunum

Ileum — Intestinal contents in ileum: indigestible carbohydrate (fiber), bile acids, and vitamin B_{12}-IF

Specialized transport systems for bile acids and vitamin B_{12}-IF in distal ileum

BA $B_{12} \cdot IF$

FIGURE 2-8.

Macronutrient digestion and absorption proceed at a rapid pace in the jejunum. More than 95% of ingested macronutrients are digested and absorbed in the jejunum [12]. The intestinal chyme in the ileum consists mainly of indigestible carbohydrates (fiber), bile acids, vitamin $B_{12} \bullet IF$, water, and electrolytes. Bile acids and $B_{12} \bullet IF$ are absorbed in the ileum by specialized transport systems. In addition, nutrients that escaped absorption in the jejunum can be absorbed in the ileum.

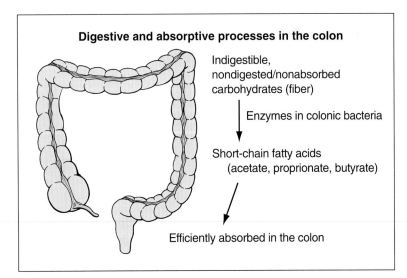

Digestive and absorptive processes in the colon

Indigestible, nondigested/nonabsorbed carbohydrates (fiber)

↓ Enzymes in colonic bacteria

Short-chain fatty acids (acetate, proprionate, butyrate)

↓

Efficiently absorbed in the colon

FIGURE 2-9.

The large bowel has a special role in carbohydrate digestion and absorption. Indigestible carbohydrates are partially broken down by enzymes in colonic bacteria to short-chain fatty acids (acetate, propionate, and butyrate), which are efficiently absorbed by the colonic mucosa [14]. The short-chain fatty acids are important metabolic substrates for the mucosal cells in the colon. In addition, the colon may serve in a reserve capacity for carbohydrate salvage in patients with carbohydrate malabsorption (*eg*, short-bowel syndrome with retained colon). About 80 g of nondigested or nonabsorbed carbohydrate can be converted to short-chain fatty acids by bacteria and absorbed by the colon.

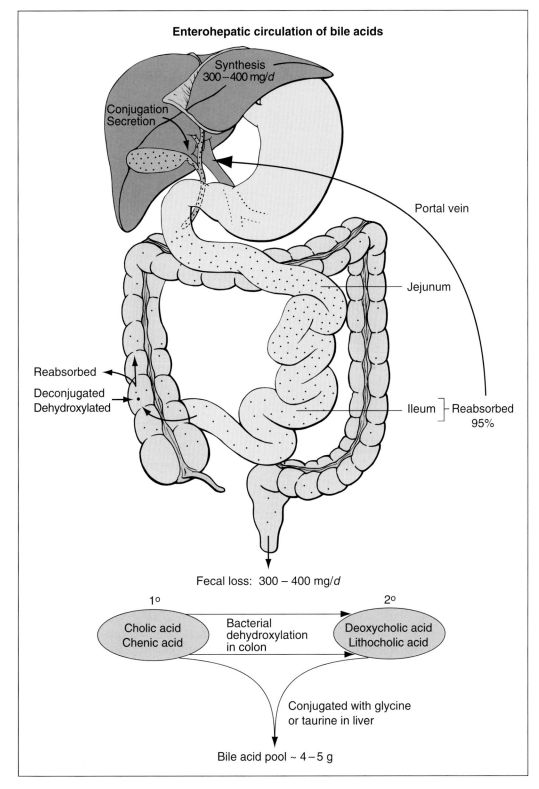

Enterohepatic circulation of bile acids

Synthesis
300 – 400 mg/d

Conjugation
Secretion

Portal vein

Jejunum

Reabsorbed

Deconjugated
Dehydroxylated

Ileum — Reabsorbed
95%

Fecal loss: 300 – 400 mg/d

1°

Cholic acid
Chenic acid

Bacterial
dehydroxylation
in colon

2°

Deoxycholic acid
Lithocholic acid

Conjugated with glycine
or taurine in liver

Bile acid pool ~ 4 – 5 g

Figure 2-10.

The primary bile acids, cholic and chenic acid, are synthesized from cholesterol in the liver. The daily synthesis is about 300 to 400 mg. The primary bile acids are conjugated with glycine or taurine before secretion into bile. The primary bile acids are deconjugated and dehydroxylated by bacterial enzymes in the distal small intestine and colon. This results in the formation of the secondary bile acids, deoxycholic and lithocholic acid, which are reabsorbed, returned to the liver, and also conjugated with glycine or taurine. The bile acid pool thus consists of eight conjugated bile acids and a small amount of the four unconjugated bile acids. The bile acid pool is about 4 to 5 g. The pool recirculates between the liver and intestine twice per meal. The bile acids are efficiently reabsorbed by an active transport system in the ileum and returned to the liver by the portal vein. The average daily fecal loss of bile acids is about 300 to 400 mg, which is balanced by hepatic synthesis to maintain a constant pool size [13].

▌LIPID DIGESTION AND ABSORPTION

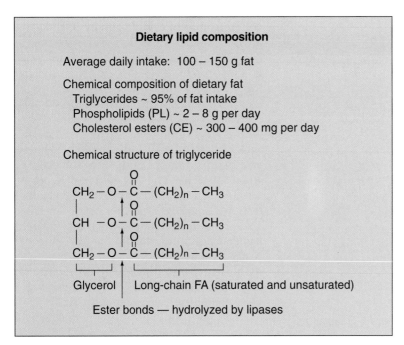

Dietary lipid composition

Average daily intake: 100 – 150 g fat

Chemical composition of dietary fat
   Triglycerides ~ 95% of fat intake
   Phospholipids (PL) ~ 2 – 8 g per day
   Cholesterol esters (CE) ~ 300 – 400 mg per day

Chemical structure of triglyceride

Glycerol | Long-chain FA (saturated and unsaturated)

Ester bonds — hydrolyzed by lipases

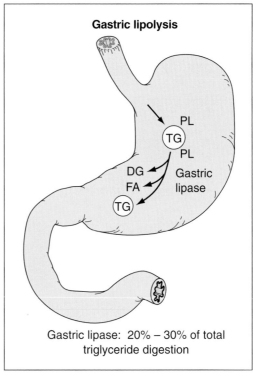

Gastric lipolysis

Gastric lipase: 20% – 30% of total triglyceride digestion

FIGURE 2-11.

Lipids have the highest energy content (9 kcal/g) of the three macronutrients. The average intake of fat by adults in the United States is about 100 to 150 g per day. The major chemical constituents of dietary fat are triglycerides, which account for about 95% of ingested lipids. Phospholipid intake is about 2 to 8 g per day. In addition, there is a daily flow of 20 to 30 g of biliary phospholipids into the small intestine. The intake of cholesterol and cholesterol esters is only 300 to 400 mg per day.

The chemical structure of a triglyceride consists of a glycerol backbone with three fatty acids (FA) attached by ester bonds. The fatty acids may be saturated or unsaturated. Only two unsaturated fatty acids, linoleic and linolenic acid, are essential.

FIGURE 2-12.

The initial event in lipid digestion in the stomach is the formation of emulsion droplets composed of triglycerides (TG) and cholesterol ester in the core of the droplet and phospholipids (PL) on the surface. The only lipolytic enzyme in gastric secretion is gastric lipase, which has a pH optimum of 4 to 5.5. Gastric lipase cleaves off a single fatty acid from triglycerides to generate diglycerides (DG) and fatty acids (FA) [15]. Gastric lipolysis accounts for about 20% to 30% of total triglyceride digestion. Gastric lipase may be substantially more important in the newborn period, when milk is the major source of ingested lipid. Gastric lipase is denatured at neutral pH, thus losing its activity in the duodenum. It may, however, attain a larger role in triglyceride digestion in patients with chronic pancreatitis because duodenal pH is lower because of decreased pancreatic bicarbonate secretion.

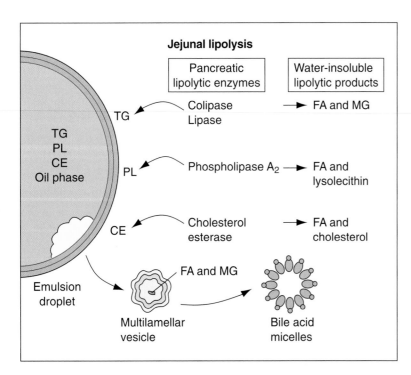

Jejunal lipolysis

Pancreatic lipolytic enzymes	Water-insoluble lipolytic products
Colipase Lipase	FA and MG
Phospholipase A$_2$	FA and lysolecithin
Cholesterol esterase	FA and cholesterol

TG
PL
CE
Oil phase

Emulsion droplet

FA and MG → Multilamellar vesicle → Bile acid micelles

FIGURE 2-13.

Lipid digestion proceeds at a rapid pace in the duodenum, where lipid emulsion droplets are attacked by pancreatic lipolytic enzymes that are secreted at a maximum rate following cholecystokinin stimulation. The four lipolytic enzymes are lipase, colipase, phospholipase A$_2$, and cholesterol esterase. Colipase is an obligate cofactor for lipase action. Colipase first attaches to a triglyceride (TG) molecule on the surface of an emulsion droplet and serves as an anchor for lipase, which then hydrolyzes ester bonds and releases fatty acids (FA) and monoglyceride (MG) [16,17]. Phospholipase A$_2$ acts on phospholipids, principally lecithin, to produce lysolecithin and fatty acids. Cholesterol esterase (CE) hydrolyzes fatty acid from cholesterol ester. The released lipolytic products are water insoluble and aggregate in multilamellar vesicles at the boundary of the emulsion droplets. Multilamellar vesicles gradually decrease in size as the lipolytic products are transferred to and solubilized by bile acid micelles [18].

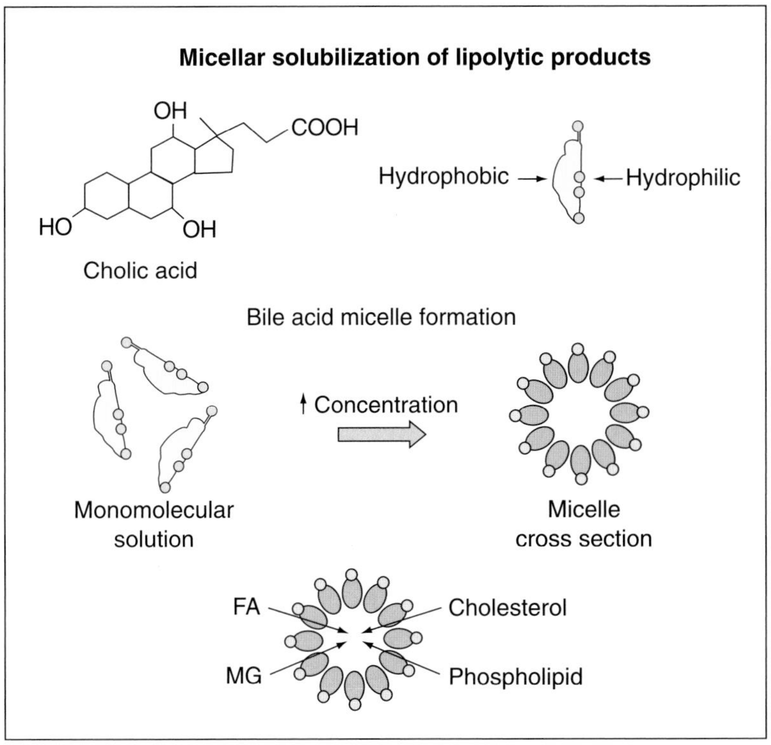

FIGURE 2-14.

Micellar solubilization of lipolytic products

Cholic acid

Hydrophobic → ← Hydrophilic

Bile acid micelle formation

↑ Concentration

Monomolecular solution

Micelle cross section

FA — Cholesterol

MG — Phospholipid

Bile acids are amphipaths (*ie*, they have both hydrophilic and hydrophobic properties). The structural formula of cholic acid, a primary bile acid, is illustrated in the upper portion of this figure. The steroid nucleus is the hydrophobic part of the molecule, and the three hydroxyl groups and one carboxylic group are the hydrophilic counterparts. A schematic illustration of cholic acid is shown where the open circles represent hydrophilic groups. Bile acids form multimolecular aggregates called *micelles*, with increasing bile acid concentration [19]. Micelles have the hydrophilic groups on the external surface facing the water phase and the hydrophobic part on the inside, as shown in the cross-section of a micelle in the middle portion of this figure. Fatty acids (FA), monoglycerides (MG), lysolecithin, and cholesterol are solubilized in the hydrophobic interior of bile acid micelles, as shown in the lower portion of this figure. The primary function of bile acid micelles is to render the lipolytic products water soluble and to transport them to the brush border of the enterocytes.

FIGURE 2-15.

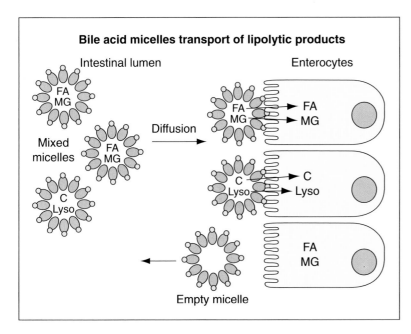

Bile acid micelles transport of lipolytic products

Intestinal lumen

Enterocytes

FA MG

Mixed micelles

FA MG

Diffusion

FA MG → FA → MG

C Lyso

C Lyso → C → Lyso

FA MG

Empty micelle

Mixed micelles diffuse from the intestinal lumen across the unstirred water layer adjacent to the brush-border membrane of the enterocytes; the lipolytic products are taken up by diffusion across the lipid bilayer of the brush-border membrane [20]. The empty micelles diffuse back into the lumen and are reused for the solubilization of lipolytic products. Bile acid micelles function as a shuttle of lipolytic products from intestinal lumen to the luminal surface of the enterocytes. There is minimal absorption of bile acids in the jejunum. Thus, a high concentration of bile acids is maintained in the proximal small intestine to facilitate lipid absorption. C—cholesterol; FA—fatty acids; Lyso—lysolecithin; MG—monoglycerides.

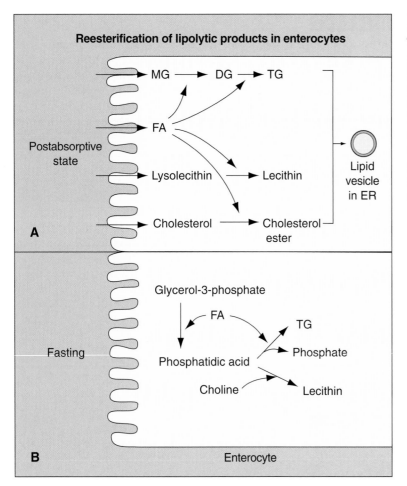

FIGURE 2-16.

The lipolytic products are resynthesized to triglycerides (TG), phospholipids, and cholesterol esters in the endoplasmic reticulum (ER) of the enterocytes by two different pathways [21,22]. In the postabsorptive state, absorbed fatty acids (FA) are activated by acetyl-CoA and reesterification-absorbed monoglycerides (MG), lysolecithin, and cholesterol to form diglyceride (DG), TG, lecithin, and cholesterol ester, as illustrated in **panel A**. The products accumulate as lipid vesicles in the ER. In the fasting state, glycerol-3-phosphate from glucose metabolism is the precursor for TG and phospholipid synthesis through the formation of phosphatidic acid, as shown in **panel B**.

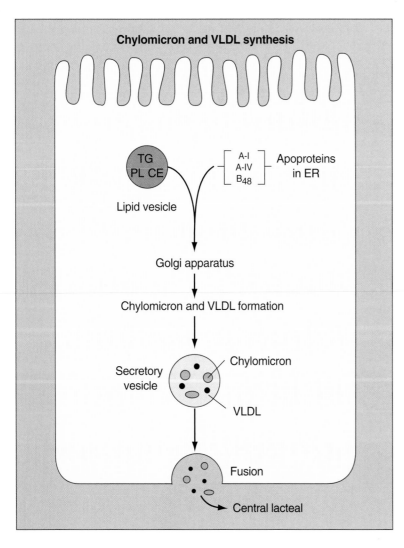

FIGURE 2-17.

The end products of lipid absorption in the enterocytes are chylomicrons and VLDL (very light density lipoproteins). Apoproteins A-I, A-IV, and B_{48} are synthesized in the endoplasmic reticulum (ER) and added to the surface of the lipid vesicles containing triglycerides (TG), phospholipids (PL), and cholesterol ester (CE) [23–26]. The lipid vesicles are transported to the Golgi, where the chylomicron and VLDL particles are formed and incorporated into secretory vesicles. These vesicles diffuse to the basolateral membrane where the chylomicron and VLDL particles are released by exocytosis. The particles diffuse to the central lacteal of the villus and are transported by lymphatics to the vascular compartment.

CARBOHYDRATE DIGESTION AND ABSORPTION

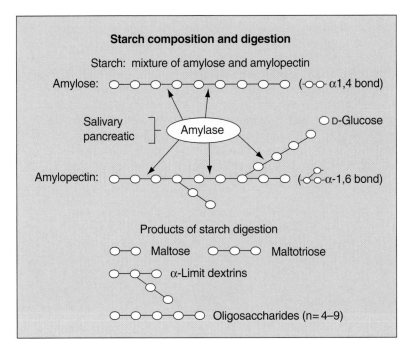

Starch composition and digestion

FIGURE 2-18.

Carbohydrate is the major energy source in the diet, and accounts for more than 50% of calories consumed per day. The major dietary sources of carbohydrates are cereals, bread, and vegetables. The average daily intake by adults by United States is about 400 g. About 50% of the daily intake is in the form of polysaccharides (large glucose polymers; MW, 10^5–10^6 kD), mainly starch and a variable amount of indigestible carbohydrate (fiber). The other 50% is accounted for by two disaccharides, sucrose and lactose, in varying proportions [27].

Starch is a mixture of amylose and amylopectin. Amylose is a straight chain of glucose molecules linked together in α-1,4 linkages. Amylopectin is a branched molecule with both α-1,4 and α-1,6 bonds where the α-1,6 bonds are the branch points. Starch digestion starts in the mouth with salivary amylase and continues in the duodenum with pancreatic amylase. The two amylases are very similar in chemical composition. They are endoglucosidases and attack only α-1,4 bonds. They do not attack the bonds at the end of the molecule; therefore, glucose is not generated, nor do they attack bonds next to an α-1,6 linkage. The products of starch digestion are maltose, maltotriose, α-limit dextrins, and oligosaccharides [28].

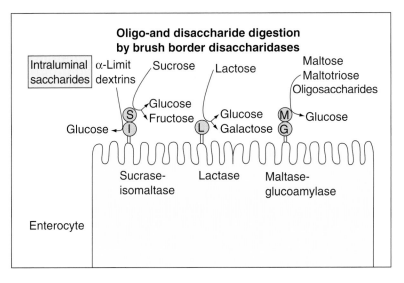

Oligo-and disaccharide digestion by brush border disaccharidases

FIGURE 2-19.

The products of starch digestion and the two dietary disaccharides, sucrose and lactose, are readily water soluble and diffuse from the intestinal lumen up to the brush-border membrane, where further digestion proceeds by the three major disaccharidases inserted in the membrane, as illustrated in this figure. Sucrase-isomaltase (SI) and maltase-glucoamylase (MG) are dimers whereas lactase (L) is a monomer as indicated by the circles [29–31]. Sucrose and lactose are split to their respective monosaccharides by sucrase and lactase, respectively. Maltose, maltotriose, and short oligosaccharides are digested by maltase-glucoamylase, but can also be digested by sucrase and isomaltase. The α-1,6 bond in α-limit dextrin can only be hydrolyzed by isomaltase. The final digestive products are three monosaccharides: glucose, galactose, and fructose.

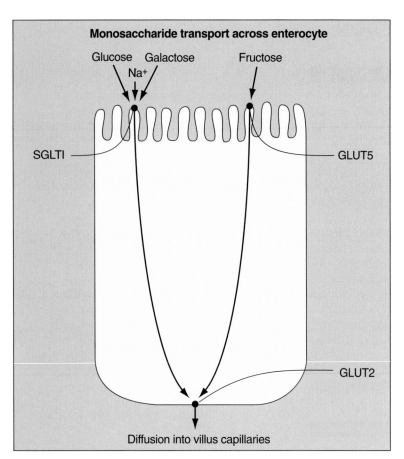

Monosaccharide transport across enterocyte

Diffusion into villus capillaries

FIGURE 2-20.

Glucose, galactose, and fructose are not lipid soluble, and therefore require specific transporters to cross the brush-border and basolateral membrane of the enterocytes. Glucose and galactose transport across the brush-border membrane in a sodium-coupled process (secondary active transport) where the energy is provided by the sodium gradient across the membrane. The transporter, SGLT1, has a high affinity for glucose and galactose, which accounts for rapid and efficient glucose and galactose absorption in the jejunum [32]. Fructose is transported across the brush-border membrane by another transporter, GLUT 5, by facilitated diffusion (no sodium requirement) [33]. The three monosaccharides are transported across the basolateral membrane by another facilitated glucose transporter, GLUT 2, and diffuse into the capillaries of the villus [34,35].

■ PROTEIN DIGESTION AND ABSORPTION

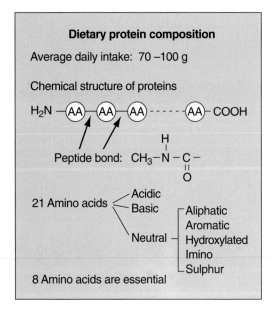

Dietary protein composition

FIGURE 2-21.

The average daily protein intake is about 70 to 100 g in adults, which is more than the recommended daily allowance (0.8 g/kg). Proteins are single strands of amino acids (AA) connected by peptide bonds. The complexity of proteins derives from the fact that there are 21 different amino acids. Amino acids are divided into three major groups on the basis of charge: acidic, basic, and neutral. The neutral amino acids are further divided into aliphatic, aromatic, hydroxylated, imino, and sulphur-containing amino acids. Eight of the 21 amino acids are essential (*ie*, they cannot be synthesized by humans) [36].

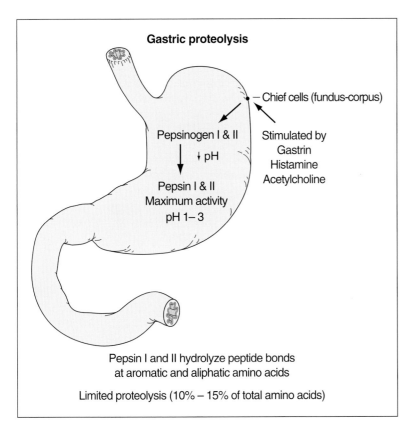

Gastric proteolysis

Chief cells (fundus-corpus)

Pepsinogen I & II

↓ pH

Pepsin I & II
Maximum activity
pH 1– 3

Stimulated by
Gastrin
Histamine
Acetylcholine

Pepsin I and II hydrolyze peptide bonds
at aromatic and aliphatic amino acids

Limited proteolysis (10% – 15% of total amino acids)

FIGURE 2-22.

Protein digestion begins in the stomach. The mediators of acid secretion —acetylcholine, histamine, and gastrin—also stimulate chief cells and mucous neck cells in the fundus and corpus of the stomach to secrete pepsinogen I and II [7]. Pepsinogen I and II are converted to the active enzymes, pepsin I and II, by the low pH in the stomach. They have maximal enzymatic activity at pH 1 to 3, but are inactive at pH more than 4.5. They preferentially cleave peptide bonds next to aliphatic or aromatic amino acids and generate oligopeptides and amino acids. Gastric proteolysis is limited and accounts for only 10% to 15% of total protein digestion. The generation of amino acids is important because amino acids are a potent stimuli of gastrin and cholecystokinin release.

Pancreatic proteolytic enzymes

Inactive Endopeptidases	Activated by	Active enzymes	Peptide-bond specificity
Trypsinogen	Enteropeptidase	Trypsin	Basic AA
Chymotrypsinogen	Trypsin	Chymotrypsin	Aromatic AA
Proelastase	Trypsin	Elastase	Aliphatic AA
Exopeptidases			
Procarboxypeptidase A	Trypsin	Carboxypeptidase A	Neutral AA
Procarboxypeptidase B	Trypsin	Carboxypeptidase B	Basic AA

FIGURE 2-23.

The proteolytic enzymes secreted by pancreatic acini upon cholecystokinin stimulation are released as proenzymes and are activated in the duodenal lumen. Three of the enzymes are endopeptidases (trypsinogen, chymotrypsinogen, proelastase) and two are exopeptidases (procarboxypeptidase A and B). Trypsinogen is activated to trypsin by enteropeptidase, which is a brush border peptidase. Trypsin, in turn, further activates trypsinogen conversion and also activates all the other proteolytic proenzymes [11]. The five proteolytic enzymes have different peptide bond specificities, as shown in this figure. AA—Amino acids.

TABLE 2-2. BRUSH-BORDER OLIGOPEPTIDE HYDROLYSIS

BRUSH-BORDER ENZYMES	SUBSTRATE	PRODUCTS
Endopeptidases		
Enteropeptidase	Trypsinogen	Trypsin
Endopeptidase 24.11	Hydrophobic AA	Peptides
Neutral endopeptidase	?	Peptides
Exopeptidases		
Aminopeptidase N	Neutral AA	Neutral AA
		Di- and tripeptides
Aminopeptidase A	Acidic AA	Acidic AA
Dipeptidylpeptidase IV	Penultimate proline	Dipeptides
Gly-Leu peptidase	Dipeptide (Aliphatic)	AA
Asp-Lys peptidase	Dipeptide (Basic)	AA
Folate Conjugase	Polyglutamated Folates	Folic Acid

V

V

TABLE 2-2.

The oligopeptides and amino acids (AA) generated by intraluminal proteolysis diffuse to the brush border of the enterocytes where oligopeptides must undergo further hydrolysis to amino acids, dipeptides, and tripeptides before absorption can take place. Several brush-border endopeptidases and exopeptidases have been identified, as outlined in this table. The presence of so many different peptidases is required because of the chemical diversity of amino acids. The substrates for the enzymes and the products generated by hydrolysis are also outlined in this table [38,39].

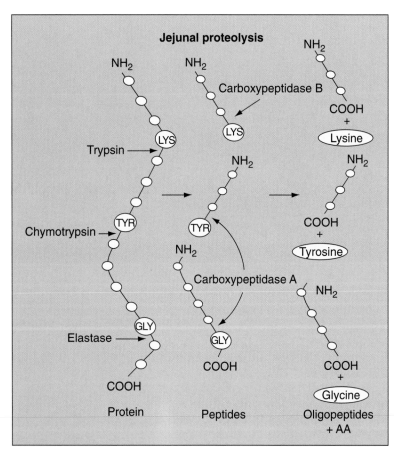

FIGURE 2-24.

The proteolytic enzymes are secreted in vast excess by the pancreas, and intraluminal proteolysis proceeds at a fast rate in the proximal small intestine. The endopeptidases attack peptide bonds inside the protein molecule. Trypsin hydrolyzes peptide bonds next to basic amino acids (AA) (lysine [LYS]); chymotrypsin attacks peptide bonds next to aromatic amino acids (tyrosine [TYR]) and elastase next to aliphatic amino acids (glycine [GLY]) to generate shorter peptides (oligopeptides). Oligopeptides are further hydrolyzed by the two exopeptidases that attack peptide bonds at the ends of the peptide fragments: carboxypeptidase A, which has broad specificity for neutral amino acids, and carboxypeptidase B, which cleaves off basic amino acids to generate free amino acids and short oligopeptides [37–39].

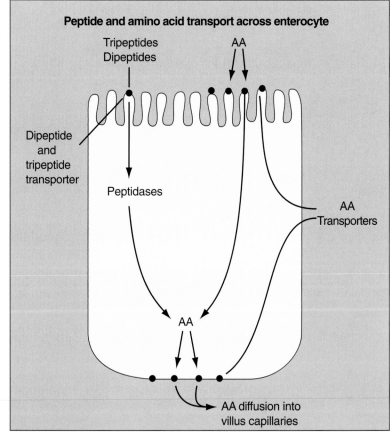

FIGURE 2-25.

The dipeptides, tripeptides, and amino acids (AA) are transported across the brush-border membrane into enterocytes by an array of transporters. Dipeptides and tripeptides are taken up by a single peptide transporter. The transport process is active and sodium coupled [40]. The dipeptides and tripeptides are hydrolyzed by cytosolic peptidases to amino acids. Amino acid transport across the brush border and basolateral membranes is facilitated by a number of different transporters, which are described in Table 2-3. Amino acids transported across the basolateral membrane diffuse into villus capillaries to reach the portal circulation.

TABLE 2-3. AMINO ACID TRANSPORT SYSTEMS IN ENTEROCYTES

BRUSH BORDER	BASOLATERAL MEMBRANE	AMINO ACID SPECIFICITY	SODIUM COUPLED
A	A	Neutral	+
ASC	ASC	Neutral	+
B		Neutral	+
$B^{O,+}$		Neutral	+
$b^{O,+}$	$b^{O,+}$	Neutral	-
Imino		Proline	+
L	L	Branched AA	-
X^-		Asp, Glut	+
y+AG	y+	Arg, Lys	-

TABLE 2-3.

The amino acid (AA) transport systems in the brush-border and basolateral membranes are outlined in this table. There are, so far, nine different transport systems identified and characterized in the brush-border membrane; five of these transport systems are also found in the basolateral membrane. The transport systems are named with capital or lower-case letters to indicate their dependence on sodium coupling (upper case) or independence (lower case). The naming of system L is an exception because this system is sodium independent, as indicated in this table. The amino acid specificity of the transporters is also outlined [41,42].

MICRONUTRIENT ABSORPTION

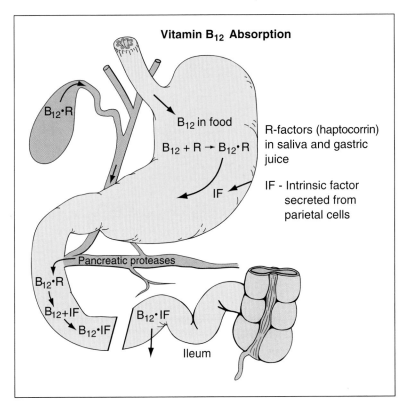

Vitamin B$_{12}$ Absorption

B$_{12}$·R

B$_{12}$ in food

B$_{12}$ + R → B$_{12}$·R

R-factors (haptocorrin) in saliva and gastric juice

IF

IF - Intrinsic factor secreted from parietal cells

Pancreatic proteases

B$_{12}$·R

B$_{12}$+IF

B$_{12}$·IF

B$_{12}$·IF

Ileum

FIGURE 2-26.

Vitamin B$_{12}$ (cobalamin) is one of the water-soluble vitamins; its digestion and absorption have been well characterized. Vitamin B$_{12}$ in food is liberated in the stomach and is bound in a tight complex to R factors (haptocorrin), which are glycoproteins secreted in saliva and gastric juice. R factors have a much higher affinity for B$_{12}$ than intrinsic factor (IF), which is secreted from the parietal cells in the stomach. B$_{12}$ is also secreted in bile complexed to R factors. The B$_{12}$•R factor complex is degraded by pancreatic proteases in the duodenum; the liberated B$_{12}$ is then complexed to IF. This complex is resistant to pancreatic proteases and travels to the ileum, where a specific transport system is responsible for uptake of the B$_{12}$•IF complexes. The daily need for absorbed vitamin B$_{12}$ has been estimated to be about 1 μg [43].

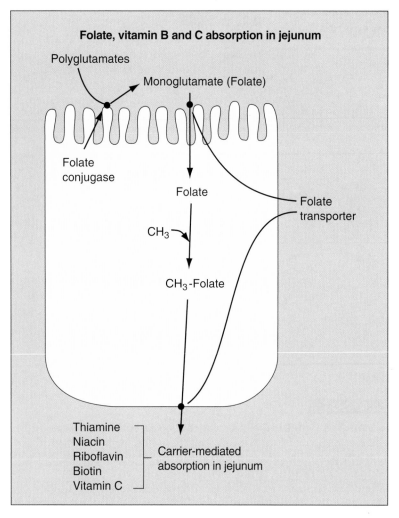

Folate, vitamin B and C absorption in jejunum

FIGURE 2-27.

Folate is present in food, primarily in polyglutamate form. The glutamic acid residues are removed from polyglutamates by folate conjugase, an exopeptidase, in the brush-border membrane. Polyglutamates are converted to monoglutamate, which is the moiety of folic acid that is transported by a folate transporter in the brush-border membrane. Folate is methylated in the enterocyte before transport out of the cell across the basolateral membrane [44].

The transport of the other water-soluble vitamins, such as thiamin, niacin, riboflavin, biotin, and vitamin C, appear to be carrier mediated and sodium coupled; the individual transporters have not yet been identified [45]. The absorption of the fat-soluble vitamins (A, D, E, and K) follows the same steps as described under lipid absorption.

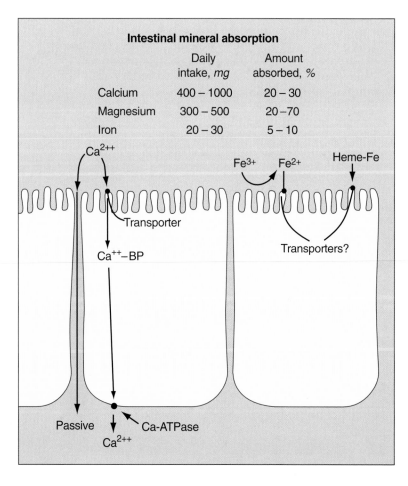

Intestinal mineral absorption

	Daily intake, mg	Amount absorbed, %
Calcium	400 – 1000	20 – 30
Magnesium	300 – 500	20 –70
Iron	20 – 30	5 – 10

FIGURE 2-28.

The daily intake of three major minerals in the diet (calcium, magnesium, and iron) is in the milligram range. The percentage absorbed of the daily intake is much lower than for macronutrients, as shown in this figure.

Calcium (Ca) is absorbed by both passive and active mechanisms. The active transport system consists of Ca transporters in the brush-border membrane. Ca is bound to calcium-binding proteins in the cytosol (VBP). The transport out of the cells is presumed mediated by a Ca-ATPase in the basolateral membrane. The passive route is presumed to be calcium diffusion across tight junctions and through the intercellular spaces [45,46].

The absorption of iron is still not well characterized. Iron is present in food as ionized iron, primarily ferric Fe^{3+} and heme-iron. Some ferric iron is reduced to ferrous iron Fe^{2+} in the stomach, which increases its solubility. Unreduced ferric iron must be converted to ferrous iron at the brush-border membrane before absorption. The uptake of ferrous iron and heme-iron across the brush border is mediated by two different transporters, which have not been identified [47,48].

TABLE 2-4. TRACE ELEMENT ABSORPTION

	DAILY INTAKE, MG	AMOUNT ABSORBED, %
Zinc	10–15	20–50
Copper	1–3	30–70
Selenium	0.1–0.2	?
Manganese	2–5	15–25

Uptake processes of trace elements are poorly defined—presumably both carrier-mediated transport and passive diffusion play a role.

TABLE 2-4.

Trace elements are important constituents of the diet. They are essential because they are integral parts of important molecules in many biochemical pathways. The intake of zinc, copper, selenium, and manganese is in the low milligram to microgram range. The uptake of these trace elements is relatively inefficient, as indicated, but deficiency rarely develops on a well-balanced diet. The characterization of the uptake process of trace elements is still in its early stages [48–52].

REFERENCES

1. Brown ML: *Present Knowledge in Nutrition.* Washington, DC: International Life Sciences Institute; 1990.

2. *Recommended Dietary Allowances,* edn. 10. Washington, DC: National Academy Press; 1989.

3. Aggett PJ: Trace element status of the human diet. *Proc Nutr Soc* 1988, 47:21–25.

4. Feldman M, Richardson CT: Role of thought, light, smell, and taste of food in the cephalic phase of gastric acid secretion in humans. *Gastroenterology* 1986, 90:428–433.

5. Lerner A, Rosenthal MA, Liebow C, Lebenthal E: Salivary secretion. In *Textbook of Gastroenterology.* Edited by Yamada T. Philadelphia: JB Lippincott; 1991:218–233.

6. Goldschmiedt M, Feldman M: Gastric secretion in health and disease. In *Gastrointestinal Disease.* Edited by Sleisenger M, Fordtran J. Philadelphia: WB Saunders; 1993:524–544.

7. Samloff IM: Pepsins, peptic activity and peptic inhibitors. *J Clin Gastroenterol* 1981, 3:91–94.

8. Abrams CK, Hamosh M, Lee TC, *et al.*: Gastric lipase: Localization in the human stomach. *Gastroenterology* 1988, 95:1460–1464.

9. Meyer JH: The physiology of gastric motility and gastric emptying. In *Textbook of Gastroenterology.* Edited by Yamada T. Philadelphia: JB Lippincott; 1991:137–157.

10. Mayer EA: The physiology of gastric storage and emptying. In *Physiology of the Gastrointestinal Tract.* Edited by Johnson LR. New York: Raven Press; 1994:929–976.

11. Pandol SJ: Pancreatic physiology. In *Gastrointestinal Disease.* Edited by Sleisinger M, Fordtran J. Philadelphia: WB Saunders; 1993:1585–1600.

12. Johansson C: Studies of gastrointestinal interactions: Characteristics of the absorption pattern of sugar, fat and protein from composite meals in man. *Scand J Gastroenterol* 1975, 10:33–42.

13. Hofmann AF: The enterohepatic circulation of bile acids in health and disease. In *Gastrointestinal Disease.* Edited by Sleisenger M, Fordtran J. Philadelphia: WB Saunders; 1993:127–150.

14. Read NW: Dietary fiber and the gut. In *Gastrointestinal Disease.* Edited by Sleisenger M, Fordtran J. Philadelphia: WB Saunders; 1993:2097–2108.

15. Gargouri T, Pieroni G, Riviere C, *et al.*: Kinetic assay of human gastric lipase on short- and long-chain triacylglycerol emulsions. *Gastroenterology* 1986, 91:919–925.

16. Borgstrom B: The importance of phospholipids, pancreatic phospholipase A_2 and fatty acid for the digestion of dietary fat. *Gastroenterology* 1980, 78:954–962.

17. Blachberg L, Hernell O, Olivecrona T: Hydrolysis of human milk fat globules by pancreatic lipase: Role of colipase, phospholipase A_2 and bile salts. *J Clin Invest* 1981, 67:1748–1752.

18. Rigler M, Honkaneu RE, Patton JS: Visualization by freeze fracture, in vitro and in vivo, of the products of fat digestion. *J Lipid Res* 1986, 27:836–857.

19. Carey MC, Small DC: The characteristics of mixed micellar solution with particular reference to bile. *Am J Med* 1970, 49:590–608.

20. Westergaard H, Dietschy JM: The mechanism whereby bile acid micelles increase the rate of fatty acid and cholesterol uptake into the intestinal mucosal cell. *J Clin Invest* 1976, 58:97–108.

21. Brown JL, Johnston JM: The utilization of 1- and 2-monoglycerides for intestinal triglyceride biosynthesis. *Biochem Biophys Acta* 1964, 84:448–457.

22. Mansbach CB, Parthasarathy S: A reexamination of the fate of glyceride-glycerol in neutral lipid absorption and transport. *J Lipid Res* 1982, 23:1009–1019.

23. Sabesin SM, Frase S: Electron microscopic studies of the assembly, intracellular transport, and secretion by rat intestine. *J Lipid Res* 1977, 18:496–511.

24. Davidson NO, Glickman RM: Apolipoprotein A-1 synthesis in rat small intestine: Regulation by dietary triglyceride and biliary lipid. *J Lipid Res* 1985, 26:368–379.

25. Davidson NO, Kollmer ME, Glickman RM: Apolipoprotein B synthesis in rat small intestine: Regulation by dietary triglyceride and biliary lipid. *J Lipid Res* 1986, 27:30–39.

26. Apfelbaum TF, Davidson NO, Glickman RM: Apolipoprotein A-IV synthesis in rat intestine: Regulation by dietary triglyceride. *Am J Physiol* 1987, 252:G662–G666.

27. MacDonald I: Carbohydrates. In *Modern Nutrition in Health and Disease.* Edited by Shils ME, Young VR. Philadelphia: Lea & Febiger; 1988:38–71.

28. Olsen WA, Lloyd ML: Carbohydrate assimilation. In *Textbook of Gastroenterology.* Edited by Yamada T. Philadelphia: JB Lippincott; 1991:334–353.

29. Hunziker W, Spiess M, Semenza G: The sucrose-isomaltase complex: Primary struture, membrane orientation, and evolution of a stalked, intrinsic brush-border protein. *Cell* 1986, 46:227–234.

30. Naim HY, Sterchi EE, Lentze MJ: Biosynthesis and maturation of lactase-phlorizin hydrolase in the human small intestine epithelial cells. *Biochem J* 1987, 241:427–434.

31. Naim HY, Sterchi EE, Lentze MJ: Structure, biosynthesis and glycosylation of human small intestinal maltase-glucoamylase. *J Biol Chem* 1988, 263:19709–19717.

32. Hediger MA, Coady MJ, Ikeda TS, Wright EM: Expression, cloning and cDNA sequencing of the Na+/glucose co-transporter. *Nature* 1987, 330:379–381.

33. Davidson NO, Hausman AM, Ifhovits A, *et al.*: Human intestinal glucose transporter expression and localization of GLUT 5. *Am J Physiol* 1992, 262:C795–C800.

34. Thorens B, Sarkar HK, Kaback HR, Lodish HF: Cloning and functional expression in bacteria of a novel glucose transporter present in liver, intestine, kidney and β-pancreatic islet cells. *Cell* 1988, 55:281–290.

35. Wright EM, Hirayama BA, Loo DD, *et al.*: Intestinal sugar transport. In *Physiology of the Gastrointestinal Tract*. Edited by Johnson LR. New York: Raven Press; 1994:1751–1772.

36. Munro HN, Crim MC: The proteins and amino acids. In *Modern Nutrition in Health and Disease*. Edited by Shils ME, Young VR. Philadelphia: Lea & Febiger; 1988:1–51.

37. Silk DBA, Grimble GK, Rees RG: Protein digestion and amino acid and peptide absorption. *Proc Nutr Soc* 1985, 44:63–72.

38. Ahnen DJ: Protein digestion and assimilation. In *Textbook of Gastroenterology*. Edited by Yamada T. Philadelphia: JB Lippincott; 1991:381–392.

39. Alpers DH: Digestion and absorption of carbohydrates and proteins. In *Physiology of the Gastrointestinal Tract*. Edited by Johnson LR. New York: Raven Press; 1994:1723–1749.

40. Silk DBA: Peptide transport. *Clin Sci* 1981, 60:607–615.

41. Ganapathy V, Brandsch M, Leibach FH: Intestinal transport of amino acids and peptides. In *Physiology of the Gastrointestinal Tract*. Edited by Johnson LR. New York: Raven Press; 1994:1773–1794.

42. Mailliard ME, Stevens BR, Mann GE: Amino acid transport by small intestinal, hepatic and pancreatic epithelia. *Gastroenterology* 1995, 108:888–910.

43. Seetharam B: Gastrointestinal absorption and transport of cobalamin (vitamin B_{12}). In *Physiology of the Gastrointestinal Tract*. Edited by Johnson LR. New York: Raven Press; 1994:1997–2026.

44. Mason JB, Rosenberg IH: Intestinal absorption of folate. In *Physiology of the Gastrointestinal Tract*. Edited by Johnson LR. New York: Raven Press; 1994:1979–1996.

45. Schron CM: Vitamins and minerals. In *Textbook of Gastroenterology*. Edited by Yamada T. Philadelphia: JB Lippincott; 1991:392–409.

46. Civitelli R, Avioli LV: Calcium, phospate and magnesium absorption. In *Physiology of the Gastrointestinal Tract*. Edited by Johnson LR. New York: Raven Press; 1994:2173–2181.

47. Simpson RJ, Raja KR, Peters TJ: Mechanisms of intestinal brush border iron transport. *Adv Exp Med Biol* 1989, 249:27–34.

48. Turnberg LA, Riley SA: Digestion and absorption of nutrients and vitamins. In *Gastrointestinal Disease*. Edited by Sleisinger M, Fordtran J. Philadelphia: WB Saunders; 1993:977–1008.

49. Sandstrom B: Factors influencing the uptake of trace elements from the digestive tract. *Proc Nutr Soc* 1988, 47:161–167.

50. Steel L, Cousins RJ: Kinetics of zinc absorption by luminally and vascularly perfused rat intestine. *Am J Physiol* 1985, 248:G46–G53.

51. Lee HH, Prasad AS, Brewer GJ, Owyang C: Zinc absorption in human small intestine. *Am J Physiol* 1989, 256:G87–G91.

52. Reasbech PG, Barbezat GO, Weber FL, *et al.*: Selenium absorption by canine jejunum. *Dig Dis Sci* 1985, 30:489–494.

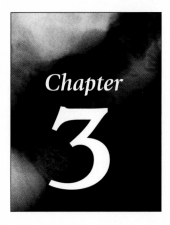

Chapter 3

Small-Bowel Motility

ROBERT W. SUMMERS

When at rest, the intestinal lumen collapses passively, but it remains a potential channel or conduit for chyme. Active wall motion causes the gut to function as both a mixing apparatus and a pump. The muscular wall of the intestine contracts and relaxes to accomplish its purposes of mixing and propulsion of the luminal contents. The contractile process is carried out through the biochemical processes of the muscle and orchestrated by the closely related interstitial cells of Cajal. It is modified by various chemical, neural, and humoral influences. The nutrient *chyme* is mixed after a meal by muscular action with enzymes and gastrointestinal secretions to begin the processes of digestion. In addition, mixing exposes the simplified nutrients to the mucosal epithelial cells permitting absorption. Mixing is accomplished by nonmigrating or short-migrating contractions originally called *segmenting waves*. As water, electrolytes, and nutrients are extracted by the epithelium, the chyme eventually becomes a non-nutrient residue that is normally emptied into the colon and eliminated from the digestive tract, through the action of longer propulsive waves that produce aboral flow or transit from one segment to the next. In the fasting state, a repetitive pattern of powerful contractions continually empties the intestine, keeping it free from bacterial contamination and other residual contents. Small intestinal motility is a complex process accomplished by many integrated components acting together to produce normal function.

TABLE 3-1. PEOPLE AND DEVELOPMENTS IN THE STUDY OF INTESTINAL MOTILITY BEFORE 1990

1857—Meissner [1] and Auerbach identified and described the submucosal and myenteric plexuses that respectively carry their names.

1899—Bayliss and Starling [2] defined the *law of the intestine*, in which a contraction develops above, and relaxation below, a distending bolus.

1902—Cannon [3] began a series of studies of the movements of the intestine using roentgenography with bismuth as a contrast agent. He described segmental and peristaltic contractions.

1905—Langley [4] recognized the enteric nervous system as a distinct entity and proposed that it was capable of functioning independently from the central nervous system; Boldyreff [5] observed periodic phenomena in the digestive tract, including pancreatic secretions and contractions of the stomach, inferring that the latter also occurred in the intestine.

1914—Alvarez [6] described electrical *action currents* (slow waves) and observed a frequency gradient along the length of the intestine.

1921—Payne and Poulton [7] began their studies of visceral pain using motility-monitoring balloons in the gastrointestinal tract.

1947—Ambache [8] noted the association of slow waves and phasic intestinal contractions.

1953—Bülbring [9] established that the peristaltic reflex was due to the action of intrinsic nerves.

1961—Bortoff [10] recorded intestinal slow-wave potentials intracellularly from smooth muscle cells in vitro with microelectrodes.

1962—Dewey and Barr [11] described the nexus (gap junction) in circular muscle, a low-resistance pathway important for cell-to-cell communication.

1964—Brown [12] discovered, purified, and later, sequenced *motilin*, a hormone that stimulates gastric antral movement and activity fronts.

1966—Christensen [13] recorded the slow-wave frequency gradient in intact healthy humans.

1968—Szurszewski and Code [14] reported the migrating myoelectric complex in fasting dogs.

1970—Wood [15] and Prosser initiated studies of the *intracellular* potentials from a variety of intrinsic intestinal nerves using microelectrodes.

1974—Gabella [16] used light and electron microscopy to describe the ultrastructural details of intestinal smooth muscle cells, their innervation, and supporting structures.

1985—Furness and Costa [17] embarked on a series of elegant studies to define the neurochemistry and circuitry of the enteric nerves. Thuneberg restated that the interstitial cells of Cajal are intestinal pacemakers and pointed out their intimate structural and functional relationships to neurons and smooth muscle cells.

TABLE 3-1.

Important people and developments in intestinal motility up to the 1990s.

ANATOMY

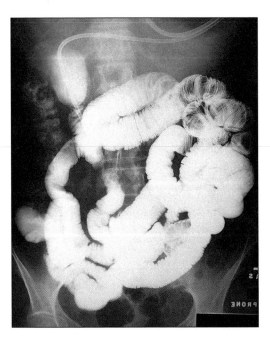

FIGURE 3-1.

The small intestine is approximately 5 m in length, depending on the degree of contraction or relaxation. It is clearly defined on this small bowel enteroclysis study. The duodenum extends about 25 cm from the pylorus to the ligament of Treitz. It has the largest diameter and the thickest wall, but the shortest length of all of the three intestinal regions. The jejunum is about 2 m long, with a proximal diameter about twice that of the distal ileum. The ileum is about 3 m long; its wall is thinner than that of the jejunum. Although the jejunum differs structurally from the ileum, no sharp anatomic distinction exists between the two. In the duodenum and jejunum, the mucosa is redundant and arranged so that it produces circular folds (valvulae conniventes). These folds probably act as baffles to disrupt laminar flow and contribute to more turbulence, enhancing mixing of intestinal contents with digestive secretions and exposure to the absorbing surface. Valvulae do not exist in the ileum, giving it a smoother contour. (*Courtesy of* Dr. Charles Lu, University of Iowa.)

Layers of the intestinal wall

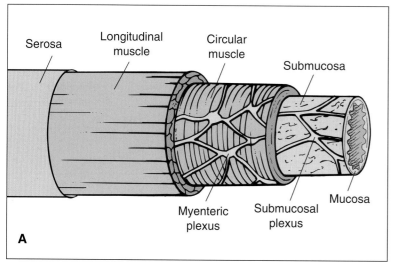
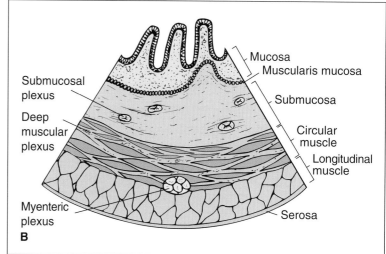

FIGURE 3-2.

A–B, The small bowel is made up of an outermost serosa, a muscular coat (consisting of an outer layer of smooth muscle oriented in the longitudinal axis and an inner circular muscle layer arranged at right angles to the longitudinal muscle), a loose connective tissue submucosa, and the innermost mucosa. The circular muscle layer is also divided by a nerve plexus (the deep muscular plexus) into two parts, a thin inner layer and a thicker outer layer. Another very thin muscle layer, known as the *muscularis mucosae,* also exists at the inner margin of the submucosa. It produces some movement of the mucosa and may affect absorption, but it probably has minimal effects on overall flow of the intestinal contents. (*Adapted from* Gabella [18,19].)

Components of the contractile process

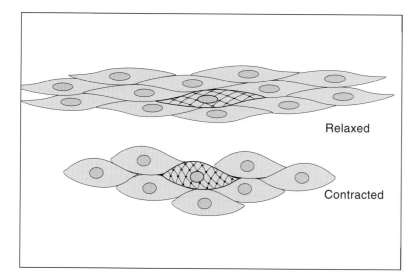

Relaxed

Contracted

FIGURE 3-3.

Gastrointestinal smooth muscle. Intestinal smooth muscle cells are thin, elongated cells that assume a spindle shape when they are isolated and dispersed. They are about 5 to 20 µm in diameter, 400 to 700 µm in length, and their volume is about 2000 to 4000 cubic µm. When they contract they become shorter and plumper. Muscle cells as a tissue are joined together mechanically through cell-to-cell junctions called *intermediate junctions* and *gap junctions*. They are also surrounded by and attached to the stroma, which is made up of elastic and collagen fibers [18]. When the individual muscle cells are coordinated in contractile activity, the mechanically joined cells produce movement of the entire intestinal wall.

Gap junctions

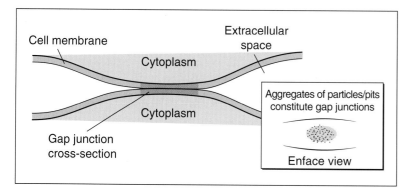

FIGURE 3-4.

The more specialized gap junctions provide not only mechanical adhesion between the cell membranes of adjacent smooth muscle cells, but also cell-to-cell communication [19]. Gap junctions are confined to the circular muscle and are composed of special channels, which allow exchange of ions and other small molecules from cell to cell. They are important in facilitating the spread of electrical excitation along and around the muscle layer. Freeze fracture preparations show that gap junctions are composed of aggregates of intramembrane particles on the surface of one cell. Corresponding aggregates of pits are found on the membranes of adjacent cells. Communication between cells is also provided by the interstitial cells of Cajal through their multiple processes, which also form gap junctions with myocytes [20].

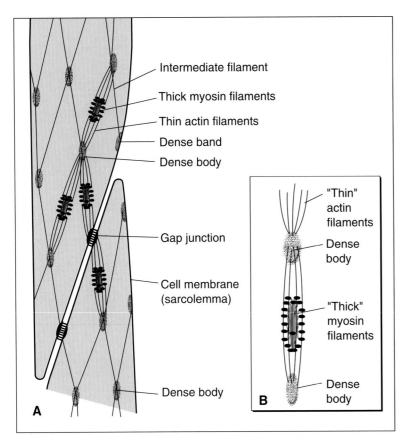

A

B

FIGURE 3-5.

A, In addition to the ordinary organelles common to all cells, smooth muscle cells contain myofilaments of various thickness [21]. So-called *intermediate filaments* (10 nm) are composed of the protein desmin. They connect dense bands on the cell membrane and dense bodies in the cytoplasm to serve as a cytoskeleton on which the contractile filaments can exert their action. **B**, Thin filaments (7 nm) consist of actin and tropomyosin whereas thick filaments (15–17 nm) consist of aggregates of myosin molecules. The actin filaments are arranged in bundles and penetrate and attach to the dense bodies. The myosin molecules are more cable-like and have side polar filaments with cross-bridges, which are essential in the contraction-relaxation process [22].

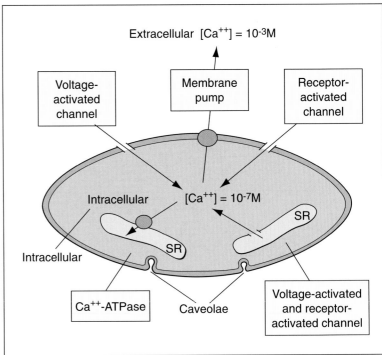

FIGURE 3-6.

Intracellular calcium. The process of contraction is initiated by an increase in intracellular calcium ions [23–25]. Intracellular calcium concentration partly depends on extracellular concentrations of calcium. The low concentration of calcium (10^{-7}M) within the cell at rest is maintained by a membrane pump, which extrudes calcium and maintains the concentration gradient across the cell membrane (sarcolemma). A pump on the endoplasmic reticulum also acts to reduce cytoplasmic calcium by sequestering calcium within the endoplasmic reticulum. Influx of calcium may occur through voltage-sensitive calcium channels that may be activated during membrane depolarization. Calcium influx can also occur through receptor-specific channels that may be activated by neurotransmitters, hormones, or certain drugs. In the latter case, contractions can occur without membrane depolarization. The main source of intracellular calcium ions for initiating contraction, however, appears to be from stores within the sarcoplasmic reticulum. Acetylcholine, cholecystokinin, and substance P (all binding to membrane receptors) have the capacity to release calcium from the sarcoplasmic reticulum through second messengers. ATPase—adenosine triphosphatase; SR—sarcoplasmic reticulum.

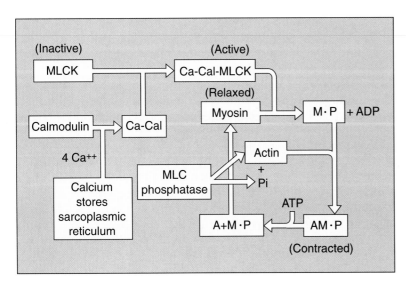

FIGURE 3-7.

Calcium and contractions. When the intracellular calcium rises to a critical level, it activates the contractile apparatus. Four calcium ions react with one molecule of calmodulin, a high-affinity, calcium-binding protein. The calcium-calmodulin complex combines with and activates myosin light-chain kinase (MLCK). This phosphorylating enzyme causes one of the MLC heads to bind with an actin filament. These attachments of myosin to actin, their release, and reattachments are termed *cross-bridge cycling*; this process is responsible for shortening or contraction of the muscle cell [26–31]. A—actin; M—myosin; P—phosphate.

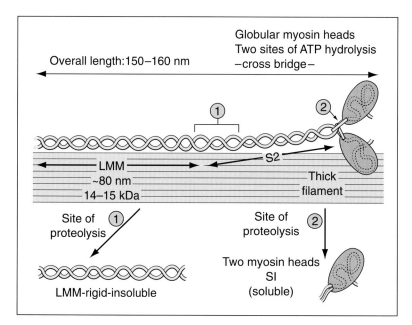

FIGURE 3-8.

Myosin cross-bridges. Myosin filaments are made up of an insoluble core or rope-like tail (LMM) with several soluble cross-bridge heads (SI) that project laterally. The heads are hinged and have the capability of changing the angle at which they project from the tail. This change in configuration occurs through ATP hydrolysis, release of Pi, and a change in binding affinities between actin and myosin. The process results in the relative movement of actin and myosin filaments, shortening of the muscle cell, and the generation of force. (*Adapted from* Hartshorne [32].)

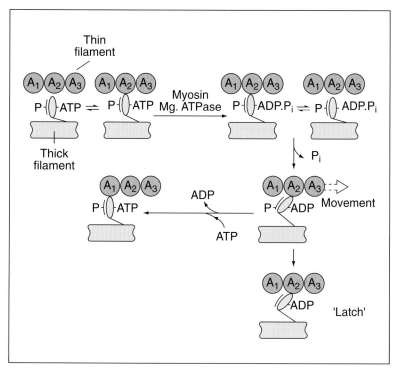

FIGURE 3-9.

Actin and myosin filament interaction. When the globular myosin heads are phosphorylated and ATP is bound, the cross-bridge heads are in an unattached or weakly attached state (*upper left*) until myosin-Mg-ATPase cleaves ATP into ADP and Pi. This enzyme can work on both attached and unattached myosin cross-bridge heads. Force is generated when the myosin heads pivot as Pi is released and movement is generated. Replacement of ADP by ATP restores the angle between the cross-bridge heads, and the cycle can begin again. When the calcium concentration falls, the processes reverse. Dephosphorylation of the myosin head requires the enzyme *myosin phosphatase*. This step stops cross-bridge cycling to allow relaxation. Various drugs can decrease calcium concentration through induction of the second messengers cyclic adenosine monophosphate (cAMP) or cyclic guanosine monophosphate (cGMP). Through the activation of protein kinases, appropriate enzymes are phosphorylated; calcium is either transported out of the cell or bound to intracellular storage sites. The entire process in phasic intestinal contractions takes about 1 to 2 seconds. In the sphincters, and possibly in the intestine, muscles can remain tonically contracted with low rates of energy consumption. These muscles are said to be in the *latch state*. Dephosphorylated cross-bridges remain attached to the actin filaments, even with low calcium concentrations. (*Adapted from* Hartshorne [32].)

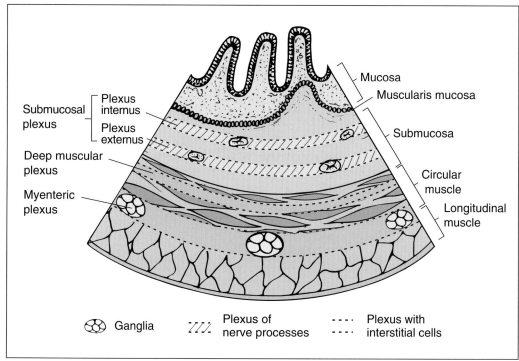

FIGURE 3-10.

The interstitial cells of Cajal [ICC] are only found in certain locations of the layers of the gastrointestinal tract. In the small intestine, ICCs are found in the submucosal plexus (Meissner's plexus internus and Schabadasch's plexus externus), the myenteric (Auerbach's) plexus between the longitudinal and circular muscle layers, and the deep muscular plexus within the inner circular muscle layer. Interstitial cells are closely surrounded by many neurites, and their own multiple branching processes interface with multiple smooth muscle cells as well as with nerves. It is unknown whether these variably shaped cells are derived from the mesenchyme (muscle cells or fibroblasts) or from neural or glial cells. (*Adapted from* Christensen [33].)

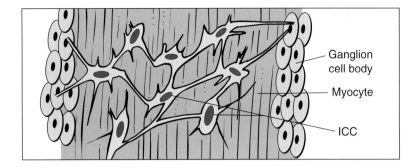

FIGURE 3-11.

One of the most striking features of interstitial cells is that they have multiple processes which form intimate relationships with networks of neurons and muscle cells. Although they have been recognized in the gastrointestinal tract for many years, only recently has the function of the interstitial cells been established. Studies strongly suggest that they play a key role in the origin and propagation of slow waves. The presence of gap junctions and intermediate desmosome-like junctions supports the hypothesis that interstitial cells of Cajal [ICC] and myocytes are coupled electrically and mechanically. Their close proximity to neurons and axons form an interconnecting plexus providing a system to permit neural modulation of intestinal motility. It is likely that these cells play a key role not only in initiating rhythmic pacemaker activity, but also in communicating information between nerves and muscle cells, and in coordinating groups of muscle cells [34].

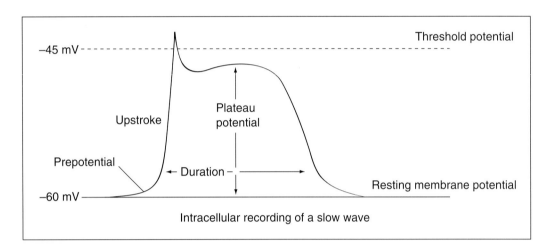

FIGURE 3-12.

Slow waves. More than 50 years ago, recordings from gastric extracellular electrodes revealed rhythmic spontaneous depolarizations that were called *basic electrical rhythm* [36]. They were also observed in the intestine, and are now usually called *slow waves*; other terms are *pacemaker potentials* and *electrical control activity*. The resting transmembrane potential of the smooth muscle is between -40 and -80 mV with respect to the extracellular space. Intracellular recordings show that the membrane potential fluctuates in a rhythmic, regular, and fairly stereotypical fashion; a rapid depolarization is followed by partial repolarization, a more prolonged repolarization or plateau phase, and finally complete repolarization to the baseline resting potential. These "slow waves" are probably generated from the interstitial cells of Cajal within the circular muscle layer.

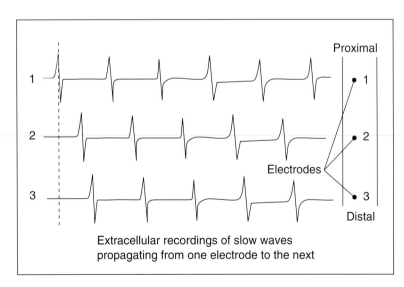

FIGURE 3-13.

Slow waves determine the frequency of contractions and the direction of their propagation. Slow waves are very regular, occurring at a rate of 11 to 12 per minute in the human duodenum, and propagating aborally along the intestine at a velocity of about 7 to 10 cm per second. Circumferentially, slow waves are even more rapidly propagated so that if they are associated with spike bursts, phasic contractions create a moving ring of muscle shortening. The rate of slow-wave depolarization decreases progressively to about 7 to 8 per minute in the distal ileum. The velocity of propagation slows as well. Proximal muscle cells "drive" the cells that are distal to them at a faster rate than they would depolarize if the intestine were physically divided. It appears that both the circular and longitudinal muscle layers are required for normal propagation of slow waves.

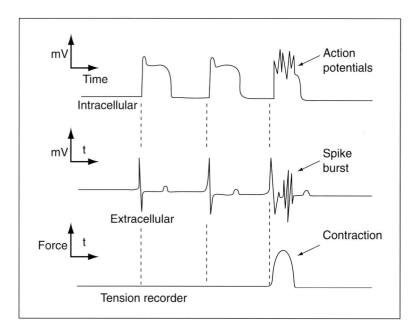

FIGURE 3-14.

Spike bursts. When the membrane depolarization exceeds a threshold level, another more rapid series of membrane depolarizations occurs during the plateau phase of the slow wave. These are called *action potentials* or *spike bursts*; they are associated with phasic contractions of the muscle. Because the timing of these depolarizations is controlled by the rate of slow-wave depolarization, they have also been termed *electrical response activity*. The changes in potential and excitability depend on the permeability of membrane channels to ions, such as sodium, potassium, chloride, and calcium. Permeability is modified by excitatory agonists, such as acetylcholine, from the enteric nerves to enhance contractile activity. Under the influence of inhibitory agonists, such as norepinephrine or nitric oxide, the membrane becomes hyperpolarized and less excitable. In this situation, slow waves continue but do not achieve threshold potentials to initiate spike potentials, and contractions are less likely to occur. Determinants of membrane excitability other than neural input include stretch or mechanical influences and humoral substances, such as hormones, drugs, or other circulating substances.

THE SMALL INTESTINAL NERVOUS SYSTEM

The extrinsic innervation of the intestine

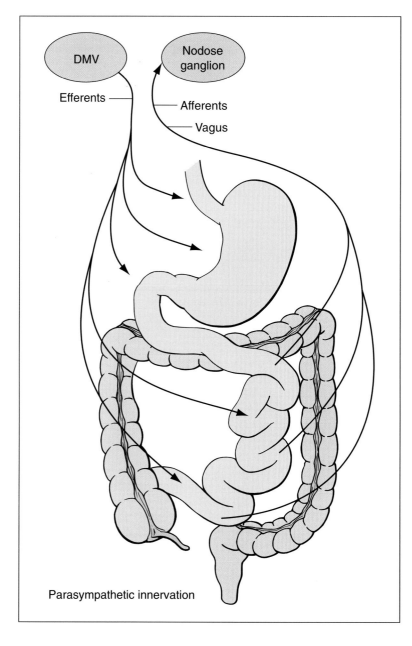

FIGURE 3-15.

The intestinal smooth muscle receives and sends neural messages that modulate its function [37]. The extrinsic nerves relay information to and from the brain, spinal cord, and the extraintestinal ganglia. The intestine can function quite well without the extrinsic nervous system; however, extrinsic nerves serve an important role to modify the activity of the intrinsic nervous system and the motor function of the intestine. In addition to modulating the local enteric reflexes, extrinsic nerves serve to integrate and coordinate widely separate regions of the gastrointestinal tract through its own reflexes. The extrinsic nervous system has three major subdivisions: the parasympathetic pathways, the sympathetic pathways, and the sensory pathways.

The parasympathetic system to the intestine is provided entirely by the tenth cranial nerve, the vagus. The efferent nerve cell bodies arise in the dorsal motor nucleus of the vagus (DMV), and their axons pass directly to synapse mainly with the enteric ganglia. The vagus is made up of four types of nerve fibers: excitatory preganglionic cholinergic nerves, inhibitory preganglionic cholinergic nerves, sympathetic fibers from the cervical ganglia, and afferent fibers from the intestinal wall. In fact, 80% to 90% of the vagal fibers are afferent nerves that terminate on neurons of the nodose ganglia. The excitatory neurotransmitter released from the intramural nerves is acetylcholine; the inhibitory substance is probably nitric oxide. Bilateral section of the vagus has little long-lasting effect on the intestinal motility patterns whereas the response to vagal stimulation usually causes a mixture of excitation and inhibition.

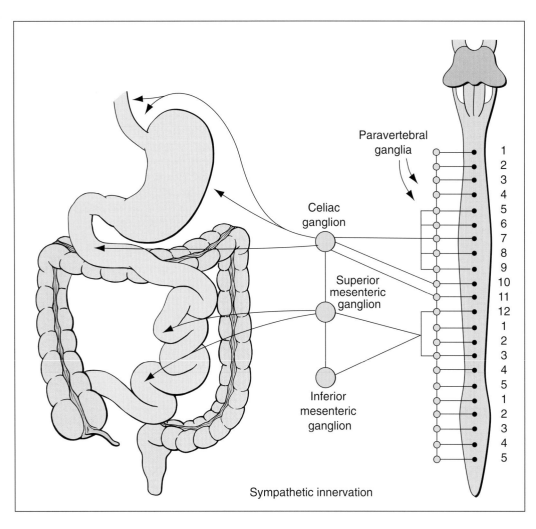

Paravertebral
ganglia

Celiac
ganglion

Superior
mesenteric
ganglion

Inferior
mesenteric
ganglion

1
2
3
4
5
6
7
8
9
10
11
12
1
2
3
4
5
1
2
3
4
5

Sympathetic innervation

FIGURE 3-16.

The thoracolumbar pathways form the sympathetic system. Cholinergic preganglionic cell bodies emanate from the lower thoracic and upper lumbar segments of the cord. Spinal roots T9 and T10 provide the main sympathetic supply to the intestine. Their axons pass through the splanchnic nerves via the celiac, superior mesenteric, and inferior mesenteric ganglia; from there, they pass mainly to the intrinsic enteric ganglia. Noradrenergic postganglionic neurons originate in either the paravertebral ganglia or the prevertebral ganglia (celiac, superior mesenteric, inferior mesenteric); their postganglionic fibers synapse with enteric neurons. Stimulation of the efferent splanchnic nerves inhibits motility through release of norepinephrine. Section of the splanchnic nerves markedly increases motor activity. Thus, this system plays an important inhibitory role in the regulation of motor activity.

Sensory nerves

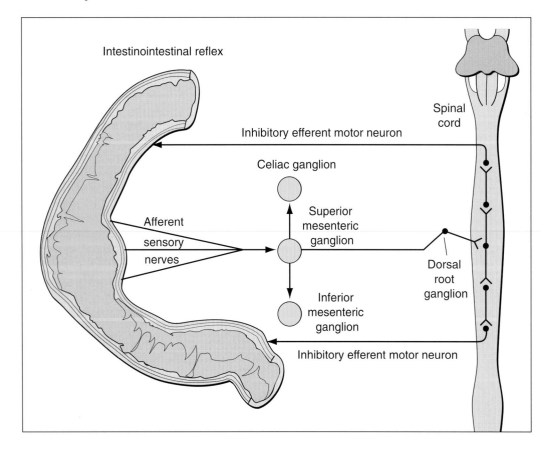

Intestinointestinal reflex

Inhibitory efferent motor neuron

Spinal
cord

Celiac ganglion

Afferent

sensory

nerves

Superior
mesenteric
ganglion

Dorsal
root
ganglion

Inferior
mesenteric
ganglion

Inhibitory efferent motor neuron

FIGURE 3-17.

Vagal afferents project mainly to the nucleus tractus solitarius. Splanchnic nerves enter the cord via the dorsal roots, and second order neurons ascend to the brain via spinal thalamic tracts, spinal reticular tracts, and the dorsal columns. These so-called visceral sensory afferent nerves participate in transmitting conscious sensations, such as satiety, fullness, nausea, discomfort, and pain; however, this is not their only important role, for they also perform regulatory functions that do not evoke any conscious sensations. They participate in modifying intestinal motor functions, such as propulsion, evacuation, and continence. Moderately severe distention of the intestine produces poorly localized pain, which is mostly sensed in the periumbilical region. It also induces a marked inhibition of motility both proximal and distal to the site of the distention; this is known as the *intestinointestinal reflex*. The degree and extent of the inhibition is proportional to the length of intestine distended and the severity of the distention. If intestinal distention affects the colon, it is known as the *intestinocolonic inhibitory reflex*. Distention of the duodenum also has been shown to inhibit gastric contractions. These reflexes are not affected by bilateral vagotomy, but are abolished by splanchnic nerve section.

INTRINSIC INNERVATION

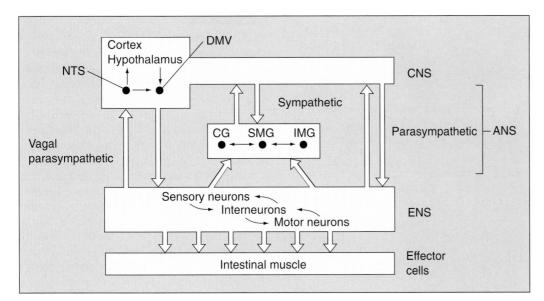

FIGURE 3-18.

The intrinsic nerves are more numerous than the extrinsic nerves, and they communicate largely to modify local motor function through an extensive network of interconnected ganglion cells called *plexuses* [38]. These nerves communicate with sensory nerves from all layers of the intestine and coordinate the patterns of contraction in response to stimuli. This system is called the *enteric nervous system* (ENS) or *gut brain*. It is estimated that it contains one million nerves, about the same number as the spinal cord. ANS—autonomic nervous system; DMV—dorsal motor nucleus of the vagus; NTS—nucleus of the solitary tract. (*Adapted from* Furness and Costa [38].)

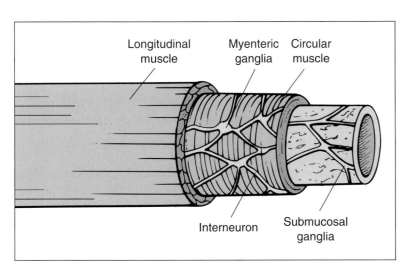

FIGURE 3-19.

The submucous and myenteric plexuses are composed of multiple ganglia, which are collections of nerve cell bodies. All of the ganglia are interconnected by bundles of axons to form a mesh-like arrangement. These include axons from the extrinsic nerves, axons from other intrinsic neurons (interneurons), axons projecting to neurons outside the enteric nervous system, and afferent nerves [39]. The interstitial cells of Cajal are an integral part of this network, and they appear to distribute and amplify the effects of the enteric nerves.

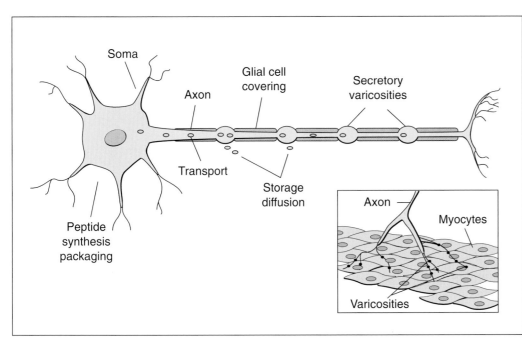

FIGURE 3-20.

The axons have multiple branches, which spread diffusely over sheets of muscle cells. The fine terminals have multiple varicosities which store one or more than one transmitter substance in membrane-bound vesicles. Activated nerves release these substances from the membrane vesicles through interruptions in the glial cell coverings over the neurites. The transmitters diffuse out to influence many muscle cells. Excitatory neurochemical transmission may be perpetuated by electrochemical effects relayed from cell to cell through low-resistance gap junctions. Most axons contain two or more neurotransmitters or neuromodulators. Peptidergic nerves differ from conventional nerves in that the secretory substance is synthesized in the cell soma in peptidergic nerves rather than at the nerve terminal. Peptidergic nerves tend to act more slowly and over greater distances. Finally, secretory substances are secreted in "families" producing a wider range of biologic activities.

Local reflexes

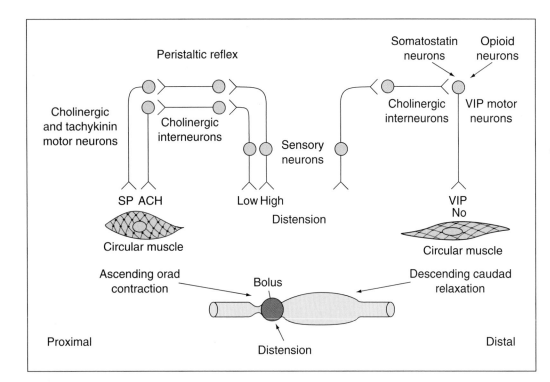

FIGURE 3-21.

Mild distention at a single site induces circular muscle contraction proximal to the distention and inhibition distal to it. Excitatory neurons mostly run in a cephalad direction whereas inhibitory neurons are mainly directed in a caudad direction. This arrangement is responsible for the peristaltic reflex or "law of the intestine." Two predominant types account for approximately 80% of intrinsic motor neurons. Excitatory motor neurons contain acetylcholine (ACH) and tachykinins (neurokinin A and substance [SP]). They are responsible for the contractile phase of the peristaltic reflex. Inhibitory motor neurons contain nitric oxide synthase, vasoactive intestinal peptide (VIP), and PHM (peptide histidine methionine), which is derived from the same precursor as VIP. They are responsible for relaxation of the bowel wall distal to the distending bolus [40,41]. The longitudinal muscle relaxes during circular muscle contraction and contracts during circular muscle relaxation. (*Adapted from* Grider [42].)

Endocrine, paracrine, and chemical regulation

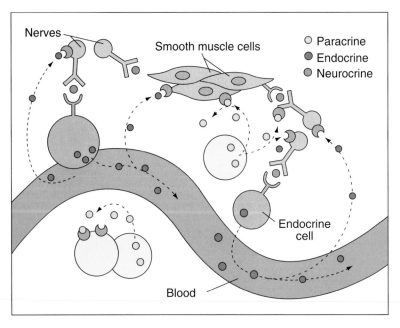

FIGURE 3-22.

Release of neuronal modulators, transmitters, and peptides into the circulation is defined as an endocrine function. Humoral substances may modify intestinal motility, but their effects on motor function are probably less important than their effects on absorption and secretion. Secretin, glucagon, and gastric inhibitory peptide have inhibitory effects when given intravenously; however, their role in the physiologic response to a meal is uncertain. The same is true for the excitatory effect of cholecystokinin. Extracellular release of substances to cause a local effect on adjacent cells is defined as a paracrine effect. Paracrine effects, however, are probably quite important in local responses to many stimuli. Not only do modulators act directly on smooth muscle targets, but they also act on neural transmitter release.

FLUID FLOW AND MOTILITY IN THE INTESTINE

Plain radiographs

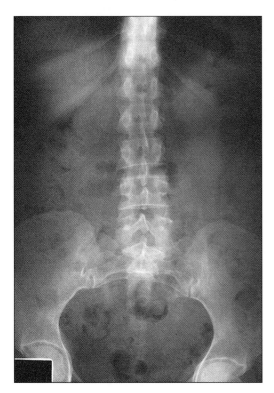

FIGURE 3-23.

Upright and supine plain abdominal radiographs without contrast are useful in assessing gastrointestinal motility. They are readily available, inexpensive, noninvasive, and indirectly provide information about normal and abnormal anatomy and motor function. Despite these benefits, they are frequently not considered in the evaluation of patients with suspected motor disorders. Normal studies, such as in this figure, show little or no air in the intestine, and no air-fluid levels are present. Indirectly, this indicates the absence of bowel obstruction and suggests that the contents of the bowel are moving adequately through the lumen. (*Courtesy of* Dr. Charles Lu, University of Iowa.)

Contrast radiographs

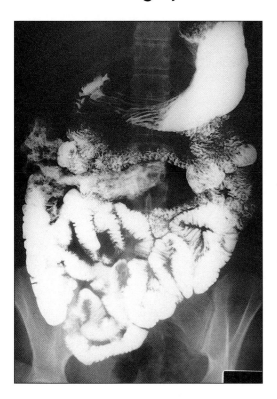

FIGURE 3-24.

One of the earliest and most readily available investigative methods is contrast radiography. Some problems exist in using barium sulfate, the most commonly used contrast medium, to analyze transit. It has a density much greater than water, its flow characteristics are unlike intestinal chyme, and it does not initiate events triggered by the biochemical constituents of food; however, the technique can yield valuable preliminary information about motor activity. The small bowel series can evaluate luminal patency, caliber, and contractile activity. In this study, no dilatation or cut-off of the barium column is present. Barium flows unimpeded through a lumen of relatively uniform caliber except where contractions narrow or obliterate it. The crisp definition of the lumen by barium allows the detailed observation of wall motion when the bowel is filled with contrast medium. Overlapping loops of bowel may, however, obscure details of individual segments, and observations can be misleading if the cavity is only partly filled. The use of cinefluorography allows repeated observations and detailed frame-by-frame analysis, although the results are qualitative. Careful observation shows that stationary ring contractions divide the bolus and produce bidirectional movement, whereas migrating annular contractions produce unidirectional movement either orad or aborad, usually for short distances of several centimeters. A small bowel series is also helpful in detecting the ability of contractions to the obliterate of the lumen. Unfortunately, because of radiation exposure, radiologic studies cannot be repeated often or used for extended periods in humans. (*Courtesy of* Dr. Charles Lu, University of Iowa.)

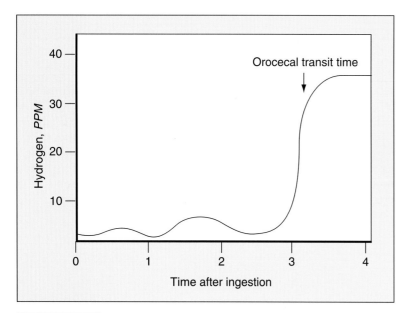

FIGURE 3-25.

Breath hydrogen test for transit. *Transit* is the movement of intestinal chyme; chemical, radioactive, or radiodense markers; or other intestinal contents between two points in the digestive tract. *Propulsion* is the active process of accomplishing that movement. The study of movement involves depositing a liquid or solid bolus at one locus and then serially detecting its arrival at another more distant locus. Most of these studies are only semiquantitative and represent the integrated end point of multiple momentary processes. Consequently, the definition and range of normal values are difficult to determine with precision. In studying transit, it is important to discontinue pharmacologic agents which affect contractility at least 24 hours before the test.

The first use of the breath test to measure orocecal transit was described by Bond and Levitt [43]. A poorly absorbed carbohydrate, such as lactulose, is administered orally to fasting patients. This sugar is not normally hydrolyzed by brush-border enzymes in the small intestine, but passes unchanged to the colon (cecum). There, bacteria act on the remaining disaccharide to form hydrogen, which readily diffuses into the mucosal blood vessels whence it is transported to the lungs and exhaled. End-expiratory air is sampled every 10 to 15 minutes after the meal and measured in electrochemical gas analyzers. An increase in hydrogen concentration of 10 to 20 parts per million above baseline is assumed to represent arrival of the

bolus in the cecum; this correlates with the arrival in the cecum of a simultaneously administered radioisotope as determined by scintigraphy. When lactulose is administered alone to normal subjects, the larger the dose, the shorter the transit time [44]. Larger doses act as osmotic laxatives and accelerate transit. When this same sugar is given with a mixed meal that includes proteins and fats, the transit time is prolonged, but results are more reproducible [45]. This is partly due to delay of gastric emptying and slower entry of the marker into the bowel. Transit is further retarded if the nonabsorbed carbohydrate is part of a solid meal, (ie, raffinose, which is the nondigested substrate in beans) [44,46]. Frequently, a brief rise in hydrogen occurs within the first hour of monitoring. This early peak is thought to result from the fermentation of ingested sugar by mouth bacteria; it may be reduced or eliminated by brushing the teeth and rinsing the mouth with an antibacterial substance, such as chlorhexidine [47]. Some of this early peak may also result from ileal emptying of residue from a previous meal, stimulated by the current meal. This can be reduced by a longer fast and elimination of nondigestible fiber and carbohydrates from the previous meal. It is also important to instruct the subject to refrain from smoking before and during the test because smoke can interfere with the measurement of breath hydrogen concentrations. The major problem with the test occurs when bacteria overgrow in the small intestine. This happens in patients with achlorhydria, which may be due to varied causes, such as potent antisecretory drugs, previous gastric surgery, or pernicious anemia. It may also occur in patients with mechanical small bowel obstruction or disordered motility. Bacterial overgrowth leads to fermentation of carbohydrates in the small bowel and an early rise in breath hydrogen levels. Administration of antibiotics may reduce the bacterial flora in the colon and prevent or delay a rise in breath hydrogen.

The breath hydrogen test is inexpensive and can safely be used repeatedly. In normal subjects reproducibility is good, provided that conditions are carefully controlled; however, there are a great number of variables that may influence the results and interfere with interpretation of the test for orocecal transit. Thus, even though it is simple, safe, and inexpensive to administer, it is not a good test for clinical decision making. Even when administered according to a controlled and standardized protocol, its inherent defects do not allow reliable interpretation. This is especially true in patients in whom delayed transit is likely. For this reason, its use has been most helpful in the study of normal physiology and the effects of stress, medications, and other related variables on transit. This test should not be relied on for the diagnosis of dysmotility [48].

Radioscintigraphy

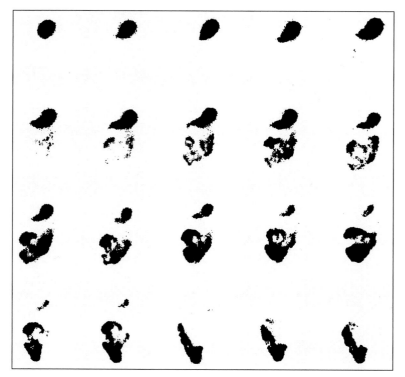

FIGURE 3-26.

The incorporation of a nonabsorbed γ-emitting radioisotope into various meals allows monitoring of the flow of fluids from one point in the intestine to another using a collimated γ camera [49]. After an overnight fast the test meal is given orally. ^{99m}Technitium-labeled sulfur colloid in scrambled eggs, ^{99m}technitium-labeled chicken liver, or ^{131}I-labeled bran are frequently used as the radioactive source. After the meal, serial abdominal images are obtained at regular intervals for up to 10 to 12 hours.

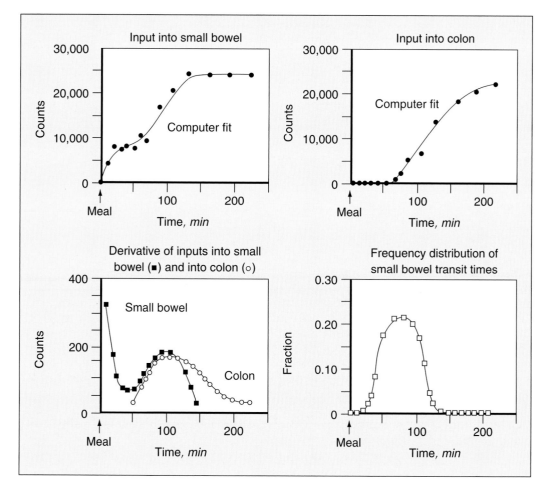

FIGURE 3-27.

Counts are corrected for decay, for movement of isotope in the anterior-posterior axis, and for overlap of the stomach, intestinal loops, and colon. Using a technique called *deconvolution*, the rate of small bowel transit can be computed using the rate of gastric emptying and colonic filling [51]. Poor resolution of the detection device prevents the precise identification of wall motion. Overlapping of bowel loops and inadequate anatomic localization of the isotope cause problems in interpreting the information obtained by using this technique. The ability to incorporate the marker into normal meals, however, provides quantitative, reproducible information not available by other methods. When the meal is given orally, the transit represents the resultant of gastric emptying and transit of the meal residue through the small bowel. Extreme delay of gastric emptying delays the passage of bowel contents through the intestine. The rate of passage of the meal is influenced not only by the motor activity of the bowel, but also by changes in either epithelial absorption or secretion. Again the hazards of radioactive materials limit the repeated use of these agents in humans. (*Adapted from* Malagelada *et al.* [50].)

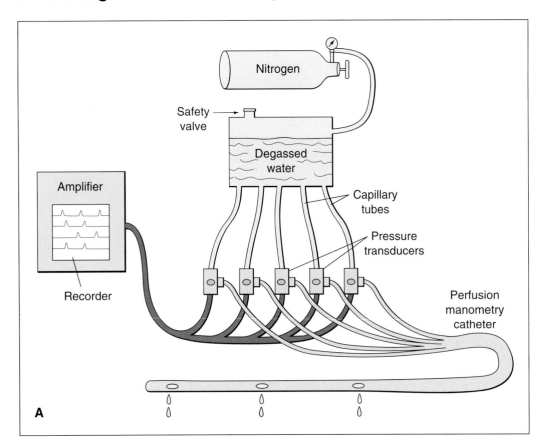

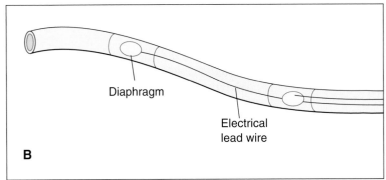

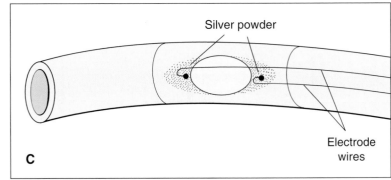

FIGURE 3-28.

Intestinal contractions cause wall motion, creating forces that increase intraluminal pressure and induce flow. Direct observation of wall motion is not feasible clinically. Highly sophisticated intraluminal sensors and modern recorders offer great accuracy, sensitivity, versatility, and portability. Two types of sensors are now common, both of which use transducers (converters of mechanical to electrical energy): perfused, open-tipped, side-hole, low-compliance catheters transmit forces to sensitive external transducers (**panel A**), or forces are transmitted directly to miniature transducers incorporated into small-diameter intraluminal catheters (**panel B**). Both of these approaches are sensitive and produce high-fidelity recordings of pressure waves within the lumen. Although the measurement of mechanical activity resulting from contractions is the more commonly performed study, the electromyogram yields additional important information about motor function. Electrical signals can be detected transmucosally using intraluminal electrodes. High-quality recordings from multiple bipolar electrodes can be made using a technique described by Coremans and associates [51]. Lead wires within the catheter are incorporated into collections of silver powder at opposite edges of holes in the catheter (**panel C**). The mucosa is aspirated into the hole by applying suction to the lumen of the catheter, creating an electrical contact between the intestine and the electrodes. This permits bipolar recordings and maintains a constant spatial relationships between the electrodes.

Intestinal manometry

Normal fasting and fed motility patterns

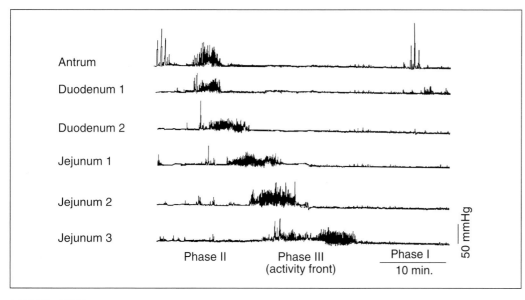

FIGURE 3-29.

The most studied intestinal motility patterns are the fasting migrating motor complex (equivalent to the migrating myoelectric complex, both of which are abbreviated MMC), and the fed or postprandial pattern [52]. The MMC is made up of three different phases: phase I lasts about 5 to 20 minutes and is characterized by absence of any spike bursts or contractions; phase II lasts from 10 to 40 minutes and exhibits intermittent contractions or spike bursts on about 50% of slow waves; and phase III (alternatively called the *activity front*) lasts from 3 to 6 minutes and consists of an intense burst of regular rhythmic contractions or spike bursts occurring at the same rate as the slow waves. The activity front begins in the stomach or the proximal jejunum and migrates along the small intestine. Only 10% of phase III activity fronts reach the ileocecal valve. When phase III begins in the stomach, it is preceded by an increase in serum motilin concentration. This complex repeats every 1 to 2 hours and recurs indefinitely until interrupted by a meal. In these recordings from normal subjects without gastrointestinal symptoms, the catheter (Gaeltec Limited, Dunvegan, Isle of Skye, Scotland) had strain gauge transducers spaced 15-cm apart with an outer diameter of 3.3 mm. Recordings were made using a 4 Mb solid-state datalogger at a sampling rate of 4 Hz (Synectics Medical, Irving, TX.)

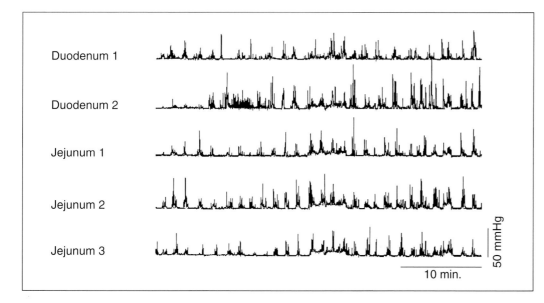

FIGURE 3-30.

Phase II activity varies considerably. This recording is characterized by prominent "clustered" contractions. This type of activity during the fasting state has been reported to occur in the irritable bowel syndrome [53]. As can be seen in this recording, clustered activity during fasting can be very prominent in a normal subject with no abdominal pain. Thus, it is not an abnormal motor pattern in the fasting period. Clustered activity within an hour of a meal is abnormal and is characteristic of partial bowel obstruction, but also has been noted to occur after meals in pseudo-obstruction syndromes [54].

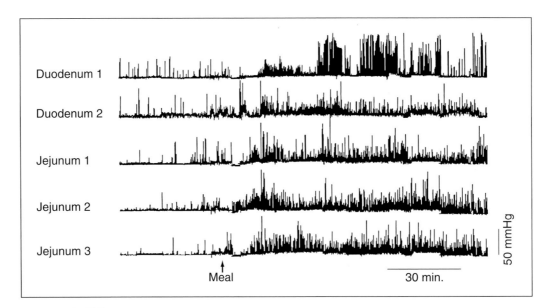

FIGURE 3-31.

After a meal, a brisk increase in motor activity occurs. The fed pattern lasts for 3 to 6 hours, depending on the size and content of the meal. During this time the fasting migrating motor complex (phases I, II, III) is not seen (*ie*, it is interrupted after meals). Meals high in fat and calories prolong the fed pattern. The fed pattern characterized by intermittent, irregular contractions or spike bursts that appear to occur randomly. All follow slow waves, but only about 30% to 60% of slow waves are followed by contractions. Spike bursts migrate from a few millimeters to 30 to 40 cm or more. Circumferential spike bursts are associated with lumen-occluding contractions. Spike bursts which do not occur in all quadrants around the bowel produce eccentric contractions and only partially occlude the lumen. The number of contractions at any one site is influenced by the content of the meal. Non-nutrient meals produce the greatest number of contractions, whereas meals mainly consisting of carbohydrates produce more contractions than meals which are high in protein and fat. Protein- and fat-rich meals not only produce fewer contractions, but the contractions also migrate shorter distances.

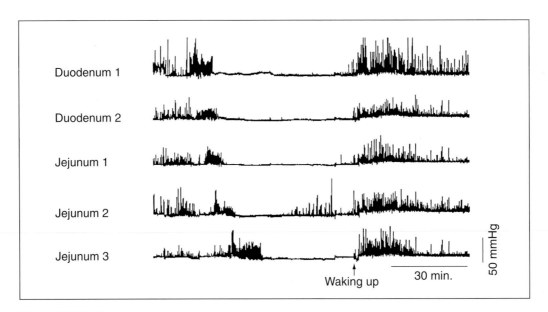

FIGURE 3-32.

During sleep, fasting motor activity is often reduced. The pattern resembles that of the awake fasting pattern, but the cycle duration is shorter. In most situations, phase II activity is markedly reduced and the duration of quiescent activity (phase I) is increased. Upon waking, a significant increase in motor activity occurs as the small bowel appears to awaken as well. It is important to recognize that a wide variety of contractile patterns occurs in normal persons.

TABLE 3-2. CLINICAL USE OF JEJUNAL MANOMETRY

Normal intestinal contraction patterns are extremely variable, and great caution must be exerted before calling results of a recording abnormal.

Manometry cannot be used to make diagnoses of cause; it only demonstrates contractile patterns. Additional studies done serially are needed to define the spectrum of contractile patterns in normal subjects and in specific diseases.

In advanced disease, manometry is often unreliable. As the intestine decompensates, it becomes dilated and changes in intraluminal pressure produce a *common-cavity* phenomenon with identical pressure waves occurring simultaneously in multiple channels.

There is great need for standardization of equipment and study protocols, in addition to consensus on what is normal and abnormal.

Catheters currently in use are limited. Not all contractions are detected by side-hole sensors because of the discrepancy between catheter and lumen diameters. No catheters capable of recording electrical activity or electrical plus mechanical activity are commercially available.

Physical exertion, mental stress, balloon distension of the intestine, the cold pressor test, pharmacologic agents, and systemic hormones affect motility patterns. These and other perturbations need to be studied in controls and various disease states.

The clinical history, physical examination, blood tests, radiography with or without contrast media, transit studies, autonomic testing, and especially histology must all be considered in interpreting manometry. It is not a stand-alone test because it is not standardized and because its limitations and variability must be considered in making clinical decisions.

TABLE 3-2.

Jejunal manometry is not well standardized. No official consensus exists on what is normal or abnormal, and recordings from normals vary considerably. Nevertheless, experience is growing, and its study provides important clinical information if a number of factors are considered.

REFERENCES

1. Meissner G: èber die Nerven der Darmwand. *Z Rat Med* 1857, 8:364–396.

2. Bayliss WM, Starling EH: The movements and innervation of the small intestine. *J Physiol (Lond)* 1899, 24:99–143.

3. Cannon WB: The movements of the intestines studied by means of the Röntgen rays. *Am J Physiol* 1902, 6:251–277.

4. Langley JN: Das sympatische und verwandt nervöse system. *Ergeb Physiol* 1903, 2:818–872.

5. Boldyreff WN: Le travail periodique de l'appareil disgestif en dehors de la disgestion. *Arch Des Sci Biol* 1905, 11:1–157.

6. Alvarez WC: Functional variations in contraction of different parts of the intestine. *Q J Med* 1914, 35:177–193.

7. Payne WW, Poulton EP: Visceral pain in the upper alimentary tract. *Q J Med* 1921, 17:53–80.

8. Ambache N: The electrical activity of the isolated mammalian intestine. *J Physiol (Lond)* 1947, 106:139–153.

9. Bülbring ER, Lin RCY, Schofield GC: An investigation of the peristaltic reflex in relation to anatomical observations. *Q J Exp Physiol* 1958, 43:26–37.

10. Bortoff A: Slow wave variations of small intestine. *Am J Physiol* 1961, 201:203–208.

11. Dewey MM, Barr L: Intercellular connection between smooth muscle cells: The nexus. *Science* 1962, 137:670–672.

12. Brown JC: The presence of a gastric motor stimulating property in duodenal mucosa. *Gastroenterology* 1967, 52:225–229.

13. Christensen J, Schedl HP, Clifton JA: The basic electrical rhythm of the duodenum in normal human subjects and in patients with thyroid disease. *J Clin Invest* 1964, 43:1659–1667.

14. Szurszewski JH: A migrating electric complex of the canine small intestine. *Am J Physiol* 1969, 217:1757–1763.

15. Wood JD: Electrical activity from single neurons in Auerbach's plexus. *Am J Physiol* 1970, 219:159–169.

16. Gabella G: Special muscle cells and their innervation in the mammalian small intestine. *Cell Tissue Res* 1974, 153:63–77.

17. Furness JB, Costa M: Types of nerves in the enteric nervous system. *Neuroscience* 1980, 5:1–20.

18. Thuneberg L: Interstitial cells of Cajal: Intestinal pacemaker cells? *Adv Anat Embryol Cell Biol* 1982, 71:1–130.

19. Gabella G, Blundell D: Gap junctions of the muscle of the small and large intestine. *Cell Tissue Res* 1981, 219:459–488.

20. Taylor AB, Kreider D, Prosser CL: Electron microscopy of the connective tissue between longitudinal and circular muscle of small intestine of cat. *Am J Anat* 1977, 150:427–442.

21. Gabella G: Structural apparatus for force transmission in smooth muscle. *Physiol Rev* 1984, 64:455–463.

22. Craig R, Megerman J: Assembly of smooth muscle myosin into side-polar filaments. *J Cell Biol* 1977, 75:990–996.

23. Somlyo AV, Somlyo AP: Strontium accumulation by sarcoplasmic reticulum and mitochondria in vascular smooth muscle. *Science* 1971, 174:990–996.

24. Henmann H-G: The subcellular localization of calcium in vertebrate smooth muscle: Calcium-containing and calcium-accumulating structures in muscle cells of mouse intestine. *Cell Tissue Res* 1976, 169:221–223.

25. Bolton TB: Mechanisms of action of transmitters and other substances on smooth muscle. *Physiol Rev* 1979 59:606–718.

26. Adelstein RS, Conti MA, Hathaway DR, Klee CB: Phosphorylation of smooth muscle myosin light chain kinase by the catalytic subunit of adenosine 3':5' monophosphate-dependent protein kinase. *J Biol Chem* 1978, 253:8347–8350.

27. Shoenberg CF, Haselgrove JC: Filaments and ribbons in vertebrate smooth muscle. *Nature* 1984, 249:152–154.

28. Eisenberg E, Hill TL: Muscle contraction and free energy transduction in biological systems. *Science* 1985, 227:999–1006.

29. Stull JT, Tansey MG, Word RA, *et al.*: Myosin light chain kinase phosphorylation: Regulation of the Ca^{2+} sensitivity of contractile elements. *Adv Exp Med Biol* 1991, 304:129–138.

30. Sanders KM: Ionic mechanisms of electrical rhythmicity in gastrointestinal smooth muscle. *Ann Rev Physiol* 1992, 54:439–453.

31. Jiang H, Stephens NL: Calcium and smooth muscle contraction. *Mol Cell Biochem* 1994, 135:1–9.

32. Hartshorne D: Biochemistry of the contractile process in smooth muscle. In *Physiology of the Gastrointestinal Tract*. Edited by Johnson LR. New York: Raven Press; 1987:431.

33. Christensen J: Gastrointestinal motility. In *Physiological Basis of Medical Practice*. Edited by West JB, Taylor. Baltimore: Williams & Wilkins; 1987:614–644.

34. Thuneberg L: Interstitial cells of Cajal: Intestinal pacemaker cells? *Adv Anat Embryol Cell Biol* 1982, 71:1–130.

35. Thuneberg L: Interstitial cells of Cajal. In *Handbook of Physiology, Section 6: The Gastrointestinal System, Volume I: Motility and Circulation*. Edited by Wood JD. Bethesda: American Physiological Society; 1989:353.

36. Richter CP: Action currents from the stomach. *Am J Physiol* 1924, 67:612–633.

37. Gonella J, Bouvier-Blanquet F: Extrinsic nervous control of motility of small and large intestines and related sphincters. *Physiol Rev* 1987, 67:902–961.

38. Furness JB, Costa M: Distribution of intrinsic nerve cell bodies and axons which take up aromatic amines and their precursors in the small intestine of the guinea pig. *Cell Tissue Res* 1978, 188:527–543.

39. Costa M, Furness JB, Pompalo S, *et al.*: Projections and chemical coding of neurons with immunoreactivity for nitric oxide synthase in the guinea pig small intestine. *Neurosci Lett* 1992, 148:121–125.

40. Brooks SJ: Neuronal nitric oxide in the gut. *J Gastroenterol Hepatol* 1993, 8:590–603.

41. Daniel EE, Haugn C, Woskowski Z, *et al.*: Role of nitric oxide-related inhibition in intestinal function: Relation to vasoactive intestinal peptide. *Am J Physiol* 1994, 266:631–639.

42. Grider JR: Peptidergic regulation of smooth muscle contractility. In *Handbook of Experimental Pharmacology: Gastrointestinal Peptides*. Edited by Brown DR. New York: Springer-Verlag; 1993:227–295.

43. Bond JH, Levitt MP: Investigation of small bowel transit time in man utilizing pulmonary hydrogen (H_2) measurements. *J Lab Clin Med* 1975, 85:546–555.

44. Read NW, Miles CA, Fisher D, *et al.*: Transit time of a meal through the stomach, small intestine, and colon in normal subjects and its role in the pathogenesis of diarrhea. *Gastroenterology* 1980, 79:1276–1282.

45. LaBrooy SJ, Male P-J, Beavis AK, Misiewicz JJ: Assessment of the reproducibility of the lactose H_2 breath test as a measure of mouth to cecum transit time. *Gut* 1983, 24:893–895.

46. Korth H, Muller I, Erckenbrecht JF, Wienbeck M: Breath hydrogen as a test for gastrointestinal transit. *Hepatogastroenterology* 1984, 31:282–284.

47. Thompson DG, O'Brien JD, Hardie JM: Influence of the oropharyngeal microflora on the measurement of exhaled breath hydrogen. *Gastroenterology* 1984, 91:853–860.

48. Thompson DG, Binfield P, DeBelder KA, *et al.*: Extraintestinal influences on exhaled breath hydrogen measurements during the investigation of gastrointestinal disease. *Gut* 1985, 26:1349–1352.

49. Read NW, Al-Janabi MN, Edwards CA, Barber DC: Relationship between postprandial motor activity in the human small intestine and the gastrointestinal transit of food. *Gastroenterology* 1984, 86:721–727.

50. Malagelada J-R, Robertson JS, Brown ML *et al.*: Intestinal transit of solid and liquid components of a meal in health. *Gastroenterology* 1984, 87:1255–1263.

51. Coremans G, Janssens H, Vantrappen G: Migrating action potential complexes in a patient with secretory diarrhea. *Dig Dis Sci* 1987, 32:1201–1206.

52. Szurszewski JH: A migrating electrical complex of the canine small intestine. *Am J Physiol* 1969, 217:742–750.

53. Kellow JE, Gill RC, Wingate DL: Prolonged ambulant recordings of small bowel motility demonstrate abnormalities in the irritable bowel syndrome. *Gastroenterology* 1990, 98:1208–1218.

54. Summers RW, Anuras S, Green J: Jejunal manometry patterns in health, partial intestinal obstruction, and pseudoobstruction. *Gastroenterology* 1983, 85:1290–1300.

Chapter 4

Secretory Diarrhea

LAWRENCE R. SCHILLER

Diarrhea, defined most comprehensively as the frequent passage of loose stools, results from reduced water absorption by the gut. This can be caused by ingestion of poorly absorbed, osmotically active molecules that obligate retention of water intraluminally, a process known as *osmotic diarrhea*, or by a reduction in the rate of solute and water absorption by the gut, a process known as *secretory diarrhea*. Despite the name, it is rare for secretory diarrhea to result from net secretion by the entire intestine. Stool volume has to exceed 10 L per 24 hours (the normal volume of fluid traversing the gut) before net secretion is present. Most patients with secretory diarrhea produce less than 2 L per 24 hours, so a reduction in global intestinal absorption rather than net secretion is present. Diarrhea can result from as little as a 1% reduction in the usual 99% efficiency of water absorption by the intestine.

Many different processes can result in secretory diarrhea. These include reduction in surface area (short-bowel syndrome, postresection diarrheas), extensive mucosal disease (Crohn's disease, celiac disease), congenital absence of an ion transport mechanism (congenital chloridorrhea), toxins produced by bacteria (cholera, enterotoxigenic *Escherichia coli*), luminal secretagogues (certain laxatives, bile acids), circulating peptides or other regulatory substances (gastrinoma, vasoactive intestinal peptidoma), some drugs and poisons (olsalazine [Dipentum], misoprostol [Cytotec], heavy metals), and a variety of medical problems that compromise regulation of the gut (vagotomy, diabetes mellitus). The differential diagnosis of secretory diarrhea, therefore, is quite extensive.

Evaluation of patients with secretory diarrhea may be limited or complex. Acute secretory diarrhea most often results from infection; therefore, diagnostic tests should be limited and directed at determining the type of infection (viral, bacterial, or protozoal). Chronic diarrhea has a broader differential diagnosis, and diagnostic tests must be selected on the basis of clues from the patient's history. Structural disease of the small bowel should be excluded by means of radiography. Analysis of a stool collection can help to confirm the secretory nature of the diarrhea by measurement of fecal electrolytes and the presence or absence of nutrient malabsorption, laxative use, or evidence of inflammation (blood, fecal leukocytes) or infection (positive bacterial cultures or ova and parasite examinations). Depending on the circumstances, mucosal biopsy of the small intestine or colon, measurement of circulating secretagogues or urinary metabolites, and tests of endocrine function may be useful.

Ideal treatment for secretory diarrhea is to make a specific diagnosis and to treat the cause of the problem. Lacking a specific diagnosis, therapy should consist of adequate rehydration (if necessary) and nonspecific antidiarrheal drugs. Rehydration can be provided intravenously or orally. Oral rehydration solutions depend on the stimulation of fluid and electrolyte absorption by ingestion of glucose or other cotransported substrates. Nonspecific antidiarrheal agents include opiates, clonidine, and octreotide. Their major effect is to retard intestinal transit, allowing more time for absorption to take place. Clonidine also may stimulate absorption rate, and octreotide may reduce the release or antiabsorptive effects of some secretagogues.

GENERAL FEATURES OF SECRETORY DIARRHEAS

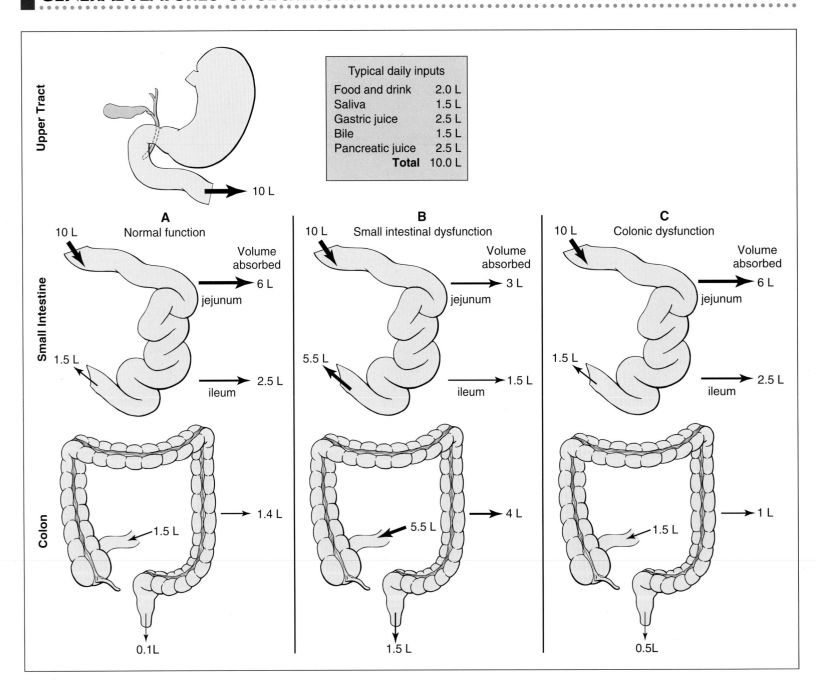

Typical daily inputs	
Food and drink	2.0 L
Saliva	1.5 L
Gastric juice	2.5 L
Bile	1.5 L
Pancreatic juice	2.5 L
Total	**10.0 L**

FIGURE 4-1.

Water fluxes through the intestine. **A,** In health, 9 to 10 L of fluid enter the intestine in the form of ingested food and drink and salivary, gastric, biliary, pancreatic, and intestinal secretions [1]. Most of this fluid is reabsorbed as it traverses the intestine, and roughly 1 to 2 L of fluid enters the colon each day. In the colon, 90% of the fluid is reabsorbed, leaving approximately 100 to 200 mL each day to be excreted in the feces. **B,** Diseases compromising absorption of water by the small intestine increase the volume of fluid entering the colon each day. Colonic reabsorptive capacity (approximately 4 L per 24 hours) has to be overcome before diarrhea will result. **C,** On the other hand, diseases compromising absorption of water only by the colon typically produce lower volume-diarrheas because most intraluminal fluid is absorbed before entering the colon.

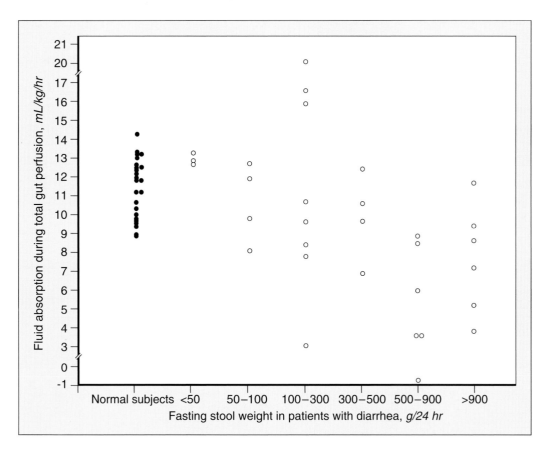

FIGURE 4-2.

Water transport rates during steady-state total gut perfusion. In this study of 31 patients with secretory diarrhea, water absorption or secretion was measured during total gut perfusion [2]. The patients are arranged by stool weight during fasting. Even patients with large fasting stool weights had net total intestinal absorption during perfusion. Only one patient had net secretion during the study. Persistent diarrhea clinically in the face of net absorption during experimental perfusion may relate to phasic transit of fluid through the intestine, which would reduce the amount of time available for absorption, or segmental secretion, especially distally in the gut, where an even more distal absorbing segment could not compensate. (*Adapted from* Fordtran *et al.* [2]; with permission.)

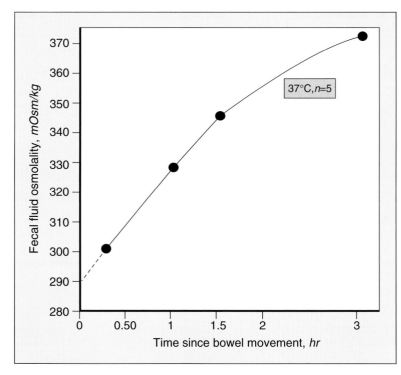

FIGURE 4-3.

Stool osmolality increases in vitro after collection. The intestinal mucosa is quite permeable to water, and this prevents the establishment of large osmotic gradients between luminal contents and body fluids. Thus, the osmolality of colon contents is the same as that of plasma, approximately 290 mOsm/kg. Once the stool sample is in a container outside the body, bacterial fermentation of stool carbohydrate generates osmoles that can no longer equilibrate with body fluids. Measurement of stool osmolality is only useful clinically to suggest contamination of the specimen with water or hypotonic urine if measured osmolality is substantially less than 290 mOsm/kg. (*Adapted from* Hammer *et al.* [3].)

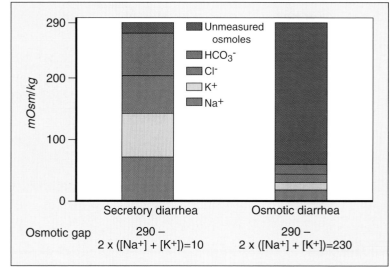

FIGURE 4-4.

Calculation of osmotic gap. Because colonic luminal contents are in osmotic equilibrium with body fluids, the sum of the concentrations of ions and small molecules contributing to osmolality must equal plasma osmolality, usually 290 mOsm/kg. In secretory diarrhea, electrolyte absorption is compromised so that sodium, potassium, and their counterions account for most of the osmoles in stool water. In osmotic diarrhea, electrolyte absorption is normal so that measured cations and their corresponding anions account for only a fraction of the osmoles in stool water. Unmeasured osmoles (*eg*, carbohydrate or magnesium ion) comprise most of the "osmotic space." Osmotic gaps more than 50 mOsm/kg are associated with ingestion of a poorly absorbed substance [4].

TABLE 4-1. TYPICAL FEATURES OF SECRETORY DIARRHEA

Voluminous, watery stools
Little or no fecal osmotic gap, stool pH near 7.0
Usually persists during fasting
Usually no pus, blood, or excess fat in stools

TABLE 4-1.

Typical features of secretory diarrhea.

DIFFERENTIAL DIAGNOSIS OF SECRETORY DIARRHEA

TABLE 4-2. MECHANISMS AND CAUSES OF SECRETORY DIARRHEA

Reduction in mucosal surface area
  Postresection diarrhea
  Short-bowel syndrome
Extensive mucosal disease and inflammation
  Viral gastroenteritis
  Celiac disease
  Whipple's disease
  Crohn's disease
  Lymphoma
Absence of ion transport mechanism
  Congenital chloridorrhea
Bacterial toxins
  Cholera
  Enterotoxigenic *Escherichia coli*
  Shigella
  Staphylococcus
  Clostridium perfringens
Luminal secretagogues
  Bile acids
  Fatty acids, hydroxy-fatty acids
  Phenolphthalein, ricinoleic acid, bisacodyl

Circulating secretagogues
  Gastrin (Zollinger-Ellison syndrome)
  Vasoactive intestinal polypeptide (VIPoma, ganglioneuroma, neuroblastoma, pheochromocytoma)
  Calcitonin, prostaglandins (medullary carcinoma of the thyroid)
  Somatostatin (somatostatinoma)
  Glucagon (glucagonoma)
  Serotonin, kinins (carcinoid tumor)
  Thyroxine (hyperthyroidism)
  Histamine (mastocytosis)
Drugs and poisons
  Misoprostol
  Olsalazine
  Colchicine
  Propranolol
  Quinidine
  Heavy metals

Abnormal circulation
  Radiation enteritis
  Mesenteric ischemia
  Mesenteric venous thrombosis
  Lymphangiectasia
Disordered regulation
  Postvagotomy diarrhea
  Postsympathectomy
  Diabetic autonomic neuropathy
  Addison's disease
Undetermined or complex mechanism
  Collagen-vascular diseases
  Giardiasis
  Tuberculosis
  Niacin deficiency
  "Idiopathic" secretory diarrhea
Secretory diarrheas of exclusively colonic origin
  Ulcerative colitis, Crohn's disease of colon
  Microscopic ("lymphocytic") colitis
  Collagenous colitis
  Secreting villous adenoma

TABLE 4-2.

Mechanisms and causes of secretory diarrhea.

Postresection diarrhea

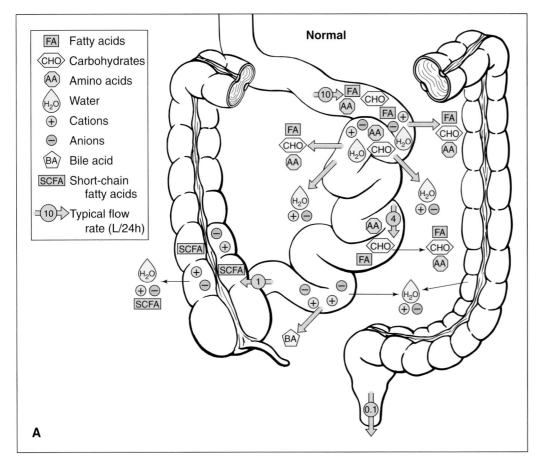

A

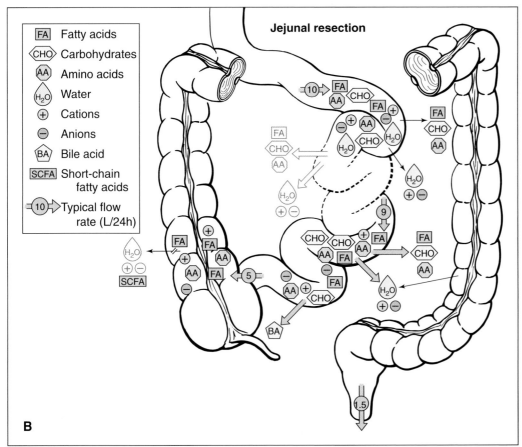

B

FIGURE 4-5.

Resection of different parts of the small intestine has differing effects, depending on the physiology of the segment removed. **A**, Under normal conditions, most nutrient absorption and nutrient-stimulated electrolyte absorption takes place in the jejunum. The ileum is responsible for absorption of residual nutrients, absorption of sodium against a concentration gradient, and completion of bile acid absorption. The colon is responsible for short-chain fatty acid absorption and the completion of fluid and electrolyte absorption. **B**, Jejunal resection compromises nutrient absorption and electrolyte absorption secondary to nutrient absorption. The ileum can compensate in part for nutrient absorption, but malabsorbed fatty acids can lead to inhibition of water absorption when they enter the colon. Because the jejunum is responsible for absorption of a substantial fraction of the water and electrolytes presented to the intestine each day, more distal regions of the bowel may not be able to compensate fully and diarrhea can be quite voluminous.

(continued on next page)

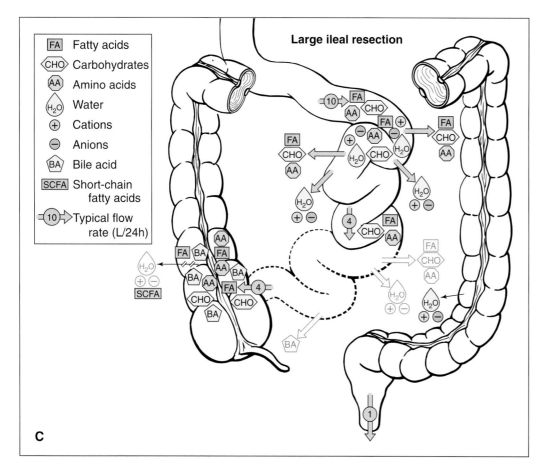

Large ileal resection

FIGURE 4-5. (CONTINUED)

C, Large ileal resections also produce substantial fluid and electrolyte malabsorption, nutrient malabsorption, and fatty acid–induced diarrhea. Bile acid malabsorption may also contribute to diarrhea, but fecal volumes are so large that the bile acid concentration in the colon may not reach a cathartic threshold (3 to 5 mmol/L). **D,** Smaller ileal resections (< 100 cm) compromise bile acid absorption and can result in bile acid–induced secretory diarrhea because less malabsorbed water is present to dilute bile acids below the cathartic threshold. Bile acid–binding resins (*eg,* cholestyramine) can reverse this mechanism of diarrhea.

(*continued on next page*)

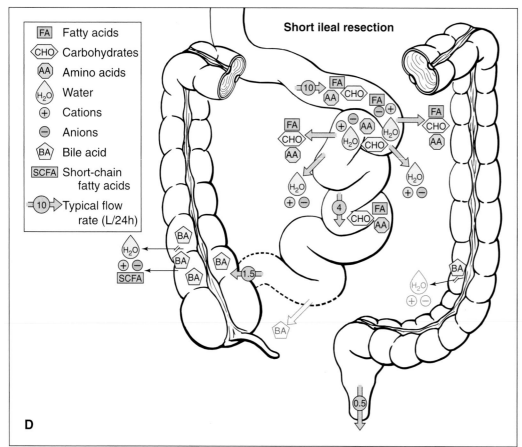

Short ileal resection

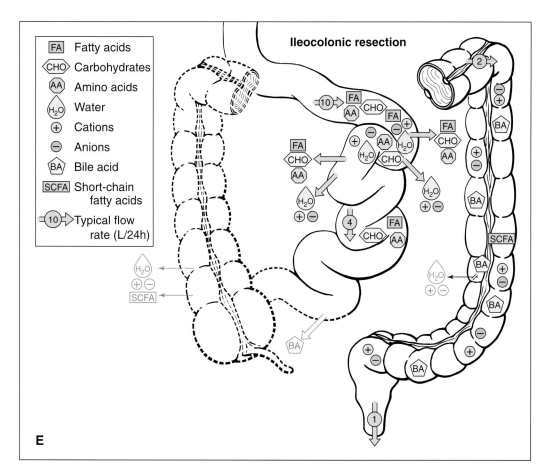

FIGURE 4-5. (CONTINUED)

E, Ileocolonic resection may produce a secretory diarrhea resistant to bile acid–binding drugs by compromising the ability to absorb sodium against a concentration gradient [5]. Unabsorbed sodium results in obligation of additional fluid within the lumen and secretory diarrhea. Slowing of transit (*eg,* by use of opiate antidiarrheals) allows more time for jejunal absorption and for the residual colon to absorb sodium against a high concentration gradient, and may be helpful.

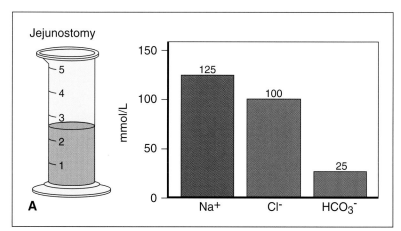

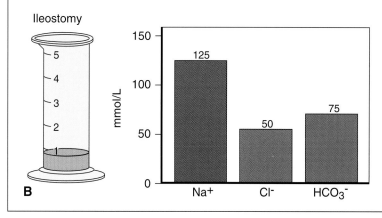

FIGURE 4-6.

Characteristics of stoma fluid. **A,** A jejunostomy usually produces 2 to 3 L of fluid per day, depending on the length of jejunum remaining in the body and dietary intake. The fluid typically has a high sodium concentration (> 100 mmol/L) and high chloride concentration (≈ 100 mmol/L) because of the lack of ability to absorb sodium against a concentration gradient and the lack of chloride-bicarbonate exchange. **B,** An ileostomy usually produces 750 to 1000 mL of fluid per day, when intestinal adaptation is complete. The fluid has a high bicarbonate concentration and pH due to chloride-bicarbonate exchange. If ileostomy volume is excessive, systemic acidosis can result.

TABLE 4-3. CAUSES OF ILEOSTOMY DIARRHEA

Ileal resection

Stenosis of ileostomy

Partial small-bowel obstruction

Recurrence of disease

Loss of ileal "brake" mechanism

Bacterial overgrowth

TABLE 4-3.

Summary of causes of ileostomy diarrhea. Several mechanisms can contribute to ileostomy diarrhea (output greater than 1000 mL/24h). Anatomical problems (*eg,* short-bowel syndrome, stenosis, obstruction, and disease recurrence) should be excluded by radiography before strictly functional problems are considered.

TABLE 4-4. MECHANISMS OF DIARRHEA IN ENTERITIS

Decreased surface area
(destruction or resection)

Disrupted mucosal
barrier (exudation)

Decreased rate of absorption, caused
by inflammatory mediators or
enteric nervous system

Diminished electrolyte absorption

Increased electrolyte secretion

Osmotic diarrhea due to malabsorption
Carbohydrates
Fatty acids, hydroxy-fatty acids
Bile acid diarrhea

TABLE 4-4.

Mechanisms of diarrhea
in enteritis. Infection
and associated inflammation can cause diarrhea in several ways.

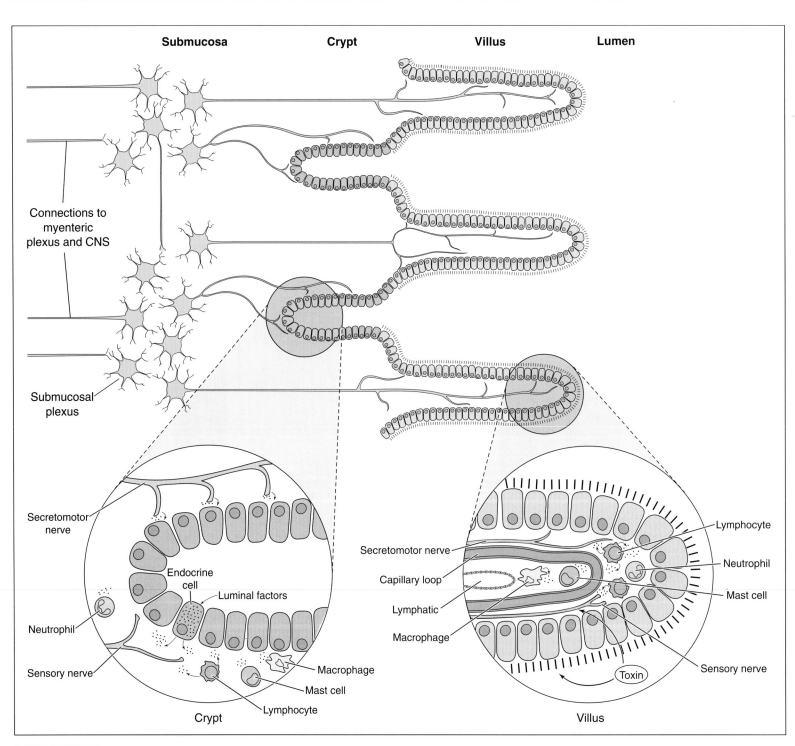

FIGURE 4-7.

The mucosal immune system, including lymphocytes, macrophages, and mast cells, interacts with mesenchymal cells (endothelium, smooth muscle, and fibroblasts) and with the enteric nervous system to produce various chemical mediators that can influence epithelial function, including various cytokines, adenosine, serotonin, histamine, bradykinin, substance P, platelet-activating factor, prostaglandins, and leukotrienes. In addition, activation of the enteric nervous system in response to these and other inflammatory chemicals (eg, bacterial toxins and other products) can also influence mucosal transport function [6].

Loss of an electrolyte transport mechanism

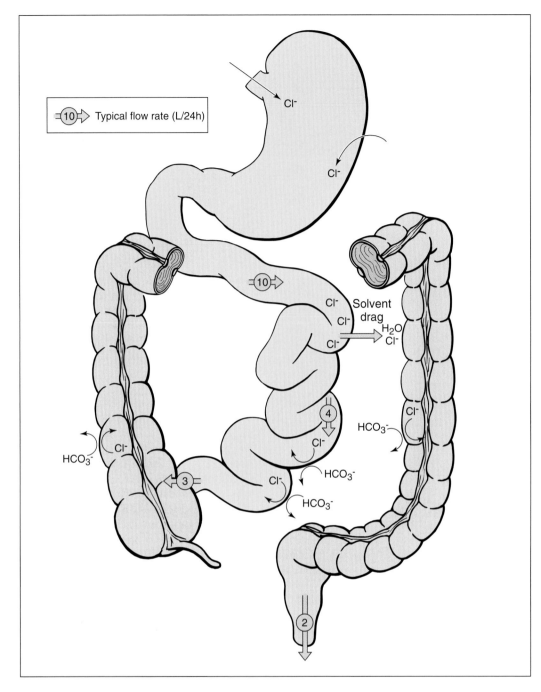

10 → Typical flow rate (L/24h)

FIGURE 4-8.

Congenital chloridorrhea, a rare but intriguing disorder, presents with diarrhea in infancy and results from an inability to exchange chloride and bicarbonate in the ileum. Chloride can be absorbed passively and in response to solvent drag, but it cannot be absorbed against a gradient. Chloride remaining within the intestinal lumen mandates water excretion. Diarrhea can be limited by reducing chloride intake; therefore, the condition may abate with fasting. Pharmacologic reduction of HCl excretion by the stomach may also be helpful [7]. Treatment consists of oral replacement of water and electrolytes to take advantage of absorption of chloride by solvent drag in the jejunum, but this does not reduce stool output.

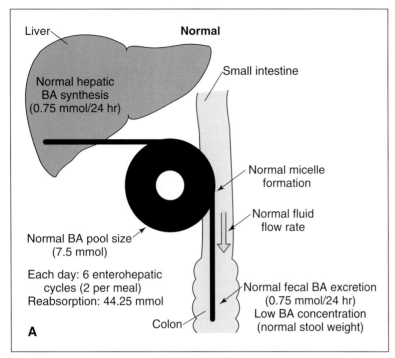

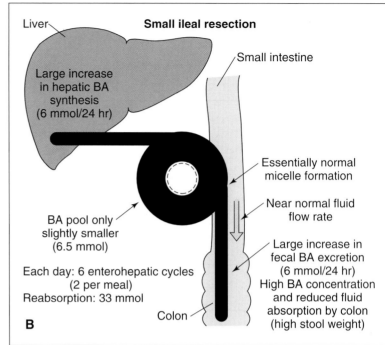

FIGURE 4-9.

Bile acid malabsorption can be caused by various mechanisms, and can result in secretory diarrhea if the concentration of bile acid in the colon becomes high enough (> 3 mmol/L) [8]. Mechanisms include rapid transit through the small intestine, which can result in delivery of excess bile acid to the colon, intestinal resection, and loss of high-affinity bile acid absorption sites due to mucosal disease in the ileum. **A**, Normal enterohepatic circulation of bile acids. **B**, Effect of a small (< 100 cm) ileal resection, which results in bile acid malabsorption but does not interrupt fat digestion or fluid absorption by the small intestine. **C**, The effects of a more substantial ileal resection, which results in malabsorption of fluid, bile acid, and fat. In this instance, the steatorrhea and fluid malabsorption may overshadow any secretory diarrhea caused by bile acid malabsorption. BA—bile acid. (*Adapted from* Fromm and Malavolti [8]; with permission.)

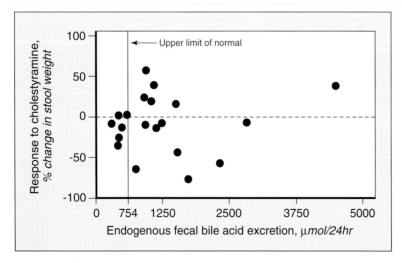

FIGURE 4-10.

Bile acid malabsorption is common in diarrhea. In this study, patients with chronic diarrhea not caused by intestinal resection had radiolabeled bile acid absorption measured [9]. Abnormal absorption was documented in most patients, but none had a complete response to treatment with cholestyramine resin, suggesting that factors other than bile acid malabsorption were contributing to diarrhea. (*Adapted from* Schiller *et al.* [9].)

TABLE 4-5. LAXATIVES AND DETECTION METHODS

Laxative	Detection Method
Phenolphthalein	Alkalinization of stool produces pink color; spectrophotometry
Bisacodyl	Thin-layer chromatography
Ipecac	Thin-layer chromatography
Senna	Urinary assay for anthraquinone
Magnesium	Osmotic gap in stool water; increased concentration of magnesium in stool water
Phosphate	Increased concentration in stool water
Sulfate	Increased concentration in stool water
Water	Creation of factitious diarrhea by addition of water to stool specimen can be detected by measurement of low-stool osmolality (<< 290 mosm/kg)

TABLE 4-5.

Laxatives and detection methods. Phenolphthalein, bisacodyl, senna, and some other laxatives reduce water and electrolyte absorption in the intestine and cause a secretory diarrhea, usually for therapeutic laxation. Some patients surreptitiously induce diarrhea using these laxatives [10,11]. Such patients can be difficult to detect unless the possibility of laxative abuse is considered and appropriate diagnostic tests are done. (*Adapted from* Schiller [10].)

TABLE 4-6. PATIENTS SUSPECTED OF LAXATIVE ABUSE

Type	Characteristics
Patients with bulimia	Usually adolescent to young adult women; concerned about weight or manifesting an eating disorder
Secondary gain	May have disability claim pending; illness may induce concern or caring behavior in others
Münchausen's syndrome	Typically, a peripatetic patient who "enjoys" being a challenge to doctors; may undergo extensive testing repeatedly
Polle syndrome (Münchausen by proxy)	Dependent child poisoned by parent with laxatives to show how effective parent can be as a caregiver; may have history of sibling who died with chronic diarrhea

TABLE 4-6.

Laxative abuse suspects.

Circulating secretagogues

TABLE 4-7. DIARRHEAL SYNDROMES RELATED TO CIRCULATING SECRETAGOGUES

Syndrome	Typical Symptoms	Main Mediators
Zollinger-Ellison	Pancreatic tumor, peptic ulcer, steatorrhea, diarrhea	Gastrin
Verner-Morrison (pancreatic cholera)	Watery diarrhea, hypokalemia, achlorhydria, flushing	Vasoactive intestinal polypeptide
Medullary thyroid carcinoma	Thyroid mass, diarrhea, hypermotility	Calcitonin, prostaglandins
Pheochromocytoma	Adrenal mass, hypertension, diarrhea	Vasoactive intestinal polypeptide, norepinephrine, epinephrine
Carcinoid	Diarrhea, flushing, wheezing, right-sided cardiac valvular disease	Serotonin, kinins
Somatostatinoma	Nonketotic diabetes mellitus, steatorrhea, diarrhea, gallstones	Somatostatin
Glucagonoma	Skin rash (migratory necrotizing erythema), mild diabetes	Glucagon
Hyperthyroidism	Diarrhea, steatorrhea, weight loss, tremor	Thyroxine, tri-iodothyronine
Mastocytosis	Flushing, dermatographism, nausea, vomiting, diarrhea, abdominal pain	Histamine

TABLE 4-7.

Diarrheal syndromes related to circulating secretagogues.

TABLE 4-8. MULTIPLE ENDOCRINE NEOPLASIA (MEN)

TYPE	COMPONENTS OF SYNDROME
MEN-1	Parathyroid tumor (hypercalcemia)
	Pancreatic tumor (gastrin, insulin, vasoactive intestinal polypeptide [VIP])
	Pituitary tumor (adrenocorticotropic hormone, prolactin)
MEN-2 (2a)	Medullary thyroid carcinoma or C-cell hyperplasia (calcitonin)
	Pheochromocytoma (epinephrine, norepinephrine, VIP)
	Parathyroid disease (parathormone)
MEN-3 (2b)	Medullary thyroid carcinoma or C-cell hyperplasia (calcitonin)
	Pheochromocytoma (epinephrine, norepinephrine)
	Ganglioneuromatosis, marfanoid habitus

TABLE 4-8.

Multiple endocrine neoplasia occurs in three patterns [12]. MEN-1 often presents with gastrointestinal symptoms due to Zollinger-Ellison or Verner-Morrison syndromes or due to hypercalcemia. Gastrointestinal symptoms in MEN-2 and -3 are often due to secretagogues released by medullary thyroid carcinoma or pheochromocytoma.

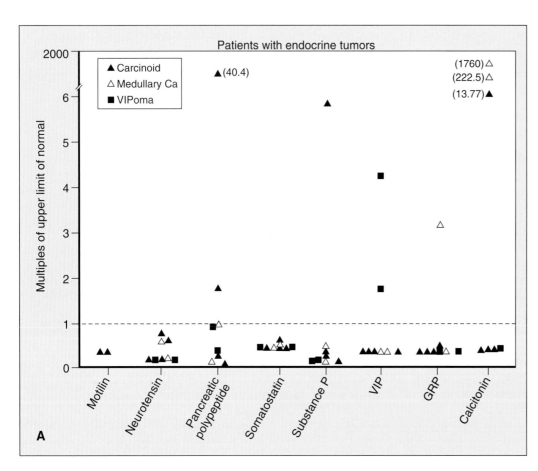

A

FIGURE 4-11.

Although tumor-induced secretory diarrhea syndromes are often considered in the differential diagnosis of chronic secretory diarrhea, these syndromes are quite rare [12]. For instance, vasoactive intestinal polypeptide (VIP)–secreting tumors have an incidence rate of approximately 1 per 10,000,000 population. Considering that chronic diarrhea severe enough to warrant diagnostic testing occurs in about 1 per 1000 population, the incidence of VIPoma in patients presenting with chronic diarrhea is only 1 in 10,000. Screening all patients with chronic diarrhea for elevated VIP levels will produce more false-positives than true-positives; this is shown in a study of more than 200 patients referred to Baylor University Medical Center for evaluation of problematic chronic diarrhea [13]. **A,** Results of a series of plasma peptide determinations in patients with known tumor-induced diarrhea. Several different peptides may be elevated in plasma in these syndromes.

(continued on next page)

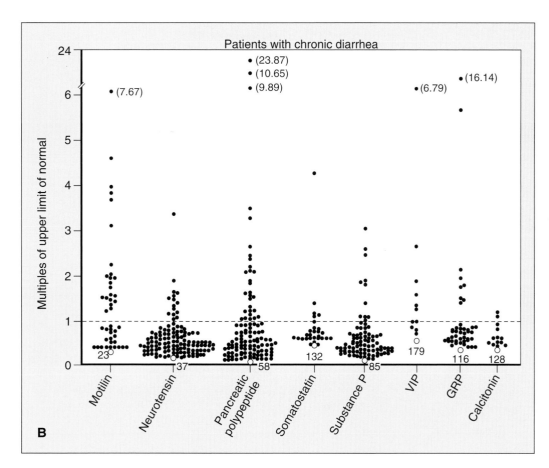

FIGURE 4-11. (*CONTINUED*)

B, The same series of plasma peptide determinations in patients without tumor syndromes. Measured levels were often as high in the group without tumors as in those with tumors. This high false-positive rate means that peptide determinations should be done selectively in patients presenting with chronic diarrhea and should probably be limited to peptides reflecting specific tumor syndromes. GRP—gastrin-releasing peptide. (*Adapted from* Schiller *et al.* [13]; with permission.)

Zollinger-Ellison syndrome

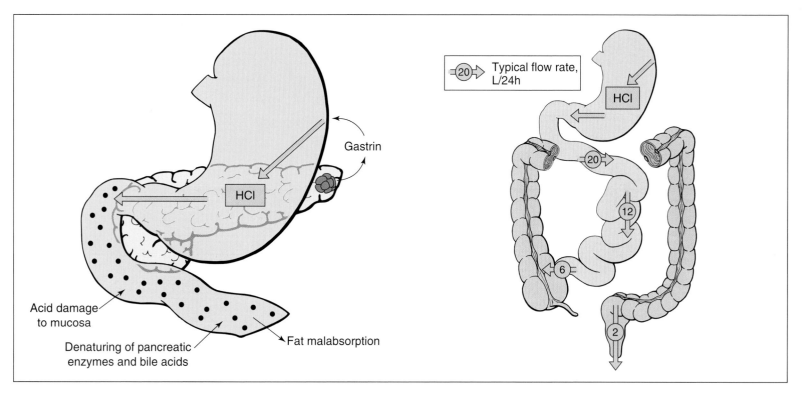

FIGURE 4-12.

Zollinger-Ellison syndrome results from secretion of gastrin by tumors in the pancreas or duodenum. This causes hypersecretion of acid by the stomach, which is responsible for the clinical manifestations of peptic ulcer disease and diarrhea. Diarrhea results from flooding the small intestine with gastric juice (up to 15 L per day), the effects of malabsorption caused by mucosal damage in the duodenum and jejunum, and the denaturing of pancreatic enzymes and bile acids.

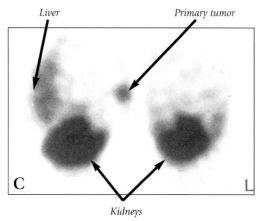

Measure and control acid hypersecretion

HCl

Goal: <10 mmol/h

A

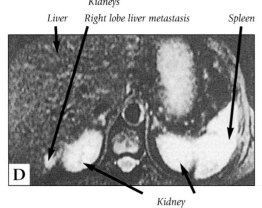

Liver

Kidneys

B

Liver   Primary tumor

Kidneys

C   L

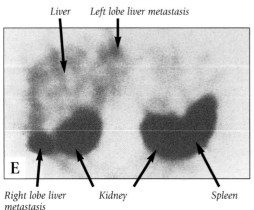

Liver   Right lobe liver metastasis   Spleen

Kidney

D

Liver   Left lobe liver metastasis

Right lobe liver metastasis   Kidney   Spleen

E

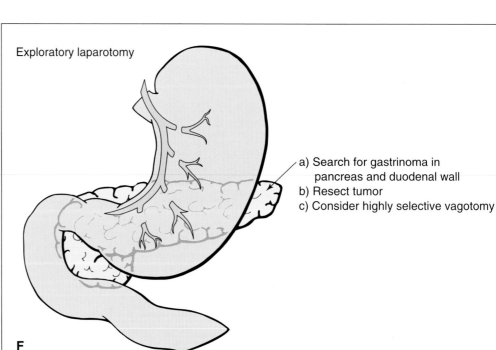

Exploratory laparotomy

a) Search for gastrinoma in
   pancreas and duodenal wall
b) Resect tumor
c) Consider highly selective vagotomy

F

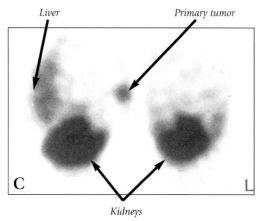

FIGURE 4-13.

Treatment of Zollinger-Ellison syndrome (ZES) involves both medical and surgical therapies [14]. Acid secretion can be effectively controlled in most patients by histamine$_2$-receptor antagonists or proton-pump inhibitors. It is essential that basal acid secretion be reduced to less than 10 mmol/hr if symptoms are to be controlled. The effectiveness of therapy needs to be measured with gastric analysis (**panel A**). After acid secretion is controlled, evidence for the resectability of tumor should be sought; computerized tomography, upper gastrointestinal endoscopy, endoscopic ultrasound, and radiolabeled octreotide scanning can be powerful tools for this purpose. **B–E**, These figures contrast findings of MR imaging (**panels B and D**) with findings of radiolabeled octreotide scanning (SRS) at the same anatomic levels (**panels C and E**) in detection of the primary tumor in one patient (**panels B and C**) and metastatic disease in another patient (**panels D and E**) with gastrinoma. The octreotide scans are clearly positive whereas the MR images do not always show the tumor [15]. If there is no evidence for metastasis, surgical exploration should be considered to identify and resect tumor (**panel F**). This is reasonable because now that acid secretion can be controlled, patients with ZES die from tumor metastasis and not acid-related complications, such as perforation. Vagotomy can be considered at the time of surgery to minimize the need for antisecretory drugs. (**B–E**, Courtesy of Dr. Robert T. Jensen, National Institutes of Health.)

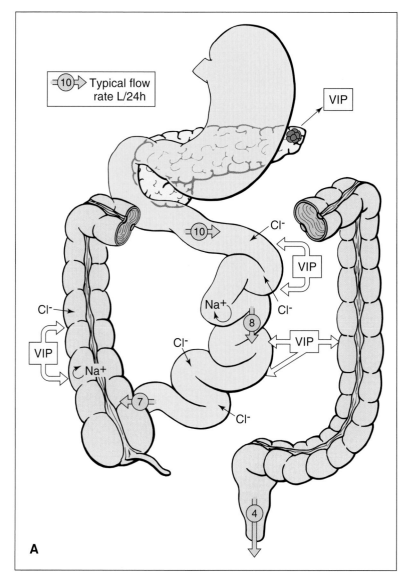

A

FIGURE 4-14.

A, Vasoactive intestinal polypeptide (VIP)–secreting tumors produce the Verner-Morrison syndrome, also known as *pancreatic cholera syndrome*, or watery diarrhea, hypokalemia, and achlorhydria syndrome. VIP produces a secretory state in the intestine by raising enterocyte cyclic AMP levels, causing chloride secretion and inhibiting sodium absorption. Stool outputs of up to 5 L per day can be observed. The tumors typically are located in the pancreas, but tumors in other locations (ganglioneuromas, pheochromocytomas) can also produce this neuropeptide. Treatment with resection is ideal, but injection of octreotide, the somatostatin analogue, has allowed good control of symptoms in many patients. **B**, A bulky VIPoma (*arrow*) in the tail of the pancreas as shown by computerized tomography. **C**, Resected tumor in the same patient. **D**, Histology of this tumor showing nest of enteroendocrine cells.

The somatostatin analogue, octreotide, often produces dramatic decreases of serum VIP levels and daily stool weights in patients with pancreatic cholera syndrome. **E–F**, These figures are from an early report and show the results of starting octreotide on day 7 on serum VIP concentration (**panel E**) and stool weight (**panel F**). (**E–F**, *adapted from* Maton *et al.* [16].)

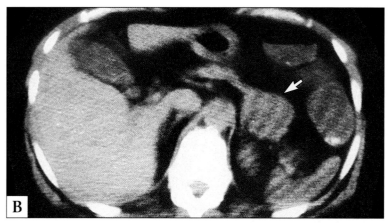

B

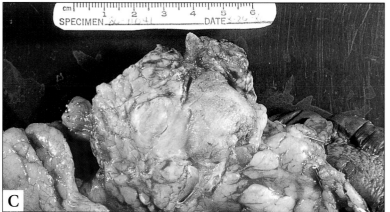

C

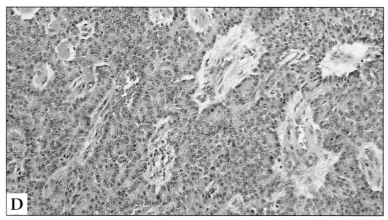

D

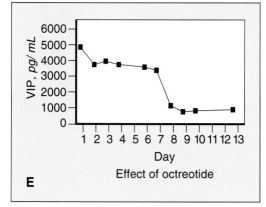

E

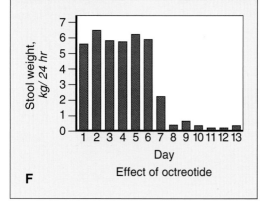

F

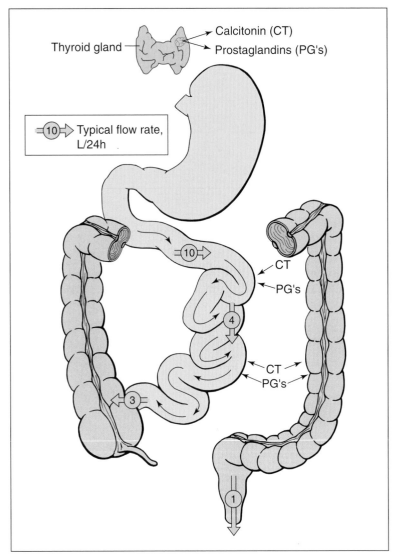

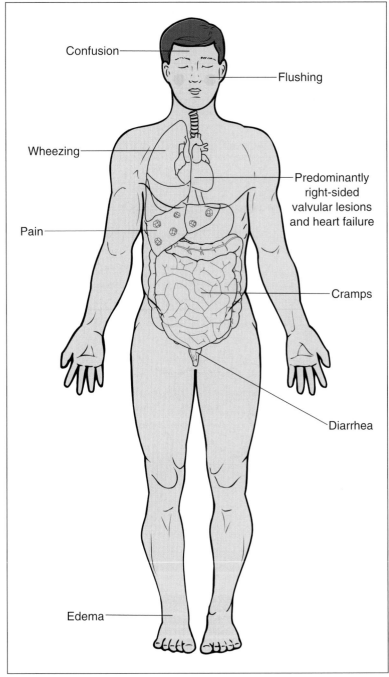

FIGURE 4-15.

Medullary carcinoma of the thyroid produces calcitonin (CT), pro-staglandins (PG), and other secretagogues. It often presents as part of multiple endocrine neoplasia type 2 (2a) or 3 (2b). Calcitonin can produce a secretory state; prostaglandins and other mediators can be associated with rapid transit, giving the diarrhea a multi-factorial etiology. Treatment with nonsteroidal anti-inflammatory drugs or opiates can control such diarrhea, but the prognosis for survival is poor when medullary thyroid carcinoma presents with diarrhea.

FIGURE 4-16.

Carcinoid tumors of the gastrointestinal tract are fairly common tumors, but carcinoid syndrome is less common [17]. To produce carcinoid syndrome, a carcinoid tumor must secrete mediators capable of producing symptoms and must be either metastatic to the liver or lung or primary at a site where direct access to the sys-temic venous circulation (bronchus, ovary) exists. The liver is capable of inactivating many of the mediators that may be produced by tumors in the intestine. After access to the systemic circulation has been achieved, the intensity of symptoms tends to be related to the tumor burden and the circulating levels of mediators. Progression of tumor is slower than that of carcinomas arising in the intestine; a course of up to 10 years from the onset of symptoms until death is not unusual. Diarrhea may be caused largely by hurried intestinal transit rather than by development of a secretory state, and usually is of only moderate volume.

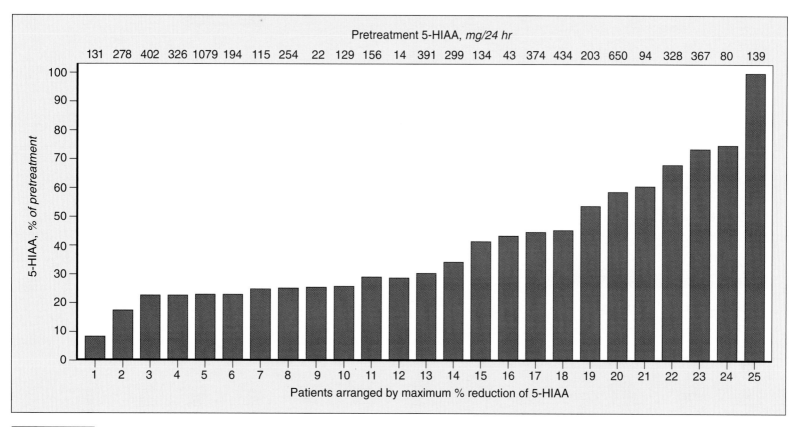

FIGURE 4-17.

Treatment for carcinoid syndrome is difficult because development of symptoms almost always indicates that metastasis is present. Partial hepatectomy has been used in some patients, but surgical options are usually limited. Reduction of tumor mass by hepatic artery embolization can reduce symptoms, at least on a temporary basis, after an acute exacerbation caused by tumor necrosis and release of mediators into the circulation. The most important therapeutic development has been the widespread use of the somatostatin analogue, octreotide, to control symptoms. Regular injection of octreotide produces control of flushing and easier management of diarrhea in most patients with carcinoid syndrome. Opiates and serotonin antagonists can be used to reduce diarrhea if control with octreotide is not satisfactory. Octreotide also has a tendency to retard tumor progression or cause regression of tumor mass, although the duration of this antineoplastic effect may be limited. This figure illustrates the reduction in urinary excretion of 5-hydroxyindole-acetic acid (5-HIAA), a serotonin metabolite, in one of the initial series of patients treated with octreotide. Tumor progression eventually kills most patients with carcinoid syndrome. (*Adapted from* Kvols *et al.* [18]; with permission.)

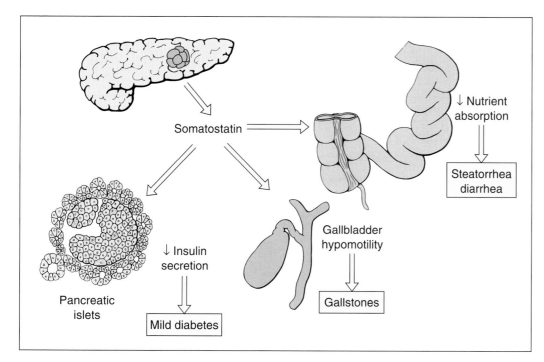

FIGURE 4-18.

Somatostatinoma is a rare syndrome in which excessive production of somatostatin by tumors of the pancreas and intestine results in mild diabetes, gallstones, steatorrhea, and diarrhea of moderate volume. Metastatic disease is common at the time of presentation, and therapeutic options are limited to symptomatic therapy.

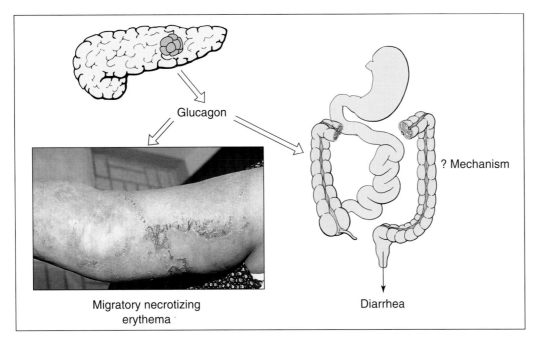

FIGURE 4-19.

Glucagonomas usually present with migratory necrotizing erythema, a skin disease. This figure shows the typical appearance of this lesion. Diarrhea occurs in a minority of patients, and its pathogenesis remains obscure. (Photograph courtesy of Dr. David A. Whiting, Dallas, TX).

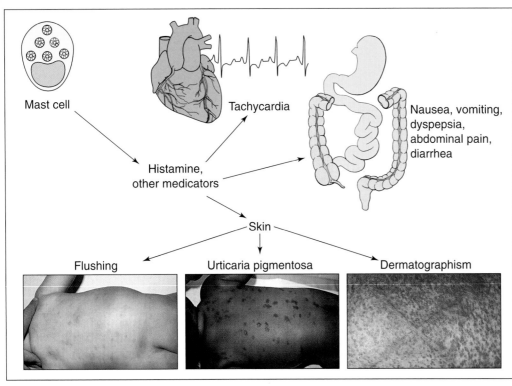

FIGURE 4-20.

Systemic mastocytosis often presents with prominent skin manifestations, including flushing, urticaria pigmentosa, and dermatographism. Gastrointestinal symptoms include nausea, vomiting, dyspepsia, and abdominal pain as well as diarrhea, usually on an intermittent basis. Diarrhea is probably caused by histamine when it occurs during the acute attacks of flushing, tachycardia, and hypotension that punctuate this illness. Chronic diarrhea may be related to increases in gastric acid secretion, infiltration of the intestine with mast cells, or release of other mediators, such as prostaglandins. (Photographs courtesy of Dr. David A. Whiting, Dallas, TX).

Drugs and poisons

TABLE 4-9. DRUGS ASSOCIATED WITH DIARRHEA

Antibiotics	Antidepressants	Hypocholesterolemic drugs	Miscellaneous agents
Antineoplastic drugs	Lithium	Lovastatin	Methysergide
Antiarrhythmics	Fluoxetine (Prozac)	Gemfibrozil	Theophylline
Quinidine	Tranquilizers	Clofibrate	Diuretics
Procainamide	Alprazolam (Xanax)	Probucol	Oral hypoglycemic
Antihypertensives	Meprobamate	Gastrointestinal drugs	drugs
Beta-blockers	Anticonvulsants	Magnesium-containing antacids	Colchicine
Angiotensin-converting	Ethosuximide	H$_2$-receptor antagonists	Thyroid hormone
enzyme inhibitors	Valproic acid	Prostaglandin analogues (misoprostal)	
Hydralazine	L-Dopa	Sulfasalazine	
		Olsalazine	
		Prokinetic drugs (cisapride)	

TABLE 4-9.

Drugs associated with diarrhea [19]. Several different categories of drugs can cause diarrhea as a side effect. Some examples are shown under each category. The mechanisms causing diarrhea are not known for most of these drugs.

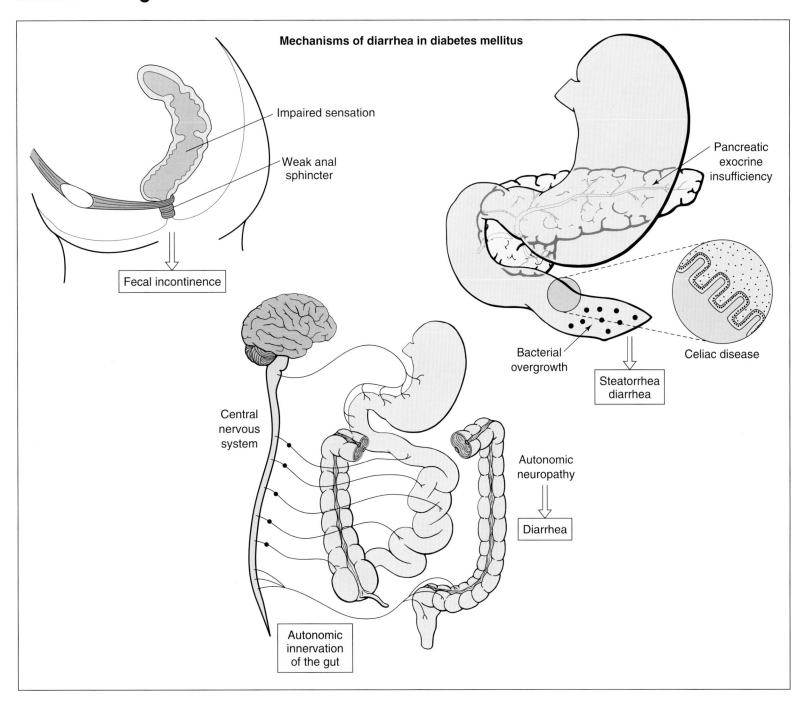

Mechanisms of diarrhea in diabetes mellitus

Impaired sensation

Weak anal sphincter

Fecal incontinence

Pancreatic exocrine insufficiency

Bacterial overgrowth

Celiac disease

Steatorrhea diarrhea

Central nervous system

Autonomic neuropathy

Diarrhea

Autonomic innervation of the gut

Longstanding diabetes mellitus is complicated by the development of chronic diarrhea in roughly 20% of patients. In some this results from fecal incontinence, misreported as diarrhea, but in others, stool weight may be abnormally high. Clinically, it is important to distinguish steatorrhea from chronic watery diarrhea in these patients. Steatorrhea may be caused by coexisting small-bowel bacterial overgrowth, celiac disease, or pancreatic exocrine insuffi-ciency. Watery diarrhea has been attributed to dysregulation by the enteric nervous system as a manifestation of diabetic autonomic neuropathy. Studies in animals suggest the possibility of adrenergic dysfunction in diabetes, but attempts to treat diabetic diarrhea in people with clonidine, an α_2-adrenergic agonist agent, have been only variably successful [20].

Idiopathic secretory diarrhea

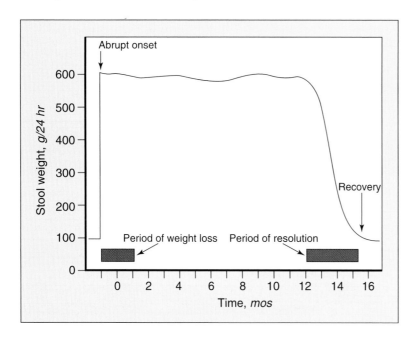

FIGURE 4-22.

Patients who have been extensively evaluated for chronic watery diarrhea without finding a cause are a remarkably homogeneous group [21]. They typically give a history of good health until the acute onset of diarrhea, often after domestic travel. This is followed by continuous diarrhea and a limited period of weight loss. Diarrhea persists at a constant intensity for 1 to 3 years and then subsides spontaneously over a few months. No causative organism has been identified, but the sudden onset and spontaneous disappearance suggest an infectious etiology. Outbreaks of a similar syndrome have been reported to be associated with consumption of milk or water, but sporadic idiopathic secretory diarrhea usually occurs in isolated individuals, even though others may have had identical food or water exposures. Nonspecific antidiarrheal therapy with opiates is helpful in most such patients.

FIGURE 4-23.

Clinical diagnostic algorithm for the approach to patients with chronic diarrhea (> 4 weeks' duration to exclude most acute infectious causes). A careful history can largely define the potential causes of chronic diarrhea. The key diagnoses that can be evaluated by history include iatrogenic diarrhea (*ie*, caused by drugs, radiation, or surgery) and systemic diseases producing diarrhea (such as hyperthyroidism, diabetes, or vasculitis). The history also provides evidence of risk factors for AIDS and the need to test for HIV infection. Physical examination and routine laboratory tests provide information on the effects of diarrhea (fluid status, electrolyte depletion) and the need for rehydration or nutritional support. Serum chemistries can disclose evidence of malabsorption, hypogammaglobulinemia, or dysgammaglobulinemia. A quantitative stool collection provides information about the severity of diarrhea, the presence of steatorrhea, the presence of an osmotic gap in stool water, indicating an osmotic component, and the presence of laxatives. If secretory diarrhea is confirmed, chronic infectious processes should be excluded by examining the stool for bacterial pathogens, parasites, and protozoa. The next step is to exclude structural and inflammatory disease with carefully conducted small-bowel radiography and colonoscopy with biopsies, even if the mucosa appears normal, to exclude microscopic and collagenous colitis. If the diagnosis remains uncertain, computerized tomography (CT) and a small-bowel biopsy with aspirate for quantitative culture are appropriate. Selective evaluation for circulating secretagogues might include serum gastrin, calcitonin, vasoactive intestinal polypeptide (VIP), and thyroid-stimulating hormone (TSH) levels, and measurement of urinary excretion of 5-hydroxyindole-acetic acid (5-HIAA), metanephrines, and histamine.

(figure on opposite page)

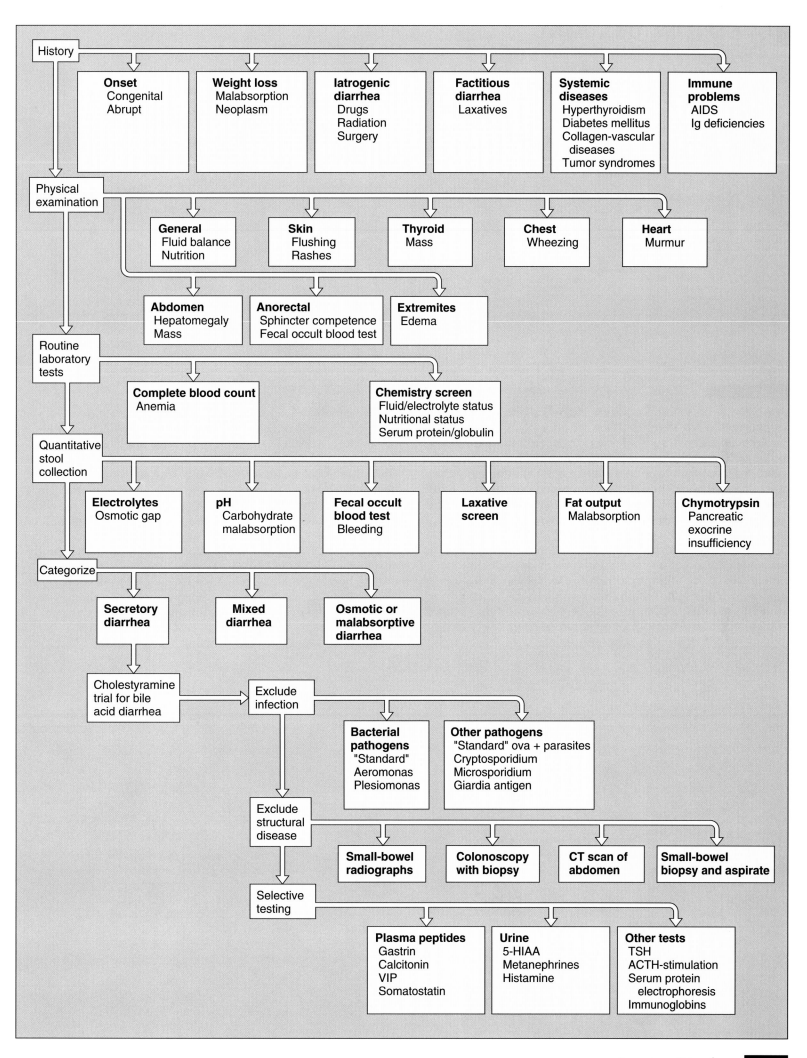

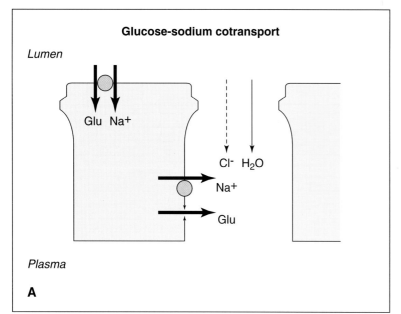

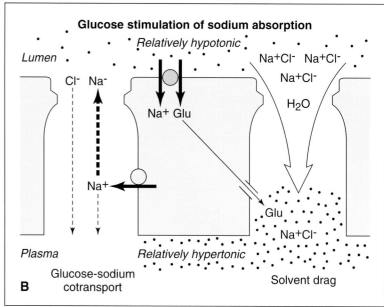

Oral rehydration solution has been a life-saving therapy for many patients with severe diarrhea. The basic principle is that glucose (and other substrates, such as amino acids) are cotransported with sodium into enterocytes in the small intestine. Unlike other mechanisms of sodium absorption, cotransport is intact in many forms of secretory diarrhea; thus, stimulation of sodium absorption by cotransport can be used to enhance sodium absorption, even in the presence of bacterial toxins. A, The usual explanation for the effectiveness of oral rehydration solution is glucose-sodium cotransport. Cotransport leads to deposition of sodium in the basolateral space as a result of glucose absorption. Chloride must enter across the tight junction for sodium to remain on the basolateral side of the enterocyte. Otherwise, sodium diffuses back to the lumen through the tight junction in response to the electrical potential generated by cotransport, and no net sodium absorption would occur. The

duodenum and jejunum are the only areas of the gut in which sufficient chloride can permeate across tight junctions to allow cotransport to result in net sodium chloride (and water) absorption. B, An alternative mechanism for glucose-stimulated sodium absorption is solvent drag. Removal of glucose from the luminal fluid by cotransport results in generation of an osmotic gradient between the lumen and the basolateral space. This generates a flux of water across the tight junctions, which entrains sodium and chloride ions by solvent drag. This mechanism also can only occur in the proximal small intestine because paracellular permeability is restricted in the ileum and glucose is not absorbed in the colon. In healthy humans, this alternative mechanism accounts for roughly two thirds of the total amount of glucose-stimulated sodium absorption. The situation may be different if paracellular permeability for water or electrolytes is altered by disease [22].

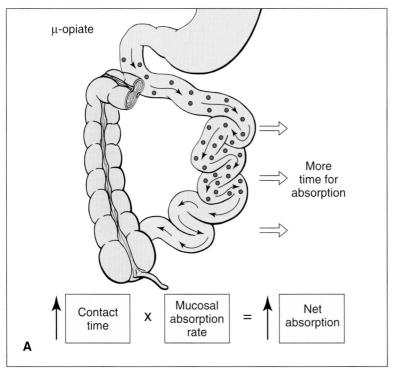

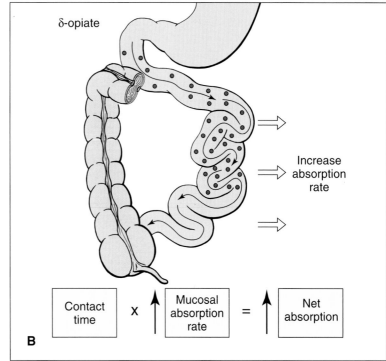

FIGURE 4-25.

A, Traditional opiates (with μ-opiate receptor selectivity) reduce diarrhea predominantly by slowing transit through the small intestine and colon, allowing more time for absorption to occur [23]. **B,** δ-Opiate receptors modulate enterocyte absorption rate; *acetorphan,* an inhibitor of enkephalinase activity, allows increased stimulation of δ-opiate receptors by endogenous opiates and reduces diarrhea without causing rebound constipation [24].

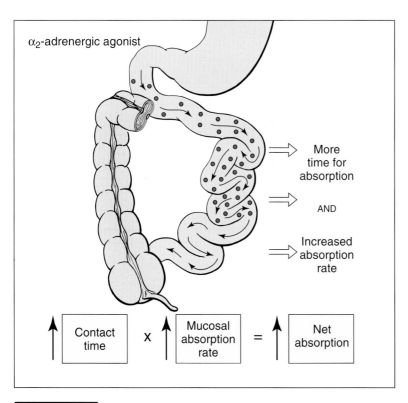

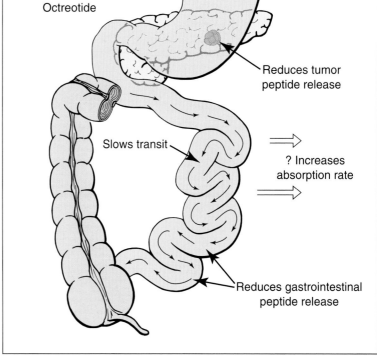

FIGURE 4-26.

Clonidine, an α₂-adrenergic agonist, has antidiarrheal activity caused both by a slowing of motility and by an increase in mucosal absorption rate [25]. The usefulness of clonidine as an antidiarrheal is limited by its antihypertensive effect.

FIGURE 4-27.

Octreotide, a somatostatin analogue, is useful in the treatment of diarrhea in carcinoid syndrome and in tumors secreting vasoactive intestinal polypeptides [26]. Controlled studies indicate that octreotide can also reduce symptoms in dumping syndrome. Clinical reports suggest some efficacy in patients with idiopathic secretory diarrhea or AIDS diarrhea, but prospective studies have been disappointing.

REFERENCES

1. Chang EB, Rao MC: Intestinal water and electrolyte transport: Mechanisms of physiological and adaptive responses. In *Physiology of the Digestive Tract*. Edited by Johnson LR. New York: Raven Press; 1994:2027–2081.

2. Fordtran JS, Santa Ana CA, Morawski SG, *et al.*: Pathophysiology of chronic diarrhea: Insights derived from intestinal perfusion studies in 31 patients. *Gastroenterol Clin North Am* 1986, 15:477–490.

3. Hammer HF, Fine KD, Santa Ana CA, *et al.*: Carbohydrate malabsorption: Its measurement and its contribution to diarrhea. *J Clin Invest* 1990, 86:1936–1944.

4. Eherer AJ, Fordtran JS: Fecal osmotic gap and pH in experimental diarrhea of various causes. *Gastroenterology* 1992, 103:545–551.

5. Arrambide KA, Santa CA, Schiller LR, *et al.*: Loss of absorptive capacity for sodium chloride as a cause of diarrhea following partial ileal and right colon resection. *Dig Dis Sci* 1989, 34:193–201.

6. Cooke HJ: Hormones and neurotransmitters regulating intestinal ion transport. In *Diarrheal Diseases*. Edited by Field M. New York: Elsevier; 1991:23–48.

7. Aichbichler BW, Zerr CH, Santa Ana CA, *et al.*: Brief report: proton-pump inhibition of gastric chloride secretion in congenital chloridorrhea. *N Eng J Med* 1997, 336:106–109.

8. Fromm H, Malavolti M: Bile acid-induced diarrhea. *Gastroenterol Clin North Am* 1986, 15:567–582.

9. Schiller LR, Hogan RB, Morawski SG, *et al.*: Studies of the prevalence and significance of radiolabeled bile acid malabsorption in a group of patients with idiopathic chronic diarrhea. *Gastroenterology* 1987, 92:151–160.

10. Schiller LR: Cathartics, laxatives and lavage solutions. In *Gastrointestinal Pharmacology and Therapeutics*. Edited by Friedman G, Jacobson ED, McCallum R. Philadelphia: Lippincott-Raven; 1997:159–174.

11. Phillips S, Donaldson L, Geisler K, *et al.*: Stool composition in factitial diarrhea: A 6-year experience with stool analysis. *Ann Intern Med* 1995, 123:97–100.

12. Rood RP, Donowitz M: Endocrine tumor-associated diarrheal syndromes. In *Diarrheal Diseases*. Edited by Field M. New York: Elsevier; 1991:397–411.

13. Schiller LR, Rivera LM, Santangelo WC, *et al.*: Diagnostic value of fasting plasma peptide concentrations in patients with chronic diarrhea. *Dig Dis Sci* 1994, 39:2216–2222.

14. Weber HC, Orbuch M, Jensen RT: Diagnosis and management of Zollinger-Ellison syndrome. *Semin Gastrointest Dis* 1995, 6:79–89.

15. Termanini B, Gibril F, Reynolds JC, *et al.*: Value of somatostatin receptor scintigraphy: a prospective study in gastrinoma of its effect on clinical management. *Gastroenterology* 1997; 112:335–347.

16. Maton PN, O'Dorisio TM, Howe BA, *et al.*: Effect of a long acting somatostatin analogue (SMS 201-995) in a patient with pancreatic cholera. *N Engl J Med* 1985, 312:17–21.

17. Kvols LK: Metastatic carcinoid tumors and the malignant carcinoid syndrome. *Ann NY Acad Sci* 1994, 733:464–470.

18. Kvols LK, Moertel CG, O'Connell MJ, *et al.*: Treatment of the malignant carcinoid syndrome: Evaluation of a long-acting somatostatin analogue. *N Engl J Med* 1986, 315:663–666.

19. Schiller LR: Drug-induced changes in bowel function. *Contemporary Gastroenterology* 1989, 2:29–35.

20. Saslow SB, Camilleri M: Diabetic diarrhea. *Semin Gastrointest Dis* 1995, 6:187–193.

21. Afzalpurkar RG, Schiller LR, Fordtran JS: The self-limited nature of chronic idiopathic diarrhea. *N Engl J Med* 1992, 327:1849–1852.

22. Schiller LR, Santa Ana CA, Porter J, *et al.*: Glucose-stimulated sodium transport by·the human intestine during experimental cholera. *Gastroenterology* 1997, 112:1529–1535.

23. Schiller LR, Davis GR, Santa Ana CA, *et al.*: Studies of the mechanism of the antidiarrheal effect of codeine. *J Clin Invest* 1982, 70:999–1008.

24. Roge J, Baumer P, Berard H, *et al.*: The enkephalinase inhibitor, acetorphan, in acute diarrhea: A double-blind, controlled clinical trial versus loperamide. *Scand J Gastroenterol* 1993, 28:352–354.

25. Schiller LR, Santa Ana CA, Morawski SG, *et al.*: Studies of the antidiarrheal action of clonidine: Effects on motility and intestinal absorption. *Gastroenterology* 1985, 89:982–988.

26. Maton PN: Expanding uses of octreotide. *Baillieres Clin Gastroenterol* 1994, 8:321–337.

Chapter 5

Nutrient Malabsorption

S AMUEL K LEIN

During the course of a normal lifetime, we ingest more than 60 million calories and more than 40 tons of water to maintain normal metabolic function and body composition. The major functions of the gastrointestinal tract are to digest and to absorb tremendous quantities of dietary nutrients. This process involves a complex and carefully integrated series of events. Luminal factors are responsible for nutrient digestion, mucosal factors for nutrient absorption, and lymphatic-vascular factors for the delivery of absorbed nutrients to other body tissues. Disruption of normal nutrient digestion and absorption at any phase of the process can cause malnutrition and serious medical complications.

The diseases that cause maldigestion and malabsorption are heterogeneous and may present with different clinical manifestations, depending on the characteristics of the disease itself and on the presence of nutritional abnormalities. Malabsorption can be specific for certain nutrients, as in patients with lactase deficiency who are unable to hydrolyze lactose and absorb its component sugars, or it can be generalized, as in patients with short-bowel syndrome who have difficulty absorbing most macro- and micronutrients. Therefore, to provide appropriate medical and nutritional therapy in patients with malabsorption, it is important to diagnose the underlying disease and to understand the impact of the disease on nutritional status.

During the past 30 years, dramatic technical advances have been made in our ability to provide nutritional support. Sophisticated use of central venous catheters and enteric feeding tubes has made it possible to feed patients with even the most complicated needs. We now realize that, when possible, patients should be fed orally and enterally rather than parenterally. Oral and enteral feeding causes fewer complications, is more physiologic, maintains better gastrointestinal structure and function, and is less expensive than parenteral feeding. However, the use of oral and enteral feeding in patients with impaired absorptive capacity can be difficult. A sound understanding of the pathophysiology of the patient's digestive and absorptive function is important to maximize the efficacy of oral and enteral nutritional therapy and to decrease the need for parenteral supplementation.

■ CLASSIFICATION

TABLE 5-1. CLASSIFICATION OF DISEASES THAT CAUSE INTESTINAL MALABSORPTION

PREMUCOSAL	MUCOSAL	POSTMUCOSAL
Pancreatic insufficiency	Celiac sprue	Congenital lymphangiectasia
Hepatobiliary disease	Tropical sprue	Secondary lymphangiectasia
Bacterial overgrowth	Whipple's disease	
Rapid intestinal transit	Eosinophilic enteritis	
Gastrectomy	Brush border enzyme deficiency	
	Lymphoma	
	Short-bowel syndrome	
	Prolonged malnutrition	
	Radiation enteritis	
	Parasitic infection	
	Mesenteric ischemia	

TABLE 5-1.

The diseases that impair nutrient absorption can be classified by the site of their primary pathophysiologic abnormality. Premucosal diseases are those that affect the digestion of nutrients in the lumen of the intestine. Mucosal diseases are those that affect the mucosal brush border digestion with or without uptake of nutrients by the small intestine. Postmucosal diseases are those that affect the systemic delivery of nutrients absorbed by the small intestine.

■ PREMUCOSAL DISEASE

Pancreatic exocrine insufficiency

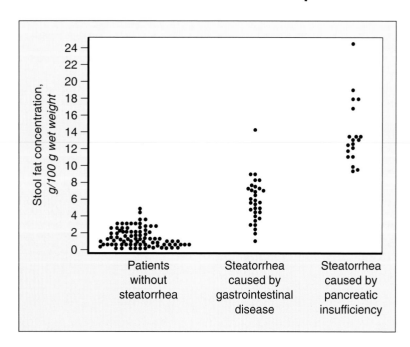

FIGURE 5-1.

Stool fat concentrations in patients without steatorrhea and in patients with steatorrhea caused by either gastrointestinal disease or exocrine pancreatic insufficiency. Fecal fat concentration is usually higher in patients with fat maldigestion (pancreatic insufficiency) than in those with fat malabsorption (small-bowel disease) because the latter group often experiences concomitant fluid malabsorption. The data from this study [1] suggest that fecal fat concentration is usually > 9.5% in patients with fat maldigestion and < 9.5% in those with fat malabsorption. Therefore, fecal fat concentration can be used as a tool to evaluate the etiology of steatorrhea. (*Adapted from* Bo-Linn and Fordtran [1]; with permission.)

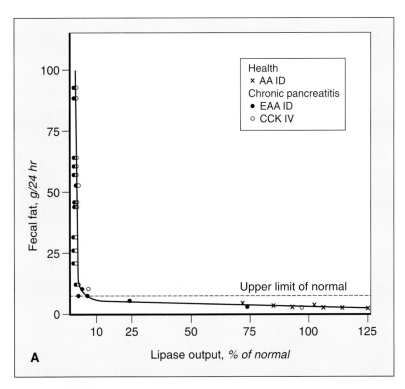

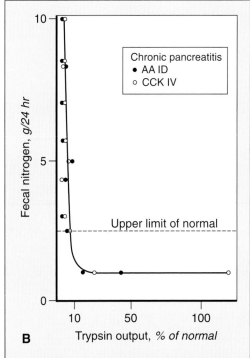

Relationships between stimulated pancreatic lipase output and fecal fat excretion (**panel A**), and between stimulated pancreatic trypsin output and fecal nitrogen excretion (**panel B**) in patients with chronic pancreatitis. Chronic pancreatitis often diminishes enzyme output. Steatorrhea and azotorrhea, however, do not occur until 90% of the pancreas is dysfunctional and pancreatic enzyme output is < 10% of normal [2]. Therefore, clinically important maldigestion usually does not occur after distal pancreatectomy and appears late in the clinical course of patients with chronic pancreatitis. AA ID—intraduodenal amino acid; CCK IV—intravenous cholecystokinin. (*Adapted from* DiMagno *et al.* [2]; with permission.)

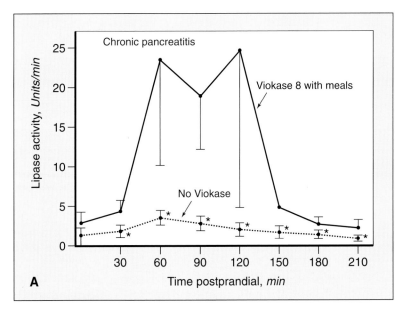

Effect of oral pancreatic enzyme replacement on intraluminal lipase activity (**panel A**) and fat absorption (**panel B**) in patients with severe pancreatic insufficiency [3]. Eight pancreatin (Viokase, A.H. Robins, Richmond, VA) tablets containing a total of 28,000 units of lipase were ingested with each meal. In these patients, enzyme therapy decreased, but did not completely normalize, fecal fat excretion. Protecting oral enzyme preparations from acid denaturation by using enteric-coated products, administering concomitant antacid treatment, or inhibiting gastric acid secretion with H_2 blockers may deliver a greater percentage

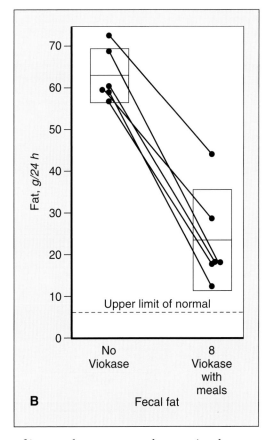

of ingested enzymes to the proximal small intestine. (*Adapted from* DiMagno *et al.* [3]; with permission.)

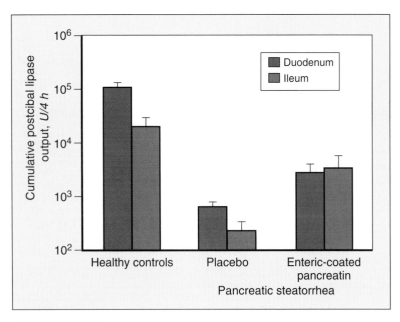

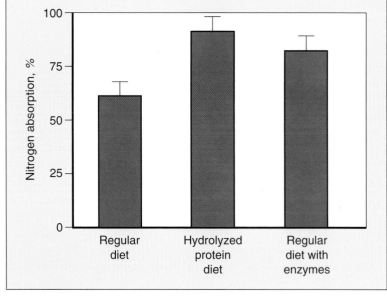

FIGURE 5-4.

Cumulative postcibal lipase output in the duodenum and ileum in normal subjects and patients with pancreatic insufficiency given enteric-coated pancreatic enzymes or placebo. Enteric-coated microspheres of pancreatic enzyme extracts protect the enzymes from destruction by gastric acid. Unfortunately, these preparations only partially correct steatorrhea in most patients. The data shown in this figure suggest that an important reason for incomplete normalization of fat absorption is inefficient use of ingested enzymes [4]. Treatment with enteric-coated preparations increases duodenal and ileal lipase activity to a similar extent. The duodenum receives a much larger nutrient load than the ileum, however, so a considerable portion of enzyme is wasted. The delayed release of enzyme in the distal small intestine is probably related to the known decrease in pancreatic bicarbonate secretion in patients with pancreatic bicarbonate secretion in patients with pancreatic insufficiency. Disintegration of the enteric coat requires a luminal pH ≥ 6. (*Adapted from* Guarner *et al.* [4]; with permission.)

FIGURE 5-5.

Effect of dietary protein composition and oral pancreatic enzyme therapy on nitrogen absorption in patients who have had a total pancreatectomy. Nitrogen absorption is markedly improved by providing a diet containing nitrogen in the form of predigested (hydrolyzed) protein compared with a regular diet containing nitrogen in the form of whole protein [5]. Similar improvement in nitrogen absorption can be achieved less expensively by administering pancreatic enzymes in conjunction with a regular diet.

Primary biliary cirrhosis

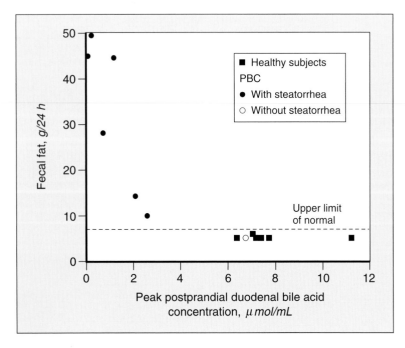

FIGURE 5-6.

Relationship between intraduodenal bile acid concentrations and fecal fat output in patients with primary biliary cirrhosis (PBC). Bile salts are essential for efficient fat absorption because they are required for mixed micelle formation. Cholestasis and biliary obstruction can cause severe fat malabsorption by decreasing delivery of bile salts into the duodenum. Patients with PBC develop steatorrhea when impaired bile acid secretion decreases peak postprandial duodenal bile acid concentration to less than 2.5 μmol/mL [6]. The severity of steatorrhea is directly correlated with the severity of cholestasis. Thus, patients with increased serum bilirubin concentrations (>4.5 mg/dL) or advanced disease (histologic disease stages III or IV) have steatorrhea. (*Adapted from* Lanspa *et al.* [6]; with permission.)

Bacterial overgrowth

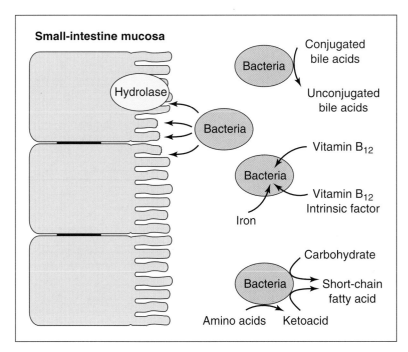

Small-intestine mucosa

FIGURE 5-7.

Diagram illustrating the pathophysiology of bacterial overgrowth. The presence of increased numbers of bacteria in the small intestine can cause malabsorption of macronutrients (fat, carbohydrate, protein) and micronutrients (vitamin B_{12}, fat soluble vitamins, iron). As shown in this figure, excess intestinal bacteria can cause structural damage to enterocytes, deconjugate and hydrolyze primary bile acids, impair mucosal brush border hydrolase activity, metabolize carbohydrates and amino acids to short-chain fatty acids, and consume vitamin B_{12} and iron.

Gastrectomy

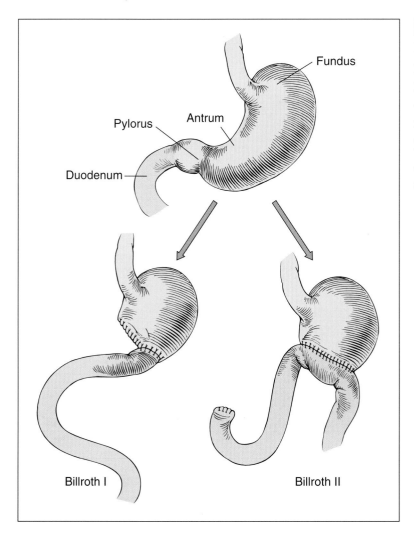

Billroth I

Billroth II

FIGURE 5-8.

Billroth I and II subtotal gastrectomy. Many patients lose weight after subtotal gastric resection with gastroduodenostomy (Billroth I) or gastrojejunostomy (Billroth II). The most important cause of weight loss is decreased food intake because of adverse gastrointestinal symptoms. Mild generalized malabsorption occurs in many patients because of accelerated gastric emptying, bypassed duodenal and proximal jejunum, rapid intestinal transit, and bacterial overgrowth. Severe anemia, caused by iron, folate, and vitamin B_{12} deficiencies, and metabolic bone disease, caused by altered calcium and vitamin D status, can occur years after surgery.

Lactase deficiency and carbohydrate malabsorption

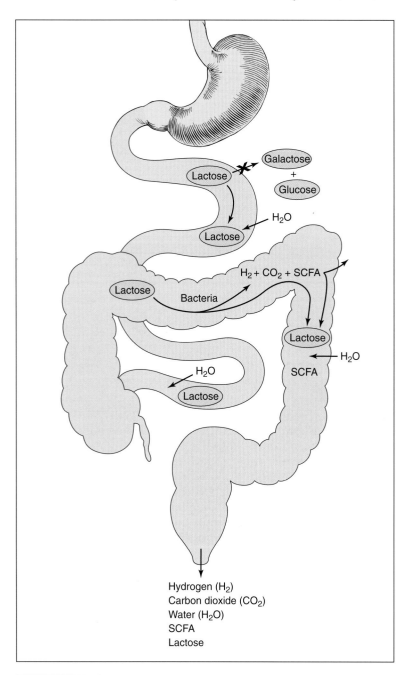

FIGURE 5-9.

Pathophysiology of lactase deficiency. Lactase deficiency is the most common mucosal brush border enzyme deficiency. Clinical symptoms of lactase deficiency include abdominal pain, bloating, flatulence, and diarrhea. These symptoms are caused by osmotic effects of unabsorbed lactose and its metabolic byproducts, increased peristalsis caused by intestinal distension, and gas (H_2, CO_2) produced by bacterial fermentations of lactose. The severity of symptoms after lactose ingestion depends on the load (amount × rate) of lactose delivered to the gastrointestinal tract and the capacity of the colon to absorb short-chain fatty acids (SCFA) produced by bacterial fermentation of lactose.

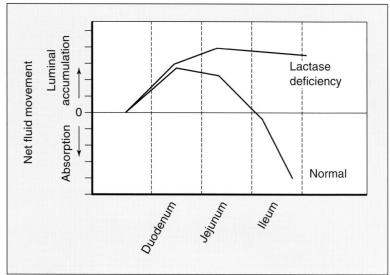

FIGURE 5-10.

Intestinal fluid accumulation after ingestion of a lactose-containing meal in normal and lactase-deficient subjects [7]. Net fluid accumulation occurs in the duodenum in both normal subjects and patients with lactase deficiency because of the hypertonicity of the meal. The hydrolysis of lactose to glucose and galactose in normal subjects stimulates monosaccharide and net fluid absorption in the jejunum and ileum. The presence of lactose in the intestinal lumen and the failure to generate glucose for sodium and glucose cotransport stimulates water secretion and impairs water absorption in patients with lactase deficiency. (*Adapted from* Chang and Binder [7]; with permission.)

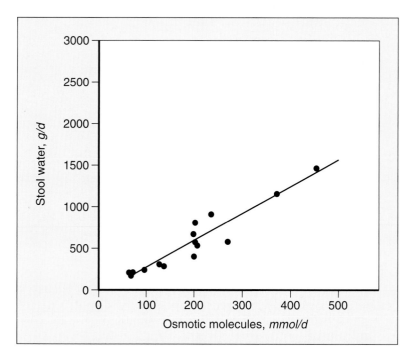

FIGURE 5-11.

Effect of unabsorbed carbohydrate on stool water output in normal subjects and patients with malabsorption. Carbohydrate that is not absorbed by the small bowel is delivered to the colon, where it can be metabolized by colonic bacteria to short-chain fatty acids, which are subsequently absorbed by colonic mucosa. However, unabsorbed carbohydrate that is not converted to short-chain fatty acids and unabsorbed short-chain fatty acids themselves represent an osmotic load that obligates water loss. The data plotted in this figure are from normal subjects with carbohydrate-induced diarrhea, and suggest that approximately 3.5 g of stool water is excreted for every millimole of unabsorbed osmotically active molecules (carbohydrate, organic acids, and cations) [8]. Carbohydrate malabsorption may be a clinically important cause of diarrhea in selected patients with gastrointestinal disease. Measurement of fecal pH, carbohydrate, and organic anions can help confirm the diagnosis of carbohydrate malabsorption. Treatment involves decreasing carbohydrate intake. (*Adapted from* Hammer *et al.* [8]; with permission.)

Enteropathies producing malabsorption

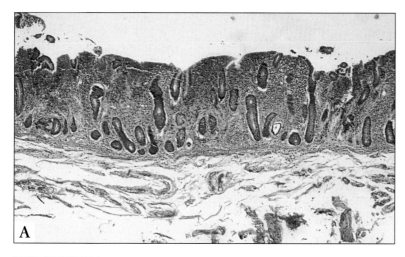

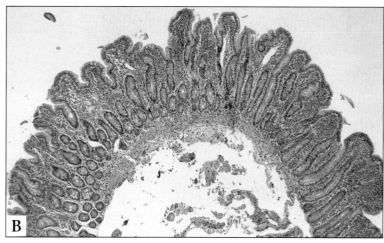

FIGURE 5-12.

Jejunal mucosal biopsy from a patient with celiac sprue before (**panel A**) and 3 months after (**panel B**) treatment with a gluten-free diet. Celiac sprue is characterized by small intestinal mucosal damage and nutrient malabsorption in susceptible persons after ingesting gluten, the water-insoluble protein component of certain grains. **Panel A** illustrates the flat mucosal surface, absence of villi, hyperplastic crypts, and increased lamina propria cellularity that are characteristic of the disease. After 3 months of treatment (**panel B**) the mucosa is markedly improved and recognizable villi are present. The villi are short, however, and crypt hyperplasia and lamina propria hypercellularity persist.

The severity of malabsorption and clinical symptoms can vary markedly in patients with celiac sprue, and are directly correlated

with the length of the intestinal lesion. Usually, the proximal intestine is most involved and disease severity decreases distally along the length of small bowel. Patients with severe disease have flatulence, progressive weight loss, and multiple nutrient deficiencies. The diarrhea is often voluminous and may float on water because of increased air and fat content. However, some patients have increased fecal mass without loose stools and complain of constipation. Removal of dietary gluten, present in wheat, rye, barely, oats, food additives, emulsifiers, and stabilizers, is essential for successful management. Patients who do not respond to a strict gluten-free diet may have refractory sprue or lymphoma.

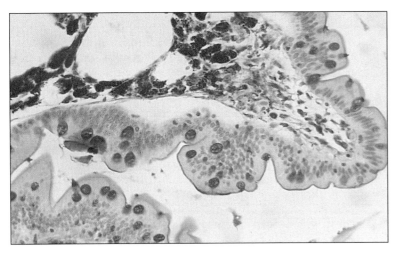

FIGURE 5-13.

Jejunal biopsy from a patient with Whipple's disease. The histologic appearance of biopsies obtained from involved small intestine is diagnostic for Whipple's disease. In this patient, the villi are flat and widened. There is also extensive infiltration of the lamina propria with large periodic acid-Schiff–positive macrophages. Whipple's disease is caused by a bacterial infection with a gram-positive bacillus. The gastrointestinal tract, musculoskeletal system, cardiovascular system, central nervous system, pulmonary system, skin, and lymph nodes may be involved, causing a broad range of symptoms. Treatment with appropriate antibiotics usually results in dramatic clinical improvement within 2 weeks. Antibiotic therapy should be continued for 1 year to decrease the risk of relapse. Short-term nutritional therapy to correct protein-calorie malnutrition and specific nutrient deficiencies, such as vitamin C deficiency, is often necessary until absorptive function improves.

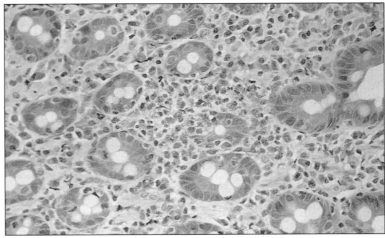

FIGURE 5-14.

Jejunal biopsy from a patient with eosinophilic gastroenteritis. A dense inflammatory cell infiltrate, composed almost entirely of eosinophils, is present in the mucosa and submucosa. Specific clinical symptoms depend on which layer of the intestinal wall is predominantly involved. Clinical manifestations of mucosal and submucosal disease include abdominal pain, nausea, vomiting, diarrhea, and weight loss. Approximately 25% of patients have steatorrhea.

Short-bowel syndrome

TABLE 5-2. PREDICTED NUTRITIONAL OUTCOME IN PATIENTS WHO HAVE HAD MASSIVE INTESTINAL RESECTION

REMAINING JEJUNAL LENGTH, CM	COLON	NUTRITIONAL OUTCOME
0–50	-	TPN
	+	TPN
51–100	-	IVFM/TPN
	+	Modified oral diet
101–150	-	Regular or modified oral diet
	+	Regular diet
151–200	-	Modified oral diet
	+	Regular diet
>200	- or +	Regular diet

TABLE 5-2.

Although the gastrointestinal tract has considerable reserve for nutrient absorption, massive small-bowel resection can cause significant malabsorption. The severity of malabsorption depends on the length and functional capacity of the remaining intestine and the site of resection. Jejunal resections are better tolerated than ileal resections because of the specialized functions of the ileum and its adaptive ability to compensate for loss of jejunal function. In addition, the status of the colon is particularly important in patients with little remaining small intestine because the colon can salvage malabsorbed carbohydrates and augment fluid absorption. The need for dietary modifications and intravenous nutritional supplementation can be difficult to predict because of the variability in absorptive capacity of the remaining intestine. This table presents reasonable guidelines that can be used in predicting nutritional outcome based on the length of remaining jejunum and the presence or absence of the colon. IVFM—Intravenous fluids and minerals; modified oral diet—regular diet plus supplemental liquid formula with or without oral rehydration solution; regular diet—table food, including high-caloric diets, frequent feedings, and modification in dietary fat levels; TPN—total parenteral nutrition; (+)—present; (-)—absent. (*Data from* Lennard-Jones [8a].)

TABLE 5-3. MACRONUTRIENT ABSORPTION IN PATIENTS WITH SHORT-BOWEL SYNDROME

STUDY	WOOLF ET AL [12] (N=8)	MESSING ET AL [10] (N=10)	COSNES ET AL [9] (N=6)	MCINTYRE ET AL [11] (N=7)
Intestinal status:				
Jejunum length, cm	approximately 100–200	0–200	90–150	80–150
Some TI remaining, n	0	5/10	0	0
Some colon remaining, n	3/8	9/10	0	0
TEST DIET	**REGULAR FOOD**	**REGULAR FOOD**	**LIQUID FORMULA**	**LIQUID FORMULA**
Nutrient absorption, %				
Fat	54 ± 4	52 ± 5	54 ± 12	59 ± 6
Carbohydrate	61 ± 7	79 ± 5	NR	NR
Protein	81 ± 5	61 ± 6	50 ± 4	66 ± 6
Total energy	62 ± 3	67 ± 4	57 ± 7	57 ± 7

TABLE 5-3.

Assessment of macronutrient balance in patients with short-bowel syndrome were remarkably similar in four studies despite considerable variability in patient populations [9–12]. Data suggest that many patients with short-bowel syndrome absorb approximately two thirds of their total calorie intake. Patients who absorb less than one third of total calories and those who have large ostomy or stool outputs are likely to require long-term intravenous support. Almost half of the patients evaluated in the studies listed required some form of parenteral supplementation. NR—Not reported; TI—terminal ileum.

TABLE 5-4. THERAPEUTIC GOALS IN PATIENTS WITH SHORT-BOWEL SYNDROME

Control diarrhea
Maximize oral and enteral nutrition
Provide parenteral nutrition when needed
Correct and prevent specific nutrient deficiencies
Prevent and treat complications
Optimize quality-of-life

TABLE 5-4.

The long-term goals of treating patients with short-bowel syndrome are listed. The specific therapeutic approach depends on the functional capacity of the patient's remaining intestinal tract; the presence of macronutrient, micronutrient, electrolyte, and fluid deficits; risk factors for future medical complications; and an evaluation of the patient's specific needs to achieve a reasonable quality-of-life. Therapy for diarrhea involves limiting endogenous secretions with H_2-receptor blockers, proton pump inhibitors, or octreotide acetate, slowing intestinal motility with the use of opiate and anticholinergic medication, and avoiding foods and medications that cause diarrhea. Oral and enteral feedings should be maximized to decrease or eliminate the need for parenteral nutrition. However, long-term parenteral nutrition can be life-saving by providing specific, but difficult to absorb, nutrients or total nutritional requirements. The treatment plan must take into consideration the patient's quality-of-life. For example, in some patients, home total parenteral nutrition given at night is more acceptable than aggressive enteral nutritional therapy, which causes a greater restriction in lifestyle.

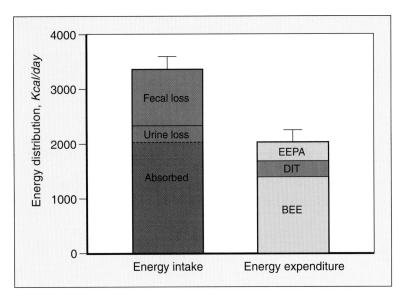

FIGURE 5-15.

Relationship between energy intake and energy requirements in patients with short-bowel syndrome. Ingestion of large amounts of food can often compensate for impaired intestinal function and can permit adequate calorie absorption to meet daily energy requirements needed for basal energy expenditure (BEE), diet-induced thermogenesis (DIT), and energy expenditure of physical activity (EEPA). This figure represents data from five patients with short-bowel syndrome [10]. Approximately 65% of ingested calories were absorbed. Energy balance was maintained by ingesting almost twice the estimated amount of calories needed for total energy expenditure. Therefore, "overfeeding" patients with short-bowel syndrome often can avoid the need for parenteral nutrition support.

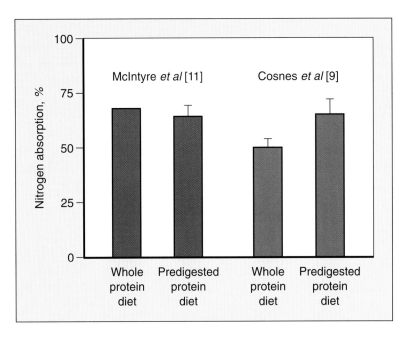

FIGURE 5-16.

Data from two studies comparing nitrogen absorption from liquid diets containing either whole protein or predigested protein in patients with severe short-bowel syndrome. Both studies evaluated patients who had jejunostomies and < 150 cm of residual jejunum [11,13]. In one study, nitrogen absorption was the same whether patients consumed a diet containing whole or predigested proteins [11]. In contrast, in the second study, nitrogen absorption was better on a predigested-protein diet than on a whole-protein diet [13]. The reason for the differences between studies is not clear, but may be related to differences in the composition of the protein hydrolysates. Despite improved nitrogen absorption, the latter study did not document any clinical or physiologic benefits of a predigested protein diet. Therefore, expensive predigested protein formulas should not be given to patients with short-bowel syndrome on a routine basis because the potential improvement in nitrogen absorption may not translate into clinical benefits, and is probably unnecessary if protein intake is increased.

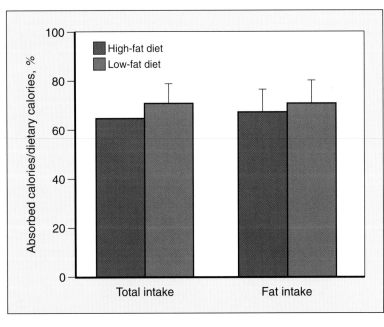

FIGURE 5-17.

Total calorie and fat absorption in patients with short-bowel syndrome ingesting either a high-fat (60% of total calories) or a low-fat (20% of total calories) diet. In this study, most patients had jejunostomies with approximately 100 to 200 cm of residual jejunum. The proportion of calories provided as fat did not affect the coefficient of either fat or total calorie absorption [14]. Because the percentage of fat absorbed remains constant over the physiologic range of dietary fat intake, ingesting a high-fat diet increases both fat absorption and fat excretion. Therefore, dietary fat should not be restricted in patients who do not have a colon. In fact, increasing fat intake often increases calorie intake because of enhanced palatability and calorie density. However, restricting dietary fat in patients who have small bowel in continuity with the colon may decrease gastrointestinal symptoms by decreasing steatorrhea.

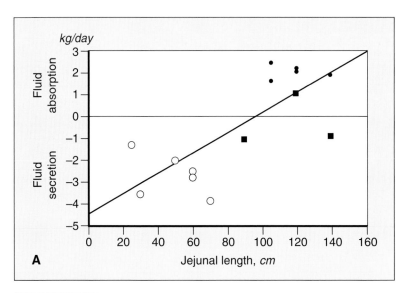

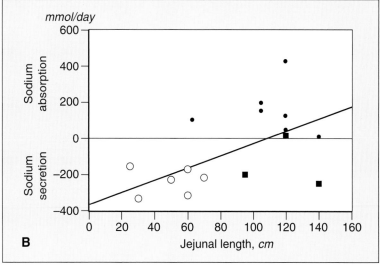

FIGURE 5-18.

A–B, Relationship between jejunal length and sodium-water absorption in patients with short bowel and a jejunostomy. Balance studies were performed while patients consumed three meals a day. The data demonstrate that sodium and water absorption are inversely correlated with intestinal length [15]. Patients with less than 100 cm of jejunum exhibited sodium and water losses that exceeded intake. Therefore, these patients cannot maintain sodium and water equilibrium without parenteral supplementation or oral rehydration formulas. (*Adapted from* Nightingale *et al.* [15]; with permission.)

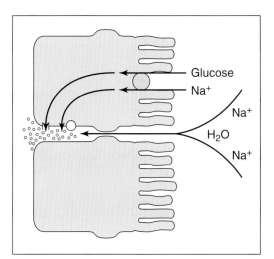

FIGURE 5-19.

Oral rehydration therapy enhances sodium and water absorption by taking advantage of the sodium-glucose cotransporter present in the brush border of the small intestine. Active absorption of glucose and sodium across the epithelial cell also stimulates passive sodium and water absorption by solvent drag in the jejunum. Oral rehydration therapy can be quite useful in maintaining sodium and fluid homeostasis in patients with severe mineral and water losses.

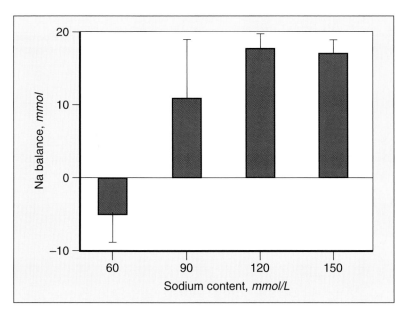

FIGURE 5-20.

Sodium balance after ingesting different sodium-containing test solutions in patients with jejunostomies and < 150 cm of residual jejunum. Net sodium loss occurred with a solution containing 60 mmol of sodium per liter, but net absorption occurred with solutions containing ≥ 90 mmol/L [16].

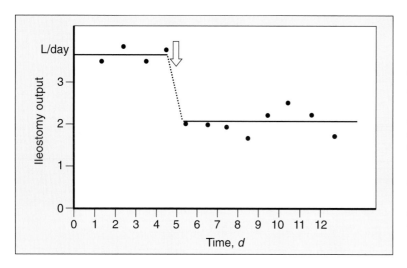

FIGURE 5-21.

Effect of oral rehydration therapy on high-volume ostomy output. Initiating treatment with glucose polymer-based electrolyte solution (indicated by the *arrow*) caused a marked decrease in ostomy output (from approximately 3.5 L/day to approximately 2 L/day) in a patient with 125 cm of remaining small bowel [17]. Oral rehydration therapy in this patient permitted maintenance of body weight and fluid status without the need for intravenous infusions. Therefore, providing a glucose-electrolyte solution which contains 100 mmol/L of sodium: 4 g of sodium chloride, 2.9 g of sodium citrate, and 20 g of glucose or 18 mg of maltodextrins dissolved in 1 L of tap water can prevent the need for home IV therapy in selected patients. (*Adapted from* Laustsen and Fallingborg [17]; with permission.)

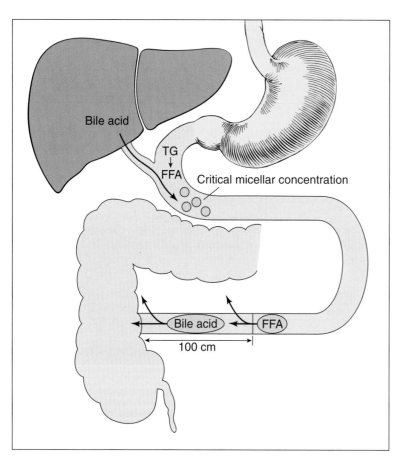

FIGURE 5-22.

Effect of ileal resection on bile acid and fat absorption. Malabsorption of bile acids occur after resection of the terminal ileum, the only site of active bile acid absorption. When resection is minimal (< 100 cm), increased bile acids are delivered to the colon, where they inhibit colonic water and electrolyte absorption and stimulate colonic motility [18]. The liver can compensate for minimal bile acid losses by increasing hepatic bile acid synthesis, thereby maintaining a normal bile acid–pool size and sufficient bile acids for micelle formation. When ileal resection is greater than 100 cm, however, the liver is unable to maintain the bile acid pool and the critical micellar concentration cannot be reached, thus causing fat malabsorption and steatorrhea. Therefore, understanding the pathophysiology of diarrhea after ileal resection has important therapeutic implications. Minimal ileal resection causes bile acid diarrhea that can be treated with cholestyramine, a bile acid binder. More marked ileal resections cause steatorrhea, which can actually be made worse by cholestyramine therapy by further depleting of the remaining bile acid pool. FFA—free fatty acids; TG—triglycerides.

TABLE 5-5. MAGNESIUM CONTENT OF SELECTED MAGNESIUM COMPOUNDS

MAGNESIUM COMPOUNDS	ELEMENTAL MAGNESIUM, MG/G	REPRESENTATIVE PRODUCT	MAGNESIUM CONTENT, MG/TABLET
Chloride	120	Slo-Mag*	64
Gluconate	54	Magonate tablet	27
		Magonate liquid	54†
Lactate	100	MagTab SR*	84
Oxide	600	Mag-Ox400	241
		Uro-Mag	85

*Sustained release caplet.
†mg/5 mL.

TABLE 5-5.

Patients with short-bowel syndrome and a jejunostomy are at high risk for magnesium deficiency because magnesium is poorly absorbed and body stores can become depleted rapidly. Magnesium is primarily an intracellular cation, so normal serum levels do not exclude the presence of magnesium deficiency. The percentage of infused magnesium excreted in urine, normally > 80% of the intravenous dose, may be a better index of body stores, but this has not been confirmed [19]. Replacing magnesium using oral supplements can be challenging because magnesium salts often increase diarrhea. Enteric-coated magnesium supplements should not be used because their delayed release reduces contact time with the intestine for absorption [20]. Soluble magnesium salts, such as magnesium gluconate (Magonate [Fleming, St. Louis, MO]), are better tolerated and absorbed than other magnesium complexes. However, magnesium content is low in magnesium gluconate supplements requiring the ingestion of a large number of tablets to meet requirements. Therefore, in some patients magnesium oxide supplements may be more effective because of increased compliance. Magnesium gluconate given in liquid form can be added to an oral rehydration solution in doses of 15 to 30 mmol (365 to 730 mg elemental magnesium) per day. Magnesium sulfate can be injected intramuscularly at a dosage of 12 mmol (290 mg of elemental magnesium) one to three times per week if attempts at oral therapy are unsuccessful. Intravenous infusion of magnesium is preferred, however, because intramuscular injections are painful and can cause sterile abscesses.

TABLE 5-6. CALCIUM CONTENT OF SELECTED CALCIUM SALTS

CALCIUM SALT	ELEMENTAL CALCIUM, MG/G	REPRESENTATIVE PRODUCTS	CALCIUM CONTENT, MG/TABLET
Acetate	250	Phos-Lo	169
Carbonate	400	Alka-Mints	340
		Caltrate 600	600
		Oscal 500	500
		Rolaids	220
		TUMS	250
Citrate	211	Citracal	200
Glubionate	64	Neo-Calglucon	115*
Gluconate	96	Generic 1000 mg	96
Lactate	130	Generic 650 mg	84
Phosphate—dibasic	234	Dical D	117
Phosphate—tribasic	400	Posture	600

*mg/5 mL

TABLE 5-6.

Supplemental calcium is given routinely to most patients with short-bowel syndrome because of both impaired intestinal absorption and the limited calcium intake associated with low-lactose diets. However, when calcium intake is inadequate, plasma levels are still maintained by mobilizing bone stores unless there is concurrent magnesium or vitamin D deficiency. Therefore, urinary calcium excretion, which should be > 2 mg/kg per 24 hours, is a more reliable index of calcium absorption than plasma concentration. Bone densitometry is helpful to assess body calcium stores. Abnormalities in calcium status indicate that more aggressive treatment needs to be initiated, such as increasing vitamin D and calcium intake or starting estrogen therapy in postmenopausal women. Most patients require 1.5 to 2 g of elemental calcium daily. As shown in this table, the amount of elemental calcium present in each calcium salt differs, influencing the number of tablets needed each day.

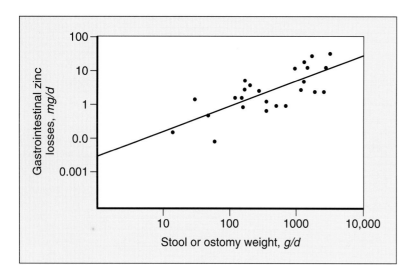

FIGURE 5-23.

Relationship between zinc losses and stool output. The gastrointestinal tract is the major route for zinc excretion. Normally, 2 to 3 mg is excreted in feces each day. This figure shows the results from a study performed in patients receiving only parenteral feeding, which demonstrated that the amount of zinc lost was proportional to stool or ostomy volume [21]. However, zinc losses also depended on the patient population. Patients who had massive small-bowel resection lost approximately 4 mg of zinc per liter or kilogram of stool or ostomy output, whereas those with intact small bowel or limited (<15 cm) small-bowel resection lost approximately 15 mg of zinc per liter or kilogram of stool or ostomy output. (*Adapted from* Wolman *et al.* [21]; with permission.)

TABLE 5-7. RECOMMENDATIONS FOR VITAMIN AND TRACE MINERAL SUPPLEMENTATION PATIENTS WITH SHORT-BOWEL SYNDROME

Supplement (representative product)	Dose	Route
Multivitamin with minerals*	1 prenatal vitamin, daily	PO
Vitamin D*	50,000 U 2–3 times per week	PO
Vitamin B$_{12}$†	1 mg daily	PO
	100–500 µg every 1–2 mo	IM
Vitamin A† (Aquasol)	10,000 to 50,000 U daily	PO
Vitamin K† (Mephyton; AquaMEPHYTON)	5 mg, daily	PO
	5–10 mg/wk	SQ/IM/IV
Vitamin E† (Liqui E)	30 U daily	PO
Zinc gluconate or zinc sulfate†	25 mg elemental zinc daily plus 100 mg/L intestinal output	PO
Ferrous sulfate†	60 mg elemental iron t.i.d.	PO
Iron dextran†	≤ 100 mg elemental iron per day based on formula or table	IV

*Recommended routinely for all patients.
†Recommended for patients with documented nutrient deficiency or malabsorption.

TABLE 5-7.

Most patients with short-bowel syndrome who are maintained on an oral diet should be given vitamin and trace mineral supplements. A daily high-dose vitamin and mineral formula (*eg*, a prenatal multivitamin with minerals), vitamin D, and calcium is recommended.

Other micronutrients should be supplemented as needed to prevent or treat specific nutrient deficiencies. IM—intramuscular; IV—intravenous; PO—oral; SQ—subcutaneous.

POSTMUCOSAL DISEASE

Lymphangiectasia

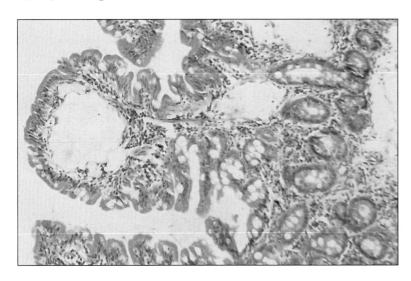

FIGURE 5-24.

Jejunal biopsy demonstrating dilated submucosal lacteals in a patient with lymphangiectasia. Congenital malformation or secondary obstruction of the lymphatic system causes dilatation of intestinal lacteals and rupture of intestinal lymphatics through the mucosa. The leakage of lymph, containing chylomicrons, protein, and lymphocytes, into the intestinal lumen causes protein, fat, and lymphocyte losses. Therefore, the clinical manifestations of intestinal lymphangiectasia include peripheral edema, chylous ascites, hypoproteinemia, lymphopenia, and impaired delayed cutaneous hypersensitivity. Treatment involves therapy of the underlying disease in patients with secondary lymphangiectasia and careful monitoring of dermatologic complications. Resection of the involved intestine can be beneficial in patients with a localized lymphatic lesion. The goal of diet therapy is to decrease intestinal lymph flow by having the patient consume a low-fat (reduced long-chain triglyceride) diet [22].

EVALUATION OF SUSPECTED MALABSORPTION

TABLE 5-8. INITIAL EVALUATION OF PATIENT WITH POSSIBLE MALABSORPTION

History and Physical Examination

Initial blood tests	Follow-up laboratory tests
Complete blood count	Serum iron
Prothrombin time	Serum folate
Standard electrolytes	Serum vitamin B_{12}
Calcium	Serum vitamin A
Magnesium	Plasma 25-hydroxy vitamin D
Blood urea nitrogen	Urinary oxalate excretion
Creatinine	Stool for Sudan stain
Alkaline phosphatase	Stool for ova and parasites
Cholesterol	
Total protein and albumin	

TABLE 5-8.

The approach to the patient with suspected malabsorption requires a careful and appropriate initial evaluation to establish the likelihood of malabsorption and to formulate a list of possible causes. The history and physical examination should assess body weight changes, appetite and food intake, generalized weakness, the presence and volume of diarrhea, stool characteristics suggestive of steatorrhea, signs and symptoms of dehydration, signs and symptoms of specific nutrient deficiencies (*see* Table 5-9), abdominal pain and other gastrointestinal symptoms, and extraintestinal manifestations. Follow-up laboratory tests are usually more expensive or more difficult to perform than the initial blood tests, and their use should be reserved for specific indications.

TABLE 5-9. SELECTED SYMPTOMS AND SIGNS OF NUTRIENT DEFICIENCIES

	SYMPTOMS OR SIGN	POSSIBLE NUTRIENT DEFICIENCY
General	Weakness, weight loss, muscle wasting	Protein, calorie
Skin	Pallor	Folate, iron, vitamin B$_{12}$
	Follicular hyperkeratosis	Vitamin A, vitamin C
	Perifollicular petechiae	Vitamin C
	Dermatitis	Protein, calorie, niacin, riboflavin, zinc, vitamin A, essential fatty acids
	Bruising, purpura	
Hair	Easily plucked, alopecia	Vitamin C, vitamin K
	Corkscrew hairs, coiled hair	Protein, zinc, biotin
Eyes	Night blindness, keratomalacia, photophobia	Vitamin C, vitamin A
	Conjunctival inflammation	Vitamin A
Mouth	Glossitis	Vitamin A, riboflavin
	Bleeding or receding gums, mouth ulcers	Riboflavin, niacin, folate, vitamin B$_{12}$, protein
	Decreased taste	Vitamin A, vitamin C, vitamin K, folate
	Burning or sore mouth and tongue	Zinc, vitamin A
	Angular stomatitis or cheilosis	Vitamin B$_{12}$, vitamin C, niacin, folate, iron
Neurologic	Tetany	Riboflavin, niacin, pyridoxine, iron
	Paresthesias	Calcium, magnesium
	Loss of reflexes, wrist drop, foot drop, loss of vibratory and position sense	Thiamine, pyridoxine
		Vitamin B$_{12}$, vitamin E
	Dementia, disorientation	
	Ophthalmoplegia	Niacin, vitamin B$_{12}$
	Depression	Vitamin E, thiamine
		Biotin, folate, vitamin B$_{12}$

TABLE 5-9.

Selected symptoms and signs of nutrient deficiencies. The history and physical examination of the patient with suspected malabsorption should involve an evaluation for specific nutrient deficiencies. In general, rapidly proliferating tissues, such as hair, skin, oral and intestinal mucosa, and bone marrow, are often most affected by nutrient deficiencies.

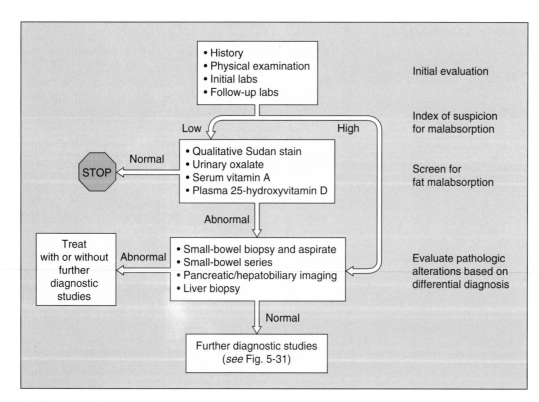

FIGURE 5-25.

Suggested algorithm for evaluating patients with suspected malabsorption. The etiology of generalized malabsorption can be diagnosed rapidly in most patients without the need for complicated studies. A small subset of patients can be much more difficult to diagnose, however, who will require extensive testing and repeating earlier studies to establish a final diagnosis (see Fig. 5-26).

The first and most important step in the evaluation is performing a careful initial assessment, which includes a history, physical examination, and simple laboratory tests (see Table 5-8). The initial assessment should provide the clinician with an index of suspicion for malabsorption and a differential diagnosis. If the index of suspicion for malabsorption is low, the evaluation can stop or simple tests to evaluate for fat malabsorption can be performed if they have not already been done. If malabsorption is suspected, an attempt should be made to diagnose the disease by identifying pathologic alterations associated with specific diseases. Studies should be performed in a logical sequence based on the clinician's suspicion of whether the cause of malabsorption is of small-bowel, pancreatic, or hepatic etiology. If one pathway of investigation (eg, small-bowel disease) is not fruitful, other diagnostic pathways (eg, pancreatic insufficiency) should be considered. A liver biopsy may be useful in patients who have cholestasis and who show no evidence of pancreatic disease.

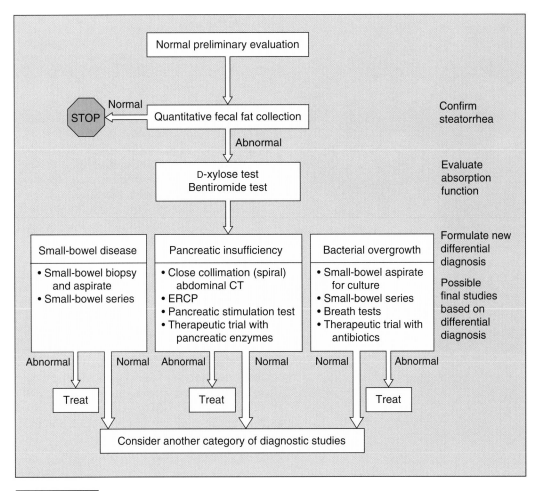

FIGURE 5-26.

If results of all studies outlined in Figure 5-25 are normal, the presence of steatorrhea should be confirmed before pursuing further diagnostic studies. Fat absorption provides a general index of intestinal digestive and absorptive function because it requires integration of premucosal, mucosal, and postmucosal processes. Quantitative fecal fat analysis usually

requires a 72-hour stool collection while the patient is consuming a diet containing 100 g of fat daily. However, collections of shorter duration are reliable in patients with rapid gastrointestinal transit. After steatorrhea has been documented, further studies should be performed, guided by the suspected etiology of steatorrhea. However, it is important to remember that diarrhea itself can cause mild steatorrhea (*see* Fig. 5-29). Results from absorptive function studies, such as fecal fat (*see* Fig. 5-1), D-xylose (*see* Fig. 5-27), and bentiromide (*see* Fig. 5-28) tests, can help formulate a new differential diagnosis. Patients with small-bowel disease usually have low fecal fat concentrations (< 9.5 g/100 g wet weight), abnormal D-xylose absorption, and either a normal or abnormal bentiromide test. Patients with pancreatic insufficiency have high fecal fat concentrations (> 9.5 g/100 g wet weight), normal D-xylose absorption, and an abnormal bentiromide test. Theoretically, patients with bacterial overgrowth who have steatorrhea should have a high fecal fat concentration, but may have either normal or abnormal D-xylose absorption. The "final" series of studies should be performed in a logical sequence based on the suspected etiology of disease. The three major categories of disease that cause steatorrhea are shown. One or more of the diagnostic studies listed in each box can be performed in addition to repeating earlier inconclusive evaluations. ERCP—endoscopic retrograde cholangiopancreatography.

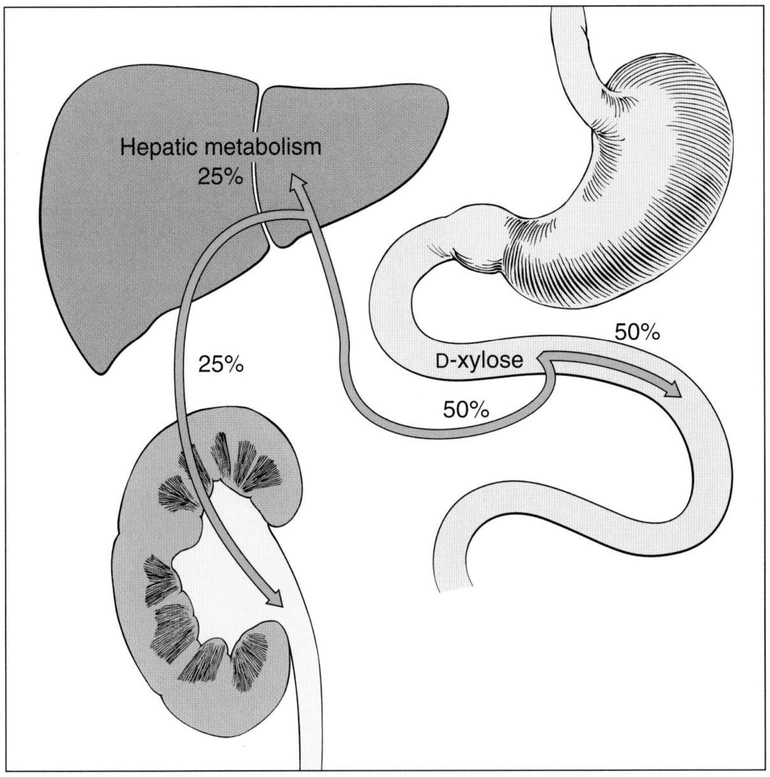

FIGURE 5-27.

Oral administration of D-xylose can be used to evaluate small-intestine absorptive function [23]. D-Xylose is a five-carbon sugar that is absorbed by both transcellular and paracellular pathways in the small intestine. Therefore, D-xylose absorption is affected by functional mucosal surface area and mucosal permeability. Normally, only 50% of ingested D-xylose is absorbed; half of this metabolized by the liver and half (25% of the ingested dose) is excreted in urine. Excreting less than 4 g in urine over 5 hours or reaching a plasma concentration of less than 20 mg/dL after ingesting a 25-g oral dose of D-xylose is considered to be abnormal. False-positive tests may occur in patients with dehydration, renal disease, ascites, portal hypertension, and bacterial overgrowth. Certain drugs, such as aspirin, indomethacin, and neomycin, may also cause false-positive results.

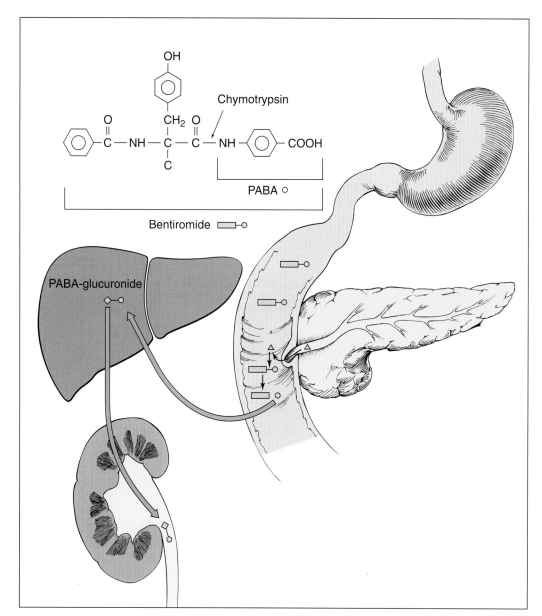

FIGURE 5-28.

Oral administration of a synthetic peptide, N-benzoyl-L-tyrosyl-*para*-aminobenzoic acid (betiromide), has been used to evaluate pancreatic exocrine function [24]. The *para*-aminobenzoic acid (PABA) moiety of bentiromide is cleaved off by pancreatic chymotrypsin. Free PABA is then absorbed, conjugated by the liver, and excreted in urine. Decreased PABA excretion after an oral load suggests the presence of pancreatic insufficiency. This test is highly sensitive and specific for patients with advanced pancreatic failure. The bentiromide test has several serious shortcomings, however. It is not very sensitive in patients with mild pancreatic insufficiency. Severe small-bowel disease, liver disease, renal disease, and diabetes diminish either PABA absorption or excretion and yield false-positive results. Many medications (such as acetaminophen, benzocaine, lidocaine, furosemide, chlorthiazide, and antibiotics containing sulfa) and certain foods (such as prunes and cranberries) may interfere with the chemical determination of PABA. However, these interfering compounds are not a problem for laboratories that measure PABA by high-performance liquid chromatography.

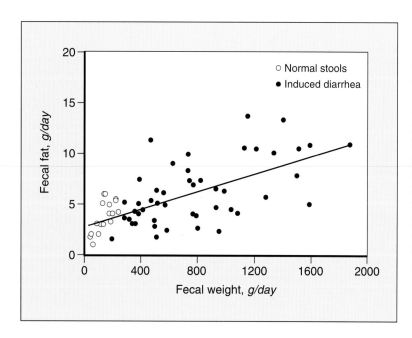

FIGURE 5-29.

Relationship between fecal weight and fecal fat in normal subjects with experimentally induced diarrhea. The presence of diarrhea itself can cause fat malabsorption and steatorrhea in persons with normal absorptive function. Fecal weight correlated closely with fecal fat when osmotic, secretory, or combined osmotic and secretory diarrhea was induced in normal volunteers [25]. However, diarrhea causes only mild steatorrhea, and even subjects with severe diarrhea (> 1600 g/day) had less than 14 g of fecal fat output per day. Therefore, mild steatorrhea (< 14 g/day on a 100 g/day fat diet) can be caused by either malabsorptive disease or other diseases that cause diarrhea. The mechanism for diarrhea-induced steatorrhea is not known, but presumably involves diluting the luminal factors involved in fat digestion and absorption, decreasing the contact time between dietary fat and small-bowel mucosa, or a combination of the two. (*Adapted from* Fine and Fordtran [25]; with permission.)

NUTRITIONAL THERAPY COMPLICATIONS

TABLE 5-10. COMPLICATIONS OF REFEEDING THE SEVERELY MALNOURISHED PATIENT

Fluid overload
Edema
Congestive heart failure
Mineral depletion
Hypophosphatemia
Hypokalemia
Hypomagnesemia
Glucose intolerance
Hyperglycemia
Dehydration
Hyperosmolar coma
Gastrointestinal dysfunction
Diarrhea
Cardiac arrhythmias
Ventricular arrhythmias
Prolonged Q–T interval
Sudden death

TABLE 5-10.

The purpose of nutritional therapy in patients with malabsorption is to correct specific nutrient deficiencies and to provide daily nutrient requirements. Refeeding the severely malnourished patient must be done with caution because of the high risk of feeding-induced complications [26]. Overzealous feeding can cause serious medical complications and death. Malnourished patients who also have limited absorptive function may require short-term parenteral therapy in conjunction with oral-enteral feeds until absorptive function and nutritional status are stabilized. In the absence of fluid overload or dehydration, fluid intake should be limited to approximately 800 mL per day plus insensible losses. Weight gain of more than 0.25 kg per day or 1.5 kg per week indicates fluid accumulation. Daily energy intake should provide 110% of resting energy requirements and contain approximately 150 g of carbohydrate and 1.2 to 1.5 g of protein per kilogram of ideal body weight. Carbohydrate feeding stimulates insulin release and intracellular uptake of phosphorus and potassium, causing a rapid decline in their plasma concentrations. Magnesium can become depleted as it is used for intracellular metabolic functions. Therefore, intravenous phosphorus, potassium, and magnesium supplementation may be needed. Sodium intake should be restricted initially to 60 mEq per day (1.5 g/day) to decrease the risk of fluid overload. During the first week of refeeding, nutritional therapy should be monitored daily and adjusted as needed to provide optimal and safe support.

REFERENCES

1. Bo-Linn GW, Fordtran JS: Fecal fat concentration in patients with steatorrhea. *Gastroenterology* 1984, 87:319–322.

2. DiMagno EP, Go VLW, Summerskill WHJ: Relations between pancreatic enzyme outputs and malabsorption in severe pancreatic insufficiency. *N Engl J Med* 1973, 288:813–815.

3. DiMagno EP, Malagelada JR, Go VLW, Moertel CG: Fate of orally ingested enzymes in pancreatic insufficiency. *N Engl J Med* 1977, 296:1318–1322.

4. Guarner L, Rodriguez R, Guarner F, Malagelada J-R: Fate of oral enzymes in pancreatic insufficiency. *Gut* 1993, 34:708–712.

5. Steinhardt HJ, Wolf A, Jakober B, Adibi SA: Nitrogen absorption in pancreatectomized patients: Protein versus protein hydrolysate as substrate. *J Lab Clin Med* 1989, 113:162–167.

6. Lanspa SJ, Chan ATH, Bell III JS, *et al.*: Pathogenesis of steatorrhea in primary biliary cirrhosis. *Hepatology* 1985, 5:837–842.

7. Chang EB, Binder HJ: *Diarrheal Diseases. The Undergraduate Teaching Project in Gastroenterology and Liver Disease.* Timonium, MD: Milner Fenwick; 1992:40.

8. Hammer HF, Fine KD, Santa Ana CA, *et al.*: Carbohydrate malabsorption: Its measurement and its contribution to diarrhea. *J Clin Invest* 1990, 86:1936–1944.

8a. Lennard-Jones JE: Practical management of the short bowel [review article]. *Aliment Pharmacol Ther* 1994, 8:563–577.

9. Cosnes J, Gendre J-P, Evard D, LeQuintrec Y: Compensatory enteral hyperalimentation for management of patients with severe short bowel syndrome. *Am J Clin Nutr* 1985, 41:1002.

10. Messing B, Pigot F, Rongier M, *et al.*: Intestinal absorption of free oral hyperalimentation in the very short bowel syndrome. *Gastroenterology* 1991, 100:1502–1508.

11. McIntyre PB, Fitchew M, Lennard-Jones JE: Patients with a high jejunostomy do not need a special diet. *Gastroenterology* 1986, 91:25–33.

12. Woolf GM, Miller C, Kurian R, Jeejeebhoy KN: Nutritional absorption in short bowel syndrome. Evaluation of fluid, caloric, and divalent cation requirements. *Dig Dis Sci* 1987, 32:8.

13. Cosnes J, Evard D, Beaugerie L, *et al.*: Improvement in protein absorption with a small-peptide-based diet in patients with high jejunostomy. *Nutrition* 1992, 8:406–411.

14. Woolf GM, Miller C, Kurian R, Jeejeebhoy KN: Diet for patients with a short bowel: High fat or high carbohydrate? *Gastroenterology* 1983, 84:823–828.

15. Nightingale JM, Lennard-Jones JE, Walker ER, Farthing MJ: Jejunal efflux in short bowel syndrome. *Lancet* 1990, 336:765.

16. Rodriguez CA, Lennard-Jones JE, Thompson DG, Farthing MJG: What is the ideal sodium concentration of oral rehydration solutions for short bowel patients? *Clin Sci* 1988, 74(suppl 18):69.

17. Laustsen J, Fallingborg J: Enteral glucose-polymer-electrolyte solution in the treatment of chronic fluid and electrolyte depletion in short-bowel syndrome. *Acta Chir Scand* 1983, 149:787–788.

18. Mekhjian HS, Phillips SF, Hoffmann AF: Colonic secretion of water and electrolytes induced by bile acids: Perfusion studies in man. *J Clin Invest* 1971, 50:1569.

19. Rude RK, Singer FR: Magnesium deficiency and excess. *Annu Rev Med* 1981, 32:245.

20. Fine KD, Santa Ana CA, Porter JL, Fordtran JS: Intestinal absorption of magnesium from food and supplements. *J Clin Invest* 1991, 88:396.

21. Wolman SK, Anderson GH, Marliss EB, Jeejeebhoy KN: Zinc in total parenteral nutrition: Requirements and metabolic effects. *Gastroenterology* 1979, 76:458–467.

22. Holt PR, Hashim SA, Van Itallie TB: Treatment of malabsorption syndrome and exudative enteropathy with synthetic medium chain triglycerides. *Am J Gastroenterol* 1965, 43:549–559.

23. Craig RM, Atkinson AJ: D-xylose testing: A review. *Gastroenterology* 1988, 95:223.

24. Heyman MD: The bentiromide test: How good is it? *Gastroenterology* 1985, 89:685.

25. Fine KD, Fordtran JS: The effect of diarrhea on fecal fat excretion. *Gastroenterology* 1992, 102:1936–1939.

26. Solomon SM, Kirby DF: The refeeding syndrome: A review. *JPEN J Parenteral Enteral Nutr* 1990, 14:90.

Chapter 6

Gastric and Small Intestinal Motility Disorders

EAMONN M.M. QUIGLEY

Gastric and small intestinal motility is fundamental to intestinal homeostasis. Gastric motility ensures the timely and orderly delivery of an appropriately processed meal to the small intestine, where the motor function of the small intestine provides for its orderly progression in a manner consistent with optimal digestion and absorption. Reflecting the various levels of control of motility, disordered motor function may result from abnormalities at several levels, including the smooth muscle cell, the enteric nervous system, the autonomic nerve supply to the gut, the spinal cord, and the brain.

Symptoms related to motor dysfunction tend to be nonspecific. Disordered gastric motility is usually described as either an acceleration or a delay in gastric emptying. Accelerated emptying is associated with the symptom constellation referred to as the *dumping syndrome*. Delayed emptying, in contrast, may cause nonspecific symptoms, such as postprandial fullness, early satiety, and epigastric discomfort, or more specific symptoms, such as delayed vomiting of undigested food. Disordered small intestinal motor function may lead to specific syndromes, which include pseudo-obstruction and malabsorption related to intestinal bacterial overgrowth, or less specific symptoms, which may mimic those commonly associated with the irritable bowel syndrome. Apart from some relatively rare and well-defined disease states, such as diabetic gastroenteropathy and systemic sclerosis, most disorders of foregut motor function are defined poorly and rarely are confirmed pathologically. Another problem that confounds the evaluation and therapy of these disorders is a poor correlation between symptoms and the extent of measurable, disordered function.

Recent years have seen an explosion of technology in the area of motility. It is, for example, now feasible to record intraluminal pressure activity from virtually any part of the gastrointestinal tract over prolonged periods; however, although the basic characteristics of normal gastric and small intestinal motility have been well-defined, criteria for the manometric diagnosis of motor disorders continue to be developed. Progress also has been made with techniques of a less invasive nature. Scintigraphic methods for the assessment of gastric emptying are well established, and have been developed for the evaluation of small intestinal transit as well. Ultrasonography, electrical impedance, MR imaging, and electrogastrography are other noninvasive techniques for the assessment of gastric motor function that continue to undergo evaluation, but have not been used widely on a clinical basis.

Among the many causes of gastroparesis, those related to earlier gastric surgery and to diabetes mellitus are among the most common. Although patients with idiopathic gastroparesis are being recognized with increasing frequency, the pathophysiology of delayed gastric emptying and gastric hypomotility observed in these patients remains elusive. Another syndrome being recognized more frequently is chronic idiopathic intestinal pseudo-obstruction, a rare disorder that typically presents with symptoms indistinguishable from those of mechanical obstruction, but is caused by disordered intestinal motility. Pseudo-obstruction may be related primarily to a neuropathy or myopathy of the gastrointestinal tract, but more commonly, may

be secondary to a wide variety of connective tissue and neuro-muscular and metabolic disorders. Many of these disorders affect the gastrointestinal tract diffusely and may involve not only the stomach and small intestine, but also the esophagus and colon.

The management of foregut motility disorders involves such general measures as rehydration, correction of electrolyte imbalance, and decompression of the distended stomach or small intestine. For many patients, nutritional therapy is paramount. Attention to the type of diet ingested and the need for enteral or total parenteral nutrition is essential. Several therapeutic agents are available for the treatment of motility disorders. These include cholinergic agonists, serotonergic agonists and antagonists, dopamine antagonists, macrolides, and somatostatin analogues. These agents have been shown to stimulate gastric and small intestinal motor activity to a variable extent; they have also been demonstrated in controlled studies to improve symptoms in patients with gastroparesis and pseudo-obstruction syndromes. Responses often are incomplete, however, and in some instances, not sustained.

EVALUATION OF GASTRIC AND SMALL INTESTINAL MOTILITY—CURRENT STATUS

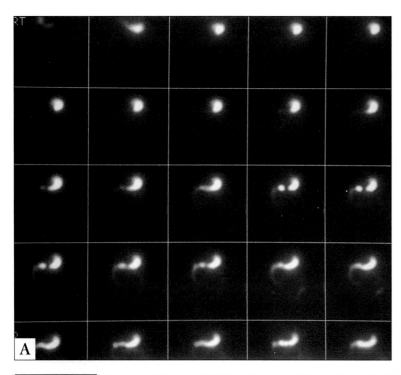

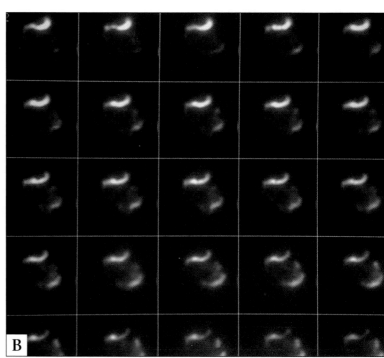

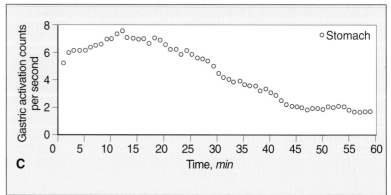

FIGURE 6-1.

Scintigraphy is the most widely accepted technique for measuring gastric emptying. **A–B,** Sequential gamma camera images from a region of interest over the fundus following ingestion of a ^{99m}technetium-labeled scrambled egg meal. Note progression of the meal from the fundus through the corpus and antrum of the stomach, into the small intestine. **C,** The graph illustrates the disappearance of counts from the region of interest. The calculated half-emptying time was normal at 33 minutes. Scintigraphy is widely available, can separately or simultaneously measure liquid and solid emptying, and is relatively noninvasive, apart from radiation exposure. Furthermore, scintigraphy is quantifiable. Various liquid and solid meals can be radiolabeled. Indigestible solids are the most sensitive in detecting gastric motor dysfunction and liquids least. Most centers employ a semisolid meal, such as radiolabeled scrambled egg or chicken liver. Each center must define its own

controls and interpret results accordingly. A limitation to gastric emptying studies is the inconsistent relationship between scintigraphic findings and symptoms.

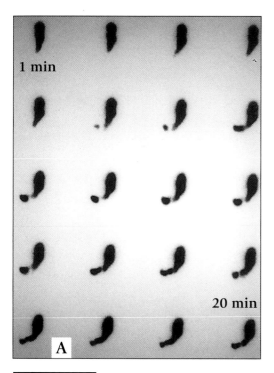
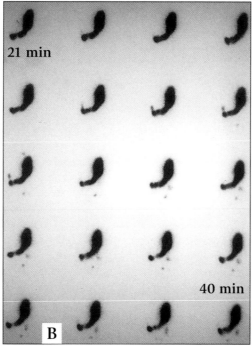
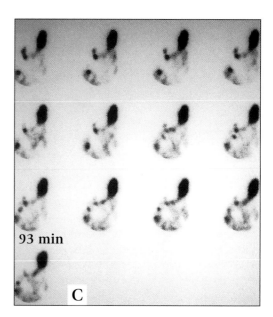

FIGURE 6-2.

A–C, Delayed gastric emptying. A sequence of images from a patient with delayed gastric emptying. Note that even at 93 minutes the major portion of the meal remains within the stomach.

TABLE 6-1. CLINICAL EVALUATION OF GASTRIC EMPTYING–ALTERNATIVES TO SCINTIGRAPHY

Barium meal	Ultrasonography
Radiopaque marker study	^{13}C or ^{14}C-octanoic acid breath test
Acetaminophen absorption study	Impedance
	Magnetic resonance imaging

TABLE 6-1.

Alternative techniques. Of the various alternatives listed, the barium meal has become obsolete because of its insensitivity and non-specificity. The radiopaque marker study, which involves taking a single plain film of the abdomen following the ingestion of radiopaque markers, has been reported as sensitive in the detection of gastroparesis. Ultrasonography can provide a measure of emptying by following a technique that evaluates changes in antral diameter, and in clinical research studies both impedance and MR imaging methodologies have been employed to measure both total and regional gastric emptying. Recently, the ^{14}C- and ^{13}C-octanoic acid breath tests have been promoted as noninvasive, but accurate, measures of gastric emptying.

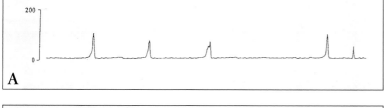
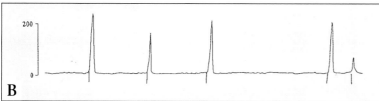
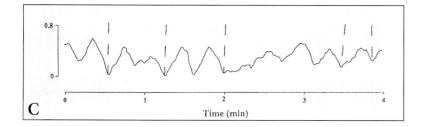

FIGURE 6-3.

Electrogastrography (EGG). These figures illustrate simultaneous recordings of surface EGG and intraluminal pressure from a normal volunteer. **A**, Antral pressure 3 cm from pylorus (mmHg); **B**, antral pressure 1.5 cm from pylorus (mmHg); **C**, EGG (mV). Note correlation between antral pressure waves and EGG signal recorded from two electrodes on the abdominal surface over the antrum and pylorus. Note also the relative variation in amplitude and contour of the EGG signal in comparison to the pressure wave (*Adapted from* Sun *et al.* [1].)

TABLE 6-2. ELECTROGASTROGRAPHY—LIMITATIONS

Low-amplitude signal

Motion artifact

Frequency data are reproducible but have unknown clinical impact

Significance of power data unclear

Clinical role uncertain

TABLE 6-2.

Though noninvasive, electrogastrography has limitations. Electrogastrograms provide a relatively low-amplitude signal that requires considerable amplification for interpretation. It is, therefore, subject to motion artifact, and subjects must be maintained relatively immobile. Using Fourier transformation, variations in the gastric frequency can be recorded in a reproducible fashion. Gastric dysrhythmias, either bradygastria or tachygastria, have been described in disease states and in response to various stimuli. Power ratios comparing fasting and postprandial signal amplitude also can be calculated, but their clinical significance is uncertain. At this time, the clinical role of electrogastrography continues to be defined.

TABLE 6-3. MANOMETRIC TECHNIQUES

PERFUSION	SOLID STATE
Intraluminal catheter perfuses side/end hole	Intraluminal miniaturized strain gauge
Continuous perfusion	Solid state system: Ambulatory recordings possible
Limits mobility	
Limits study duration	
Compliance limits utility in upper esophageal sphincter	Good dynamic performance
Initial outlay and components not expensive	Expensive
Sufficient for routine clinical purposes	

TABLE 6-3.

Comparison of the relative properties of perfused and solid-state manometric systems. Intestinal manometric devices, whether perfused or nonperfused, record lumen-occluding contractions only. Nonlumen-occluding contractions will not be registered.

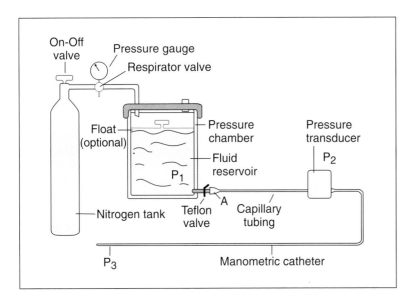

FIGURE 6-4.

Intestinal manometry—low compliance perfusion system. The low compliance perfusion system introduced by Arndorfer and colleagues [2] represented a major advance in clinical manometry. To provide reliable recordings, previous perfusion systems relied on high flow rates, which precluded prolonged studies. The newer system is also without syringes or moving parts, thereby minimizing compliance. A nitrogen gas source is connected in series to a fluid reservoir, and the pressure maintained at 1000 mm Hg (P_1). Stainless steel capillary tubing between the pressure reservoir and pressure transducer causes high resistance against flow, thereby stepping the pressure down to almost zero at the transducer. When the manometric catheter is water-filled and connected to the transducer, pressure at the transducer (P_2) will equal pressure at the catheter recording orifice (P_3), provided that the infusion rate is adequate to prevent sealing of the catheter orifice during peristalsis. The low-compliance hydraulic infusion system is based on the principle that fluid flow from the catheter is proportional to the pressure difference across the capillary. Because reservoir pressure is always high relative to catheter pressures generated by peristalsis, pressure changes in the catheter cause only small reductions in flow. (*Adapted from* Arndorfer *et al.* [2].)

FIGURE 6-5.

A, Antroduodenal manometry. This figure illustrates a conventional perfused catheter assembly with five closely spaced side holes straddling the antrum, pylorus, and proximal duodenum, and three more widely spaced recording sites positioned in the duodenum and proximal jejunum. **B**, Recording during the fasting state demonstrates the migrating motor complex. Each cycle of the migrating motor complex features a sequence of motor patterns that continue to recur as long as the individual remains fasted. Each sequence begins with phase I (motor quiescence), progresses through phase II, a period of irregular contractions, and culminates in phase III, the most distinctive pattern, which features uninterrupted rhythmic phasic contractions that migrate slowly along the intestine. In this example, recording sites in the antrum (top three), pylorus (fourth from top) and duodenum (bottom three) illustrate phase III of the migrating motor complex, a pattern of uninterrupted rhythmic contractions at the slow wave frequency for that site (three cycles per minute in the antrum and 11 to 12 cycles per minute in the duodenum).

(*continued on next page*)

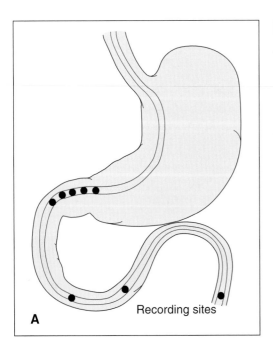

A Recording sites

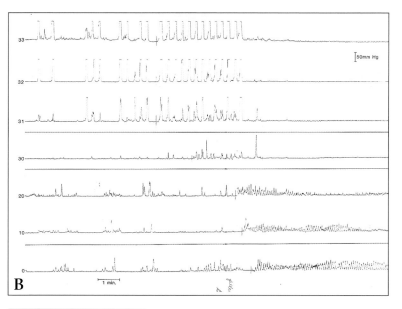

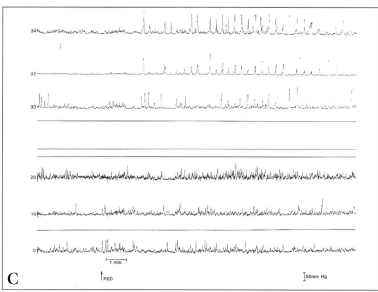

FIGURE 6-5. (CONTINUED)

C, In the postprandial motor response following meal ingestion (*arrow*), the migrating motor complex is abolished and an irregular intense motor activity develops in the antrum (top three channels) and duodenum (lower three channels). (**B–C**, *Adapted from* Quigley [3].)

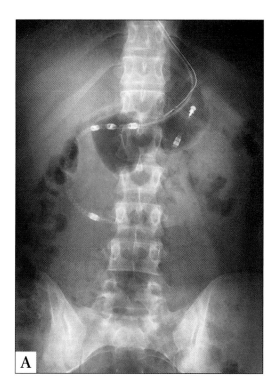

FIGURE 6-6.

Solid-state system. **A**, Radiograph illustrates a solid-state assembly in position with three solid-state pressure transducers straddling the pylorus with two more distally located transducers at the junction of the second and third parts of the duodenum and close to the ligament of Treitz, respectively.

Examples of recordings in the fasted and fed states illustrate the migrating motor complex (**panel B**) and the fed motor response (**panel C**), respectively.

For antral motility, and to record the antral post-prandial response in particular, a water-perfused system incorporating multiple closely-spaced sensors positioned across the pylorus or a sleeve is superior, given the limitations of solid-state systems in terms of sensor number and spacing. Those limitations render displacement of sensors out of the antrum likely following meal ingestion, and virtually preclude reliable antral post-prandial recordings. By permitting more prolonged (at least 24 hrs.) and ambulatory recordings, the solid state system can record many more migrating motor complex cycles than the shorter recordings provided by a typical stationary perfused catheter system.

Interpretations of antroduodenal and small intestinal motility recordings remain somewhat problematic. This must begin with agreement on what comprises a normal study and go on to consensus on the categorization of various abnormal patterns. Such an approach must take into account the extent of and the factors that may influence normal variations in the MMC. To quantify the fed response requires general agreement on the calculation of an appropriate motility index (M.I.) The categorization of abnormal patterns remains especially problematic given their subjective nature. (**B–C**, *Adapted from* Holland *et al.* [4].)

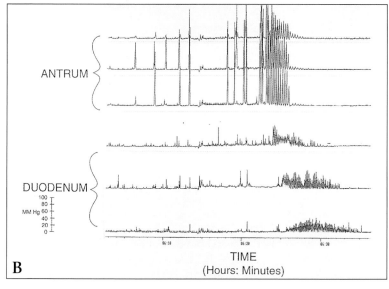

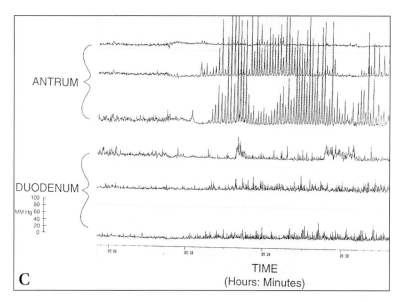

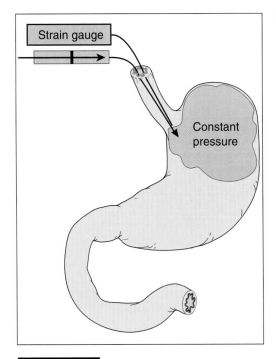

FIGURE 6-7.

Evaluation of motility of the fundus and corpus. Because of the large diameter of the fundus and corpus, conventional manometric systems will not record pressure activity accurately. This can be recorded with the barostat system, which involves the placement of an ultrathin, nondistensible polyurethane bag in the fundus and corpus. This can be maintained at a constant pressure or volume, and fluctuations in volume or pressure, respectively, are recorded.

TABLE 6-4. ASSESSMENT OF SMALL INTESTINAL MOTOR ACTIVITY

Transit	Electromyography
Breath H$_2$ excretion	Serosal
Sulfasalazine metabolites	Luminal
Scintigraphy	Research only
Problems with ROI	Manometry
definition and overlap	Perfused, stationary
of regions of interest	Ambulatory
	Need closely-spaced sensors to
	monitor antrum and pylorus.
	Intrinsic variations limit interpretations

TABLE 6-4.

Assessment of small intestinal motor activity. Three separate parameters of small intestinal motor activity are amenable to clinical evaluation—transit, electromyographic (EMG) activity, and contractile activity (by manometry).

Three techniques have been described for the assessment of small intestinal transit—breath hydrogen excretion following the administration of a nonabsorbable carbohydrate, such as lactulose; sulfasalazine metabolism following oral administration (which relies on colonic bacteria to cleave the sulfasalazine and 5-aminosalicylate and sulfapyridine moieties); and scintigraphy. While scintigraphic techniques are based on the same principles as those described for the measurement of gastric emptying, accurate definitions of small intestinal transit is more difficult: defining a region of interest (ROI) is less straightforward, and overlap of bowel loops may cause considerable confusion.

Electromyographic recordings from the small intestine have been performed from either surgically placed serosal electrodes or from electrodes mounted on an intraluminal catheter. Neither has gained a place in clinical practice, and this approach remains confined to clinical research studies.

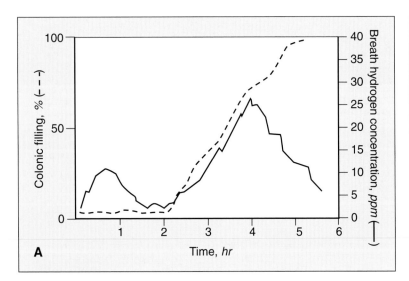

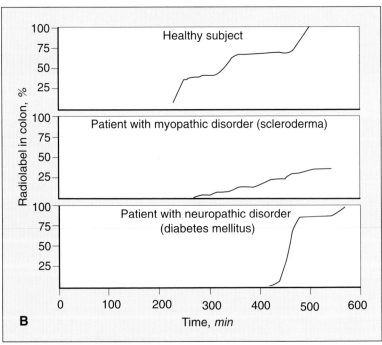

FIGURE 6-8.

A, Measurement of small intestinal transit. Relationship between breath hydrogen profile (*solid line*) and profile of cecal radioactivity (*dashed line*) after ingestion of a radiolabeled test meal containing baked beans by a normal subject. In the biphasic breath hydrogen response, the onset of the second peak corresponds to the arrival of the head of the meal in the cecum. The time from ingestion of the meal to the second rise in breath hydrogen excretion is the small-bowel transit time. B, Radioscintigraphic assessment of the small-bowel transit employing ^{111}In amberlite resin pellets. The figure illustrates the pattern of colonic filling of ingested radiolabel in a healthy subject, a patient with a myopathic disorder (scleroderma), and a patient with a neuropathic disorder (diabetes mellitus). Small-bowel transit is calculated as the difference between the onset of colonic filling and the gastric emptying time. Note the delayed onset of colonic filling in both disease groups, indicating slow small-bowel transit. The pattern of colonic filling can also be employed to differentiate between a myopathy and a neuropathy. (A, *Adapted from* Read *et al.* [5]. B, *Adapted from* Greydanus *et al.* [6].)

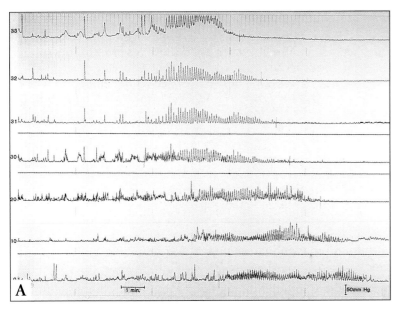

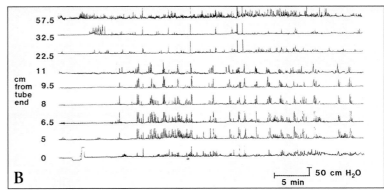

FIGURE 6-9.

Intestinal manometry. **A**, Phase III of the migrating motor complex transversing the jejunum. **B**, Motor properties of the terminal ileum and ileocolonic junction. Note the prominence of "clustered" contractions in this region. Typically, phase III of the migrating motor complex peters out before it reaches the most distal ileum. (**A**, *Adapted from* Quigley [3].)

■ CLINICAL DISORDERS

Gastric motility disorders

TABLE 6-5. GASTRIC MOTILITY CLINICAL SYNDROMES

TRADITIONAL CLASSIFICATION ACCORDING TO STATUS OF GASTRIC EMPTYING
Delayed (gastroparesis)
Accelerated (dumping)

PITFALLS
Symptoms and rate of gastric emptying may not be in correlation
One disease may initiate findings of both delayed and accelerated gastric emptying

TABLE 6-5.

Clinical syndromes of gastric dysmotility are traditionally classified according to the status of gastric emptying, whether delayed (gastroparesis) or accelerated (dumping). Gastric emptying rates and symptoms may not correlate, however, and the same disease state may, at different stages in its evolution, cause either accelerated or delayed emptying.

TABLE 6-6. GASTROPARESIS—ETIOLOGY

Acid-peptic disease
Gastroesophageal reflux
Gastric ulcer disease
Gastric mucosal disease
Gastritis
Atrophic gastritis ± pernicious anemia
Viral gastroenteritis (*eg,* cytomegalovirus)
Metabolic and endocrine
Diabetic ketoacidosis (acute)
Diabetic gastroparesia (chronic)
Hypothyroidism
Pregnancy
Uremia
Collagen Vascular Disease
Sclerodema
Pseudo-obstruction
Idiopathic
Secondary (*eg,* amyloidosis, muscular dystrophies)
Surgery
Roux-en-Y syndrome
Medications
Anticholinergics, narcotic analgesics, L-dopa
Anorexia nervosa
Idiopathic

TABLE 6-6.

Gastroparesis—etiology. This table presents some of the more common causes of gastroparesis, grouped according to broad categories of disease.

Among disorders related to *acid-peptic injury*, gastroparesis has been associated with both gastroesophageal reflux disease and gastric ulceration. *Gastric mucosal disease* has also been associated with gastroparesis. Chronic atropic gastritis such as occurs in pernicious anemia may cause delayed emptying. Acute viral gastritis, such as that related to cytomegalovirus (CMV) infection, may cause a profound gastroparesis, and a chronic post-viral gastroparesis is being increasingly recognized.

Several *metabolic and endocrine disorders* may result in gastroparesis. Diabetes may be associated with gastroparesis in a number of scenarios: acutely in relation to hyperglycemia or ketoacidosis and chronically as a consequence of diabetic gastroenteropathy. Other examples of metabolically or hormonally mediated gastroparesis include hypothyroidism, pregnancy, and uremia.

Gastroparesis may complicate *collagen vascular disorders* that involve the gastrointestinal tract, such as scleroderma, and may occur in any cause of the syndrome of intestinal pseudo-obstruction, whether idiopathic or secondary to such systemic disorders as amyloidosis or the muscular dystrophies.

Gastroparesis may be a consequence of a variety of *surgical procedures*, including Roux-en-Y gastroenterostomies, and may be a side effect of a variety of medications, including anticholinergics, narcotic analgesics, and L-dopa compounds. Gastroparesis may also be a feature of disorders of the central nervous system, including such *psychiatric disorders* as anorexia nervosa.

Finally, an ever-increasing number of patients with *idiopathic* gastroparesis are being recognized.

TABLE 6-7. POSTSURGICAL SYNDROMES

Vagotomy
    Loss of receptive relaxation
    Impaired antral function
Gastric resection
Roux-en-Y anastomoses
    Gastric stasis
    Loop asynchrony
Duodenogastric reflux

TABLE 6-7.

Post-surgical syndromes. Several factors may contribute to the pathogenesis of gastric motor dysfunction following upper

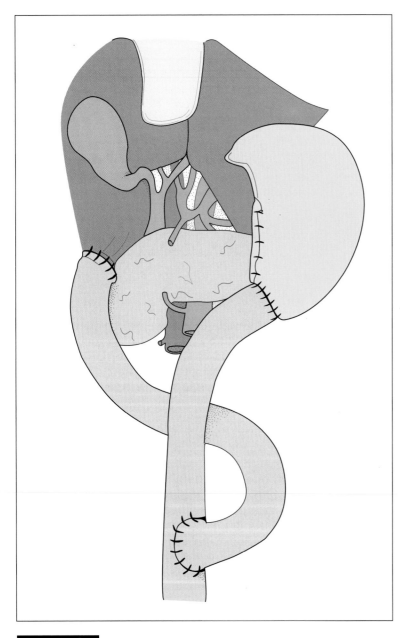

FIGURE 6-10.

A Roux-en-Y anastomosis showing a 40-cm jejunal limb (gastrojejunostomy) for the diversion of the pancreatic or biliary juices away from the residual stomach.

gastrointestinal surgery. Truncal vagotomy will tend to accelerate liquid emptying as a consequence of loss of the receptive relaxation reflex while impaired antral trituration will retard emptying of solids. In the absence of an accompanying emptying procedure, the dominant effect of vagotomy is to delay solid emptying.

The nature of the resection will clearly influence emptying. Antrectomy will lead to a loss of antral contractility, and in most circumstances, to rapid emptying of untriturated food ("gastric incontinence"). A Roux-en-Y gastroenterostomy may lead to a distinctive postoperative syndrome: the Roux syndrome. Whether post-prandial abdominal pain and vomiting in affected patients reflects stasis in the gastric remnant or the obstructing effects of motor asynchrony between stomach, Roux limb, and distal intact jejunum remains unclear.

Duodenogastric reflux related perhaps to antro-pylorus-duodenal motor dysfunction has also been implicated in the pathogenesis of symptoms following gastric surgery and cholecystectomy. Its significance, however, remains unclear.

TABLE 6-8. DIABETIC GASTROPATHY

Bezoars
    Loss of MMC Phase 3
Effects on blood sugar
    Accelerated—none
    Delayed-hypoglycemia
Typically described in long-standing, complicated Type 1
        disease, but also occurs in Type 2
Type 1, and especially Type 2, may also demonstrate
        accelerated emptying

TABLE 6-8.

Diabetic gastroparesis—clinical features. In addition to the typical symptoms of gastroparesis, patients with diabetic gastroparesis are prone to develop bezoars caused by loss of phase III of the migrating motor complex (MMC), which normally is responsible for clearing indigestible material from the stomach. Altered gastric motor activity in patients with diabetes may also upset blood sugar control. In general, accelerated emptying appears to have little effect on blood glucose levels, but delayed emptying may lead to hypoglycemia because of a failure to match insulin dosage and absorption of ingested calories. Diabetic gastroparesis typically is described in patients with long-standing complicated type 1 diabetes, but also occurs in patients with type 2 diabetes. In addition, accelerated emptying may occur at an early stage in the evolution of gastroenteropathy in patients with type 1 diabetes, and is especially common among patients with type 2 diabetes.

TABLE 6-9. DIABETIC GASTROPATHY— PATHOPHYSIOLOGY

Autonomic neuropathy
Effects of hyperglycemia
    ↓ Gastric emptying
    ↓ Gastric migrating motor complex
    ↓ Antral motility
    Tachygastria and arrhythmias
Effects of ketoacidosis

TABLE 6-9.

Diabetic gastropathy—pathophysiology. The major factor involved in the pathogenesis of the various manifestations of diabetic gastroenteropathy is autonomic neuropathy; however, hyperglycemia may also influence gastrointestinal motor function. In normal individuals, hyperglycemia has been shown to decrease the rate of gastric emptying, suppress the gastric component of the migrating motor complex, inhibit antral motility, and induce gastric dysrhythmias and tachygastria. Ketoacidosis may also be associated with a profound ileus, which includes gastroparesis.

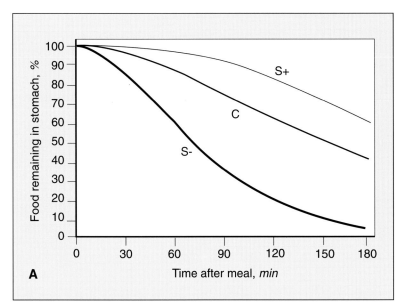

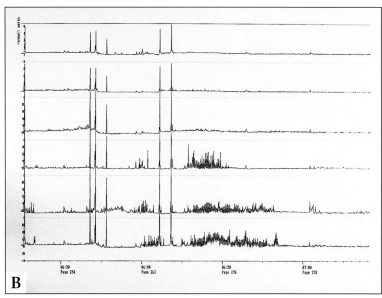

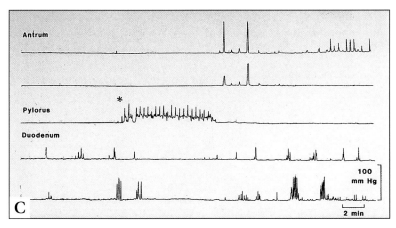

FIGURE 6-11.

A, The various types of gastric emptying curves that may occur in patients with diabetes. These observations emphasize that both accelerated and delayed emptying may occur in patients with diabetes. Emptying may be delayed, as seen in this study, in those patients with symptoms (S+) or accelerated, as noted among those without gastrointestinal symptoms (S-). A control curve (C) is shown for comparison.

  B, Simultaneous recording of antral (top three recording sites) and duodenal (bottom three recording sites) motor activity from a patient with diabetic gastroparesis. Note that phase III of the migrating motor complex is observed in the duodenal recording sites, but there is no evidence of an antral component. Note also some abnormal "phase III-type" activity preceding the normal phase III. **C,** Simultaneous recording of motor activity from the antrum, pylorus, and duodenum demonstrating a burst of intense phasic and tonic activity at the pylorus in a patient with insulin-dependent diabetes—"pylorospasm." (**A,** *Adapted from* Nowak *et al.* [7]. **C,** *Adapted from* Mearin *et al.* [8].)

TABLE 6-10. GASTRODUODENAL DYSMOTILITY IN DIFFUSE MOTILITY DISORDERS

Secondary
  Scleroderma
  Diseases of muscle and
    central nervous system
  Autonomic dysfunction
  Amyloidosis

Primary (CIIP)
  Myopathy
  Neuropathy

TABLE 6-10.

Gastroduodenal dysmotility in diffuse motility disorders. Gastro-duodenal dysmotility commonly occurs as a component of diffuse disorders of gastrointestinal motor function, whether secondary (as may occur in scleroderma) in a variety of neurological and muscle diseases (such as Parkinson's disease and muscular dystrophy), in autonomic neuropathy of any etiology and in amyloidosis, or primary (*ie*, chronic idiopathic intestinal pseudo-obstruction [CIIP]). Gastroparesis, for example, has been documented in both myopathic and neuropathic varieties of CIIP.

TABLE 6-11. DYSPEPSIA—ETIOLOGY

Acid-Pepsin
Duodenogastric reflux
Gastritis
Dysmotility
Sensation and perception
Psychopathology

TABLE 6-11.

Dyspepsia—etiology. Several hypotheses have been advanced to explain the pathophysiology of dyspepsia. These include its inclusion in the spectrum of acid-peptic disorders, duodeno-gastric reflux, gastritis, dysmotility, altered sensation, or perception and the influence of psychopathology.

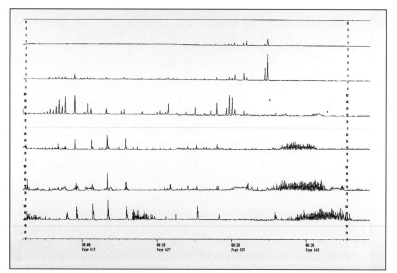

TABLE 6-12. DYSPEPSIA AND MOTILITY

Gastroparesis
Gastric fractionation
    Antral distensibility vs. fundic relaxation
Gastric electrical dysrhythmias
    Tachygastria and bradygastria
Antropyloroduodenal dyscoordination

TABLE 6-12.

Dyspepsia and motility. The relationship of motility disturbances and symptoms of dyspepsia is uncertain. The motility changes are often nonspecific and might be due to stress or could be secondary to other disturbances in the more distal parts of the gut.

FIGURE 6-12.

Antral hypomotility in nonulcer dyspepsia. This figure shows a simultaneous recording, during fasting, of motor activity from the antrum (top three recording sites) and duodenum (bottom three recording sites) from a patient with nonulcer dyspepsia. In the duodenal recording sites, phase III of the migrating motor complex can be seen to migrate in a normal fashion through the duodenum. The antral component is barely discernible.

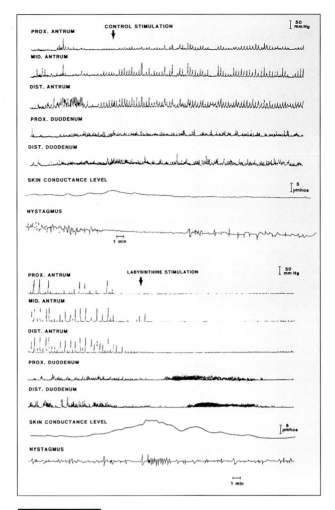

Gastric distension triggers transient lower esophageal sphincter relaxations

Role of hiatal hernia and other mechanical factors

Gastroparesis has variable prevalence with GERD disease

Duodenogastric reflux: Role of bile, alkali, and enzymes

TABLE 6-13.

Gastric motility and gastroesophageal reflux disease (GERD). In theory, any situation that leads to gastric distention could promote reflux by triggering transient lower esophageal sphincter relaxations, which are known to be initiated by gastric distention. Gastric dysfunction could also be involved in reflux through the effects of hiatal hernia on esophageal clearance and lower esophageal sphincter function. It is also possible that disruption of other gastric factors that normally contribute to the antireflux barrier may predispose to reflux. Apart from patients with primary disorders of gastric motor function, such as diabetic gastroparesis, the role of gastric dysmotility in gastroesophageal reflux disease remains controversial. Some studies have demonstrated a high prevalence of apparently unrecognized gastroparesis in patients with reflux whereas others have failed to confirm this. Duodenogastric reflux has also been implicated in gastroesophageal reflux disease, and although the status of this phenomenon remains controversial, some evidence suggests a synergistic role for bile reflux in the pathogenesis of esophagitis, and perhaps Barrett's esophagus.

FIGURE 6-13.

Dysmotility and dyspepsia. This figure illustrates the effects of stress on antroduodenal motility in a normal individual. The top panel illustrates a normal fed motor response. In the lower panel, the normal volunteer has been exposed to labyrinthine stimulation through the instillation of cold water into the ear. Note the complete suppression of antral motility and the induction of a migrating motor complex in the duodenum at a time when the individual is in the immediate postprandial period. This example illustrates the nonspecificity of antral hypomotility, induced here by stress in a normal subject. (*Adapted from* Stanghellini *et al.* [9].)

TABLE 6-14.

Gastroparesis in neuromuscular disorders. Gastric motor dysfunction and gastroparesis may result from disorders of the central nervous system (CNS). Acute gastric dilatation and chronic gastroparesis may complicate spinal cord injuries and may also occur in patients with diseases of the spinal cord, such as multiple sclerosis (MS).

Gastroparesis has also been described in such CNS disorders as epilepsy, Parkinson's disease and tumors of the brain stem and other areas. Gastroparesis may complicate any disorder that results in an elevation of intracranial pressure (ICP).

TABLE 6-14. GASTROPARESIS IN NEUROMUSCULAR DISEASES

Spinal cord disease	Peripheral nerve disorders
Spinal cord injuries	Acute peripheral neuropathies (*eg*, Guillain-Barré)
Multiple sclerosis	Chronic peripheral neuropathies
Brain disorders	Diabetes mellitus
Epilepsy	Amyloidosis
Parkinson's disease	Paraneoplastic
Brain-stem tumors, etc.	Drug-induced
Raised intracranial pressure	Vincristine
Smooth muscle diseases	Levodopa
Amyloidosis	Neurofibromatosis
Scleroderma	Multiple endocrine neoplasia-Type 2b and ganglioneuromatosis
Dermatomyositis	Autonomic neuropathies
Dystrophia myotonica	
Duchenne's muscular dystrophy	
Mitochondrial myopathy	

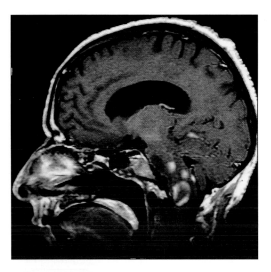

Figure 6-14.

Figure 6-14.

Sagittal view of an MR image of the head from a patient who presented with unexplained vomiting and who had been demonstrated to have gastroparesis.

Case history: This 37-year-old man presented with a 5-month history of vomiting, constipation, and weight loss; he was known to have neurofibromatosis. Evaluation revealed gastroparesis, reflux esophagitis, delayed small-bowel transit, and colonic inertia. He was assumed to have a diffuse motility disorder, but on further evaluation was noted to have asymmetric movement of the palate; MR imaging demonstrated a brain-stem tumor, which proved to be a glioma.

TABLE 6-15. VIRAL AND POSTVIRAL GASTROPARESIS

Immunosuppressed patient
Cytomegalovirus
Immunocompetent patient
Epstein-Barr virus
Herpes simplex virus
Unknown prevalence, may be common
Usually resolves

Table 6-15.

Viral and postviral gastroparesis. Acute viral gastroparesis has been most clearly documented in relation to cytomegalovirus (CMV) infection in the immunosuppressed patient.

In immunocompetent individuals, such well-defined examples of acute gastroparesis related to viral illness are rare, but have been reported in patients with documented Epstein-Barr (EBV) and herpes simplex (HSV) virus infections. More common is the patient with apparently idiopathic gastroparesis who gives a history of relatively acute onset of gastric motor dysfunction during an illness that may well have been viral. This presumed, though by no means well-defined, post-viral gastroparesis usually resolves, but may persist for months or even years in some patients.

Small intestinal motility disorders

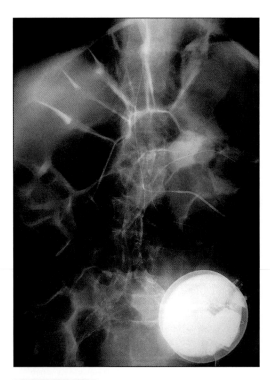

Figure 6-15.

Acute intestinal pseudo-obstruction or ileus. Although ileus is an expected consequence of abdominal and other surgical procedures, it may also occur in other non-surgical situations, such as in patients with pneumonia, pancreatitis, cholecystitis, myocardial infarction, and a variety of neurological conditions. Occasionally, ileus may occur without an obvious cause—idiopathic ileus. This figure illustrates marked dilatation of small and large intestine, a finding consistent with ileus, in a patient with multiple sclerosis. Note patient also had an implanted pump to deliver the muscle relaxant baclofen.

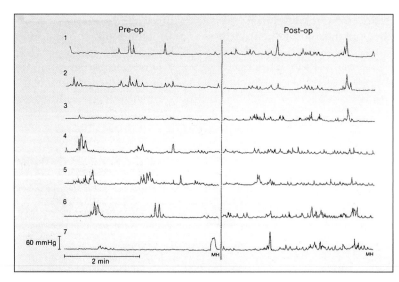

Figure 6-16.

Intestinal obstruction. Figure on left illustrates manometric features of intestinal obstruction. Note repetitive, propagated clusters of phasic contractions and rapidly propagated high-amplitude waves in the postprandial period. On right, note return of normal fed pattern in the same patient following successful operative relief of obstruction. (*Adapted from* Summers *et al.* [10].)

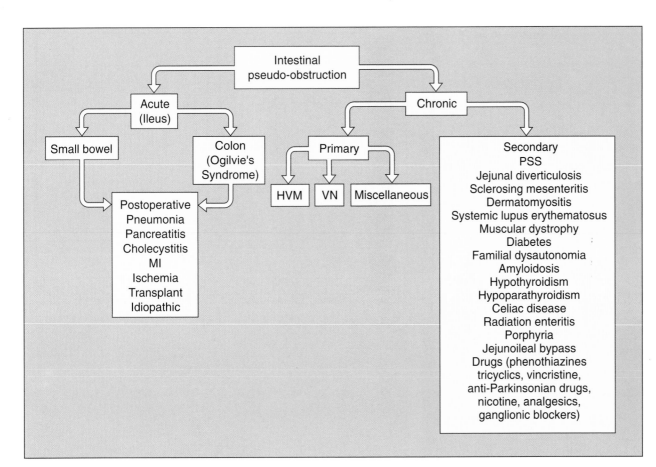

FIGURE 6-17.

Intestinal pseudo-obstruction—etiology and classification. HVM—hollow visceral neuropathy; MI—myocardial infarction; PSS—progressive systemic sclerosis (scleroderma); VN—visceral neuropathy.

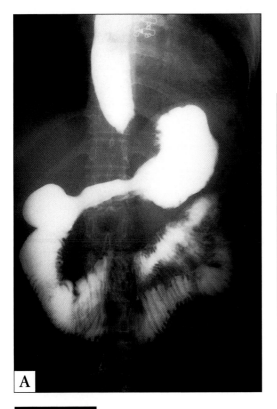

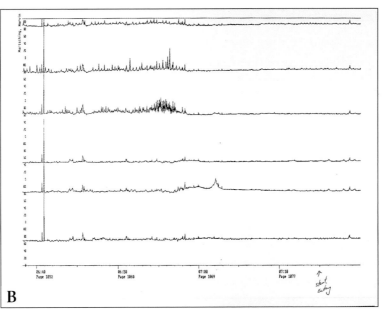

FIGURE 6-18.

Chronic intestinal pseudo-obstruction. **A,** Upper gastrointestinal barium radiography demonstrates the typical features of scleroderma involving the small intestine. Note the dilated jejunal loops with prominent valvulae conniventes, giving a "stacked coin" or "coiled spring" appearance. **B,** Simultaneous recordings of antral (top two traces) and duodenal (bottom three traces) motility from a patient with advanced scleroderma. Fasting recording demonstrates virtually complete absence of motor activity; during phase III of the migrating motor complex, a very low-amplitude phase III is evident in the antrum and duodenum. (**B,** *Adapted from* Quigley [11].)

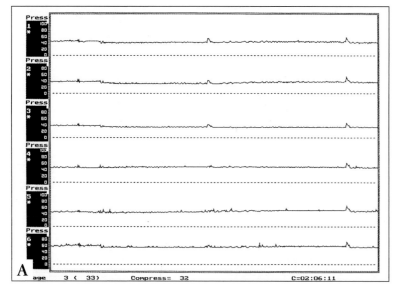

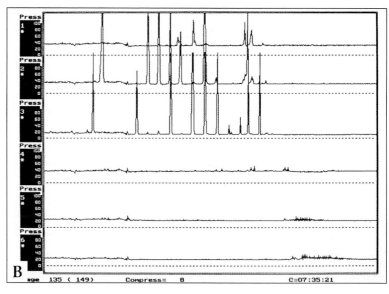

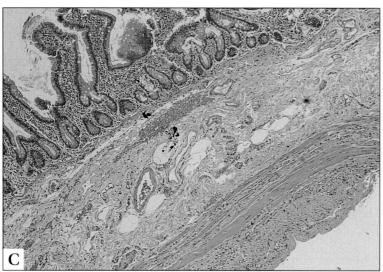

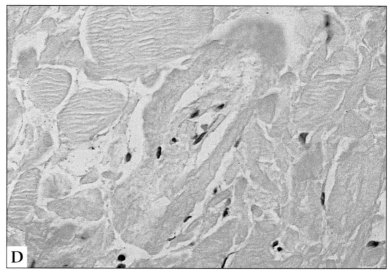

FIGURE 6-19.

Intestinal myopathy. **A,** Simultaneous recording of antral (top three traces) and duodenal (lower three traces) motor activity from a patient with an intestinal myopathy and idiopathic megaduodenum. Note marked suppression of motor activity.

B, Figure demonstrating duodenal hypomotility in a patient with an intestinal myopathy. Normal phase III of the migrating motor complex in the antrum (upper three traces), but marked suppression of the amplitude of phasic contractions during phase III in the duodenal recording sites (bottom three traces) are seen.

Pathologic features of intestinal myopathy. **C,** Full-thickness intestinal biopsy from a patient with an intestinal myopathy demonstrating essentially complete replacement of the circular muscle layer by fibrosis. Note relative preservation of longitudinal muscle layer. **D,** Amyloidosis of the small intestine. Duodenal biopsy demonstrating extensive infiltration by amyloid, seen as homogenous pink hyaline substance. (**C,** *From* Quigley [11]; with permission.)

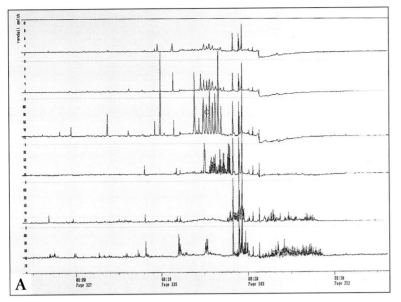

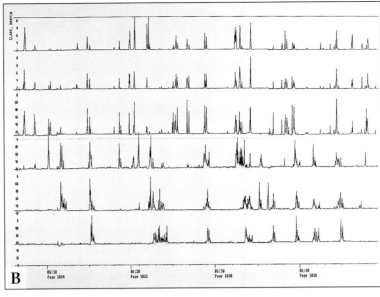

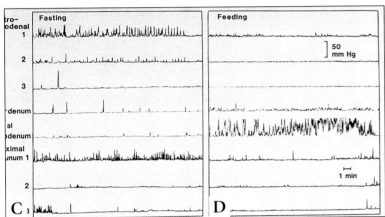

FIGURE 6-20.

Intestinal neuropathy—manometric features. **A–B,** Abnormal configuration of phase III of the migrating motor complex in the antrum (top three traces) and duodenum (bottom three traces). **B,** Intense "cluster" activity and rapidly propagated individual pressure waves from a patient with symptomatic diabetic autonomic neuropathy. **C–D,** Abnormal gastrointestinal manometric patterns characterized by marked disorganization of fasting and fed motor patterns. Note the intense burst of phasic activity at some manometric sites in the upper intestine, coexisting with almost complete quiescence at other sites.

TABLE 6-16. CHRONIC INTESTINAL PSEUDO-OBSTRUCTION— CLINICAL FEATURES AND EVALUATION

TABLE 6-16.

Chronic intestinal pseudo-obstruction— clinical features and evaluation.

Suggested evaluation by history

Tests to exclude obstruction

Transit studies

Manometry
  Small bowel
  Esophageal

Biopsy
  Surgical
  Laparoscopic
  Need special stains to demonstrate
    neural pathology

CLINICAL FEATURES

Nausea and vomiting

Pain may be severe enough to
    require opiates

Bacterial overgrowth, which may
    lead to malabsorption

Distension that may require decompression
    or venting

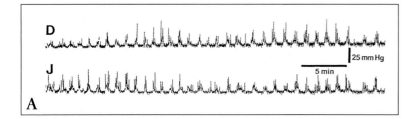

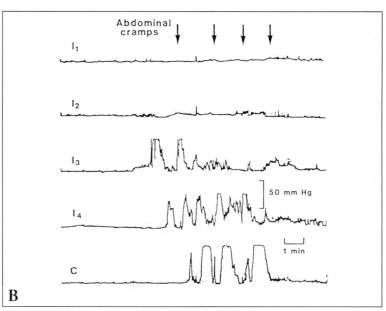

FIGURE 6-21.

Irritable bowel syndrome (IBS)—a motility disorder? **A,** Prolonged burst of "clusters" of phasic contractions from two recording sites in the jejunum in a patient with IBS. Onset of cluster activity was associated with the development of typical symptoms. **B,** Repetitive propagated high-amplitude ileal pressure waves from a patient with IBS associated with the onset of typical cramps. Although these and other manometric abnormalities have been described in patients with IBS, the role of dysmotility in the pathophysiology of IBS remains uncertain. (**A,** *Adapted from* Kellow *et al.* [12]. **B,** *Adapted from* Kellow and Phillips [13].)

■ MANAGEMENT

TABLE 6-17. GENERAL PRINCIPLES OF MANAGEMENT

GENERAL	MANAGEMENT
	Pain control
Rehydration	Suppression of bacterial overgrowth
Correct electrolytes	Symptomatic management of
abnormalities	diarrhea and constipation
Decompression	
NG tube	**NUTRITION**
PEG/PEJ	Diet low in residue and fat:
Enterotomy	emphasize liquids
	Enteral feeding (jejunostomy)
	Total parenteral nutrition

TABLE 6-17.

General principles of management. In the management of motility disorders, general principles must not be ignored. In the

acute situation this should include appropriate rehydration and correction of electrolyte deficiencies. Decompression of the stomach and intestine may play a key role in symptom relief. This may be achieved in the short term by nasogastric (NG) intubation, and in the long term by gastrostomy or jejunostomy placed endoscopically (percutaneous endoscopic gastrostomy, percutaneous endoscopic jejunostomy [PEG, PEJ]), under radiologic guidance, or laparoscopically. Surgical enterotomy may also provide decompression in appropriate cases.

Several issues deserve specific attention in the management of patients with pseudo-obstruction, and include pain control, recognition and therapy of secondary bacterial overgrowth, and the symptomatic therapy of diarrhea and constipation. Nutrition is of paramount importance in all of these patients. In some, changing from traditional solid food to a low-residue, low-fat, liquid diet may be sufficient; others may do very well with an enteral formulation delivered directly to the jejunum, thus bypassing a paretic stomach. With careful attention to formulation and delivery of enteral nutrition it should be possible to avoid total parenteral nutrition (TPN) in most patients.

TABLE 6-18. PROKINETIC DRUGS IN GASTROPARESIS

Bethanechol
Metoclopramide
Domperidone
Cisapride
Erythromycin

TABLE 6-18.

Prokinetic drugs in gastroparesis. The principal agents that have been used to exert a prokinetic effect on the gastrointestinal tract in man are the nonspecific cholinergic agonist bethanechol, the dopamine antagonists domperidone and metoclopramide, the peripheral cholinergic agonist cisapride, and the motilin agonist erythromycin.

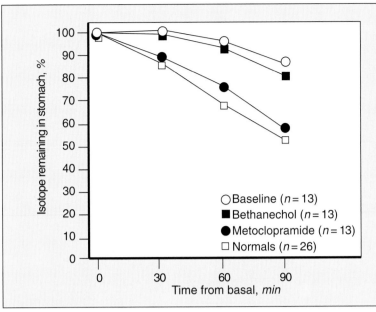

FIGURE 6-22.

Cholinergic agonists and dopamine antagonists. Comparison of the effects of metoclopramide and bethanechol on gastric emptying in patients with gastroesophageal reflux and delayed gastric emptying. Note acceleration of gastric emptying with metoclopramide, but little change with bethanechol, which is also nonspecific and produces side effects. (*Adapted from* McCallum *et al.* [14].)

TABLE 6-19. DOPAMINE ANTAGONISTS

Examples	Actions
Metoclopramide	Promote esophageal peristalsis
Domperidone	Increase lower esophageal
(Clebopride)	sphincter pressure
(Cinitapride)	Accelerate gastric emptying
(Cisapride)	**Problems**
	Central nervous system side effects
	with metoclopramide
	Hyperprolactinemia
	Tolerance

TABLE 6-19.

Dopamine antagonists and their use in gastric and small intestinal motility disorders. Agents in parentheses have some dopamine antagonist effects, but their primary mechanism of action is otherwise.

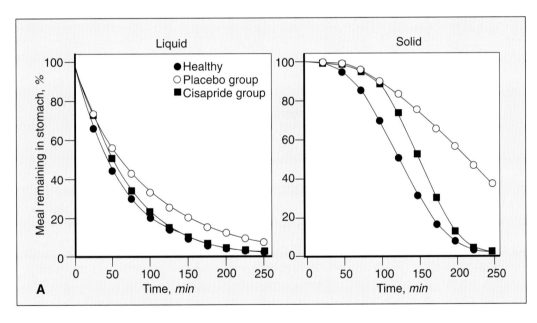

A

FIGURE 6-23.

Benzamides. Of the primary benzamides, only cisapride is available for clinical use in the United States; renzapride and zacopride have been evaluated in clinical trials in Europe. While metoclopramide and clebopride share some properties with the benzamides, their principal effects are exerted via other mechanisms. Cisapride promotes acetylcholine release in myenteric neurons most likely via a $5HT_4$ agonist effect.

A, Effects of cisapride and placebo on liquid and solid emptying in patients with gastroparesis. Note significant improvement in both liquid and solid emptying in patients treated with cisapride over a 6-week study period.

(*continued on next page*)

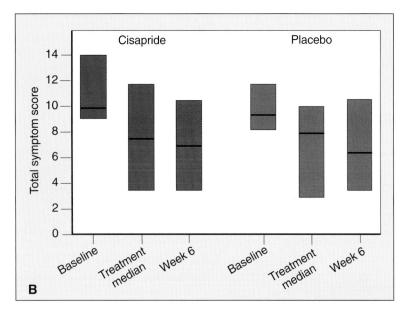

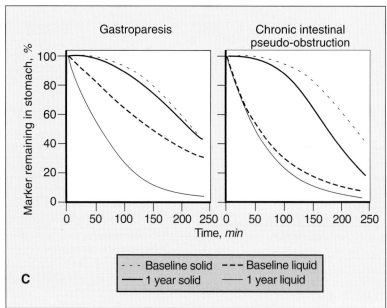

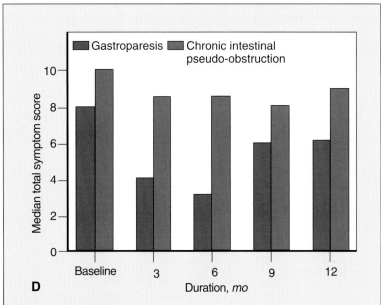

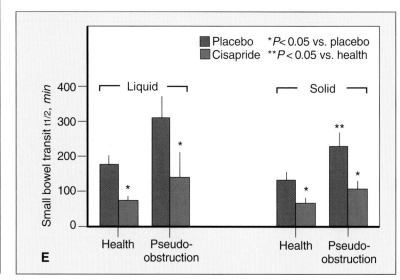

FIGURE 6-23. (CONTINUED)

B, Effect of cisapride and placebo on symptoms after a 6-week study period. Note improvement in symptoms in both cisapride and placebo groups, emphasizing the disparity that may occur between objective effects on gastroparesis on the one hand and symptoms on the other. **C,** Sustained effect of cisapride (10 mg, t.i.d.) on gastric emptying at 1 year. Note significant improvement in liquid emptying in patients with gastroparesis and solid emptying in patients with chronic intestinal pseudo-obstruction, suggesting a more prolonged effect of this agent.

D, Effect of cisapride on symptoms in patients with gastroparesis and chronic intestinal pseudo-obstruction maintained on cisapride for 1 year. Note sustained improvement in symptoms in patients with gastroparesis, but little evidence of sustained improvement in patients with chronic intestinal pseudo-obstruction. **E,** Effect of cisapride on small-bowel transit. Note significant acceleration of transit of both liquid and solid meals through the small intestine in both healthy subjects and patients with chronic intestinal pseudo-obstruction. (**A–B,** *Adapted from* Camilleri *et al.* [15]. **C–D,** *Adapted from* Abell *et al.* [16]. **E,** *Adapted from* Camilleri *et al.* [17].)

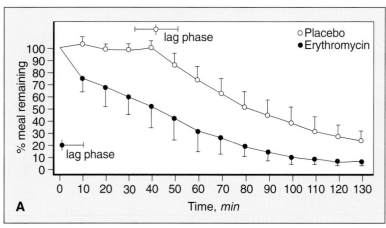

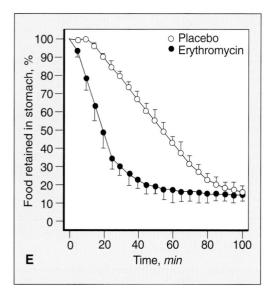

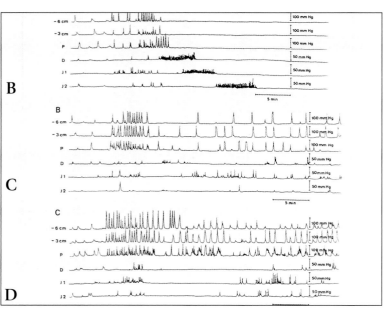

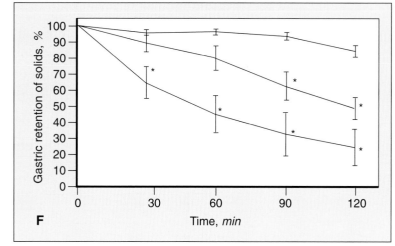

FIGURE 6-24.

Erythromycin. **A**, Effect of erythromycin on gastric emptying in normal individuals. Note significant acceleration of gastric emptying, related in large part to the abolition of the "lag" phase.

B–D, Effect of different doses of erythromycin on antroduodenal motility in normal subjects. At the lowest dose (40 mg), note the induction of normal-appearing migrating motor complex through the antrum and duodenum. At the next dose (200 mg), note intense sustained antral response with little effect in the duodenum. At the highest dose (300 mg), note extremely intense response in the antrum—again, little response in the duodenum. **E** Effect of erythromycin intravenously (200 mg) on diabetic gastroparesis. Note significant

acceleration of gastric emptying. **F**, Comparison of effects of acute intravenous (6 mg/kg) and chronic oral administration (500 mg qid) of erythromycin for 4 weeks on gastric emptying. Note significant improvement in gastric emptying following intravenous erythromycin and a modest response to chronic oral erythromycin (*top line*—baseline; *middle line*—4 weeks of oral erythromycin; *bottom line*—intravenous erythromycin; asterisks indicates significant difference from corresponding baseline value). (**A**, *Adapted from* Mantides *et al.* [18]. **B–D**, *Adapted from* Tack *et al.* [19]. **E**, *Adapted from* Janssens *et al.* [20]. **F**, *Adapted from* Richards *et al* [21].)

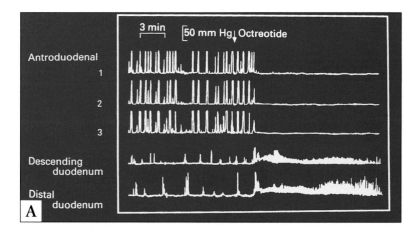

FIGURE 6-25.

Octreotide. Introduced as an antisecretory agent, octreotide appears to have a prokinetic effect, and can also modulate colorectal perception. Although the mode of action remains unclear, the agent is effective in chronic idiopathic intestinal pseudo-obstruction and irritable bowel syndrome. **A**, Figure illustrates induction of phase III of the migrating motor complex by subcutaneous octreotide.

(*continued on next page*)

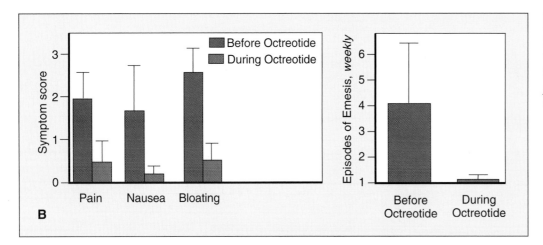

FIGURE 6-25. (CONTINUED)

B, Effect of octreotide on symptoms in patients with scleroderma. Note significant reduction in symptoms with octreotide. (**A,** *Adapted from* Haruma *et al.* [22]. **B,** *Adapted from* Soudah *et al* [23].)

TABLE 6-20. SURGERY

Completion of gastrectomy for postsurgical gastroparesis

Venting enterostomies; gastrostomy, jejunostomy tubes

Avoid bypass and resections

Transplantation

TABLE 6-20.

Surgery has a limited role in the management of gastrointestinal dysmotility. Gastric resections and gastrectomy should, in general, be avoided in patients with gastroparesis. Those with intractable post-surgical gastroparesis may, however, benefit from a completion gastrectomy. Venting enterotomies or surgically placed gastrostomy or jejunostomy tubes may relieve distension and facilitate enteral nutrition, respectively. Bypass procedures and limited resections should be avoided, and intestinal transplantation has been performed in a few patients following total enterectomy.

▮ REFERENCES

1. Sun WM, Smout A, Malbert C, *et al.*: Relationship between surface electrogastrography and antropyloric pressures. *Am J Physiol* 1995, 268:G424–G430.

2. Arndorfer RC, Stef JJ, Dodds WJ, *et al.*: Improved infusion system for intraluminal esophageal manometry. *Gastroenterology* 1977, 73:23–27.

3. Quigley EMM: Antroduodenal manometry. In *Problems in General Surgery, Vol 9: Tests of foregut function.* Edited by Hinder RA. Philadelphia: JB Lippincott; 1992:152–171.

4. Holland R, Gallagher MD, Quigley EMM: An evaluation of an ambulatory manometry system in assessment of antroduodenal motor activity. *Dig Dis Sci* 1996, 41:1531–1537.

5. Read MW, Al-Janabi MN, Bates TE, *et al.*: Interpretation of the breath hydrogen profile obtained after ingesting a solid meal containing nonabsorbable carbohydrate. *Gut* 1985, 26:834–842.

6. Greydanus MP, Camilleri M, Colemont LJ, *et al.*: Ileocolonic transfer of solid chyme in small intestinal neuropathies and myopathies. *Gastroenterology* 1990, 99:158–164.

7. Nowak TV, Johnson CP, Kalbfleisch JH, *et al.*: Highly variable gastric emptying in patients with insulin dependent diabetes mellitus. *Gut* 1995, 37:23–29.

8. Mearin F, Camilleri M, Malagelada J-R: Pyloric dysfunction in diabetics with recurrent nausea and vomiting. *Gastroenterology* 1986, 90:1919–1925.

9. Stanghellini V, Malagelada J-R, Zinsmeister AR, *et al.*: Stress-induced gastroduodenal motor disturbances in humans: Possible humoral mechanisms. *Gastroenterology* 1983, 85:83–91.

10. Summers RW, Anuras S, Green J: Jejunal manometry patterns in health, partial intestinal obstruction and pseudoobstruction. *Gastroenterology* 1983, 85:1290–1300.

11. Quigley EMM: Intestinal pseudoobstruction. In *Evolving Concepts in Gastrointestinal Motility.* Edited by Orr W, Champion MC. Oxford: Blackwell Science; 1996:171–199.

12. Kellow JE, Gill RC, Wingate DL: Prolonged ambulant recordings of small bowel motility demonstrate abnormalities in the irritable bowel syndrome. *Gastroenterology* 1990, 98:1208–1218.

13. Kellow JE, Phillips SF: Altered small bowel motility in irritable bowel syndrome is correlated with symptoms. *Gastroenterology* 1987, 92:1885–1893.

14. McCallum RW, Fink SM, Lerner E, Berkowitz DM: Effects of metoclopromide and bethanechol on delayed gastric emptying present in gastroesophageal reflux patients. *Gastroenterology* 1983, 84:1573–1577.

15. Camilleri M, Malagelada J-R, Abell TL, *et al.*: Effect of six weeks of treatment with cisapride in gastroparesis and intestinal pseudo-obstruction. *Gastroenterology* 1989, 96:704–712.

16. Abell TL, Camilleri M, DiMagno EP, *et al.*: Long-term efficacy of oral cisapride in symptomatic upper gut dysmotility. *Dig Dis Sci* 1991, 36:616–620.

17. Camilleri M, Brown ML, Malagelada J-R: Impaired transit of chyme in chronic intestinal pseudoobstruction: Correction by cisapride. *Gastroenterology* 1986, 91:619–626.

18. Mantides A, Xynos E, Chrysos E, *et al.*: The effect of erythromycin in gastric emptying of solids and hypertonic liquids in healthy subjects. *Am J Gastroenterol* 1993, 88:198–202.

19. Tack J, Janssens J, Vantrappen G, *et al.*: Effect of erythromycin on gastric motility in controls and in diabetic gastroparesis. *Gastroenterology* 1992, 103:72–79.

20. Janssens J, Peeters TL, Vantrappen G, *et al.*: Improvement of gastric emptying in diabetic gastroparesis by erythromycin. *N Engl J Med* 1990, 322:1028–1031.

21. Richards RD, Davenport K, McCallum RW: The treatment of idiopathic and diabetic gastroparesis with acute intravenous and chronic oral erythromycin. *Am J Gastroenterol* 1993, 88:203–207.

22. Haruma K, Wiste JA, Camilleri M: Effect of octreotide on gastrointestinal pressure profiles in health and in functional and organic gastrointestinal disorders. *Gut* 1993, 35:1064–1069.

23. Soudah HC, Hasler WL, Owyang C: Effect of octreotide on intestinal motility and bacterial overgrowth in scleroderma. *N Engl J Med* 1991, 325:1461–1467.

Chapter 7

Crohn's Disease of the Small Intestine

ELLEN J. SCHERL
DAVID B. SACHAR

Crohn's disease, a chronic idiopathic transmural inflammation of the bowel, may affect any portion of the gastrointestinal tract from mouth to anus; however, 80% of cases involve the small intestine, although usually not invariably including the terminal ileum. The small bowel alone (ileitis) is the site of disease in approximately one third of cases whereas nearly one half strike both small and large bowel (ileocolitis).

Defining the natural history of Crohn's disease and selecting appropriate therapy are facilitated by classifying patients into one of three clinicopathologic patterns, primarily inflammatory, stenotic, or fistulizing. The inflammatory pattern characteristically presents with recurrent episodes of right lower quadrant pain and diarrhea. A more acute presentation may mimic appendicitis, but a careful history usually discloses preexisting bowel complaints. Persistent inflammation and scarring may progress to a stenotic stage, in which thickening of the bowel wall and narrowing of the lumen ultimately produce repeated bouts of obstruction. Alternatively, deep fissures and sinus tracts may fistulize through the bowel wall to the serosa, producing a localized phlegmon with local signs of a tender right lower quadrant mass and systemic signs of suppuration. Depending upon the extent and direction of this penetrating ulceration, the process may eventuate in a psoas abscess or in enteroenteric, enterovesical, or even enterocutaneous fistulae. Another potential outcome of many years of chronic intestinal inflammation is malignant transformation to adenocarcinoma or lymphoma in the affected segments, whether bypassed or in continuity. Bowel resection ultimately proves necessary in approximately 70% of patients with Crohn's disease and it is highly rehabilitative even though there is an inexorable tendency for postoperative recurrence.

This chapter will illustrate the clinical pathophysiology, natural history, diagnosis, and differential diagnosis of Crohn's disease of the small intestine. Decades of etiologic and epidemiologic research have still not yielded the cause or cure of this perplexing disorder, but understanding its pathophysiology and natural history provides a sound framework for devising strategies of primary medical, surgical, and postoperative management.

Anatomic distribution

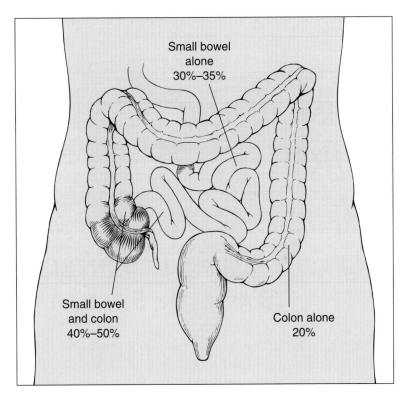

FIGURE 7-1.

Anatomic distribution in Crohn's disease. Crohn's disease affects the small bowel alone in approximately 33% of cases and the colon alone in approximately 20%; nearly 50% of the cases involve both the small and large bowels (ileocolitis).

Pathologic distribution

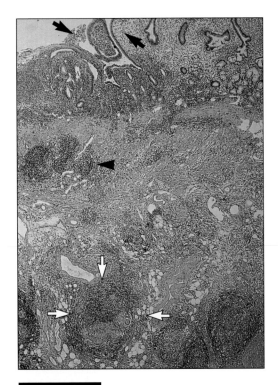

FIGURE 7-2.

Crohn's ileitis. Mucosal edema and ulceration (*closed arrows*) are early pathologic findings in Crohn's disease. Lymphoid aggregates (*arrowhead*) organize into discrete, noncaseating granulomas (*open arrows*), shown here in the deep submucosa. Although granulomas seem to be a pathognomonic feature of Crohn's disease, the absence of granulomas does not rule out the diagnosis.

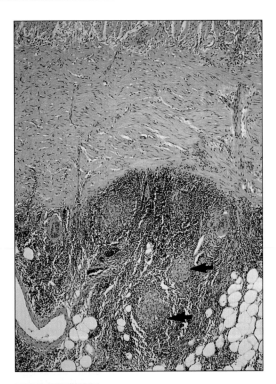

FIGURE 7-3.

Chronic subserositis. The inflammatory process spreads transmurally. Note lymphoid aggregates and granulomas in the background of chronic subserositis (*arrows*).

Classification of Crohn's disease: Staging enteric pathology

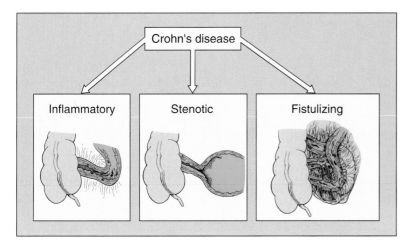

FIGURE 7-4.

It has proven useful, both for defining natural history and for selecting therapy, to think of the heterogeneous entity of Crohn's disease as comprising at least three different patterns of clinical and pathologic behavior: inflammatory, fibrostenotic, and fistulizing.

Inflammatory pattern

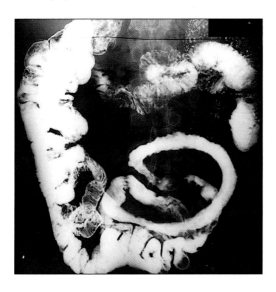

FIGURE 7-5.

Radiographic appearance of Crohn's disease of the terminal ileum. Nodularity, ulceration, narrowing, and irregularity of the lumen, characteristically affecting the terminal ileum, may result from transmural inflammation and lymphoid proliferation. Separation of involved loops of intestine from adjacent segments of bowel reflects luminal narrowing, thickening of bowel wall, and mesenteric hypertrophy.

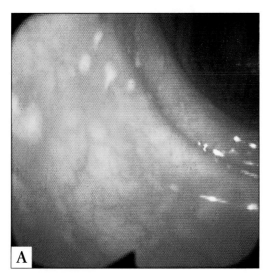

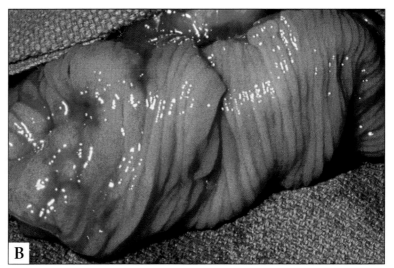

FIGURE 7-6.

A. Aphthoid ulcerations are the earliest visible mucosal lesions of Crohn's disease.

Discrete patchy ulcerations in the areas with submucosal edema (**panel B**)

(*continued on next page*)

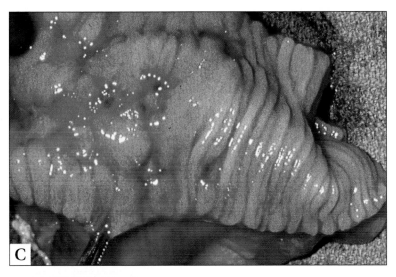

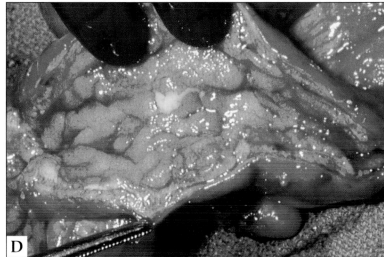

FIGURE 7-6. (CONTINUED)

progressively enlarge and spread, becoming confluent (**panel C**), until they obliterate normal mucosa entirely (**panel D**).

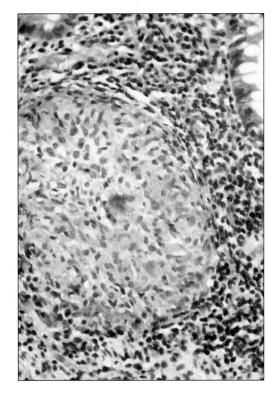

FIGURE 7-7.

Granuloma. The typical granuloma of Crohn's disease consists of one or more Langhans' giant cells and epithelioid cells surrounded by a rim of T lymphocytes.

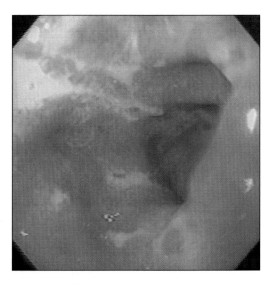

FIGURE 7-8.

Endoscopic view of ileal Crohn's disease. Edema, hyperemia, and confluent linear ulcerations are classic endoscopic findings of inflammatory Crohn's disease.

Stenosing pattern

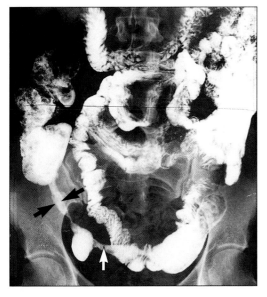

FIGURE 7-9.

In the early stages of stenosing Crohn's disease, edema and spasm produce intermittent obstructive symptoms, such as increasing postprandial pain. The spasm and edema are also responsible for the classic radiographic "string sign" (*open arrow*). Over several years the persistent inflammation progresses to scarring, narrowing, and finally, to stricture. Narrowing may be associated with asymmetric outpouchings or "pseudodiverticulae" (*closed arrows*).

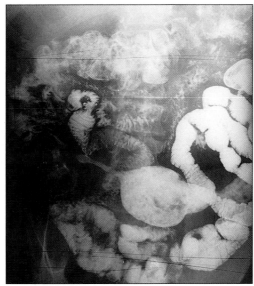

FIGURE 7-10.

Over the years, dilation proximal to fixed stenotic strictures becomes increasingly prominent.

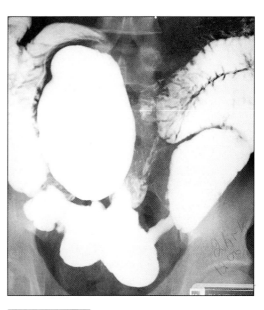

FIGURE 7-11.

When multiple strictures produce multiple areas of massively dilated proximal bowel over periods of many years, huge sacs, or "saddlebags," may develop. This saccular pattern is often accompanied by clinical sequelae of malnutrition due to impaired intake, bacterial overgrowth, and malabsorption.

Fistulizing pattern

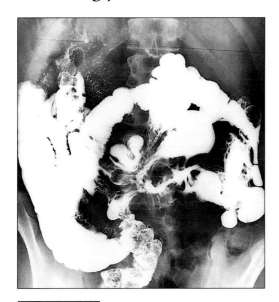

FIGURE 7-12.

Enteroenteric fistulas. Fistulization is the process in which transmural sinus tracts burrow all the way through to the serosa. These tracts often penetrate into adjacent loops of bowel to form ileoileal, ileocecal, or ileosigmoid fistulas. This figure shows complex ileal fistulas extending into adjacent ileal loops and cecum.

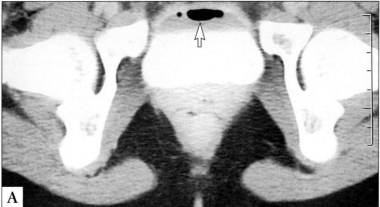

FIGURE 7-13.

Enterovesical fistulas. Enterovesical fistulization is a common complication of Crohn's disease as the distal ileum traverses the dome of the bladder. These figures show air in the bladder (**panel A**) and contrast in an ileal loop (*open arrow*) with a fistulous tract into the bladder (*closed arrow*) (**panel B**).

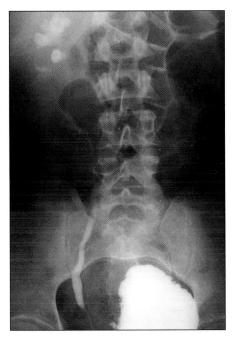

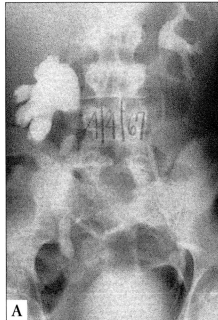

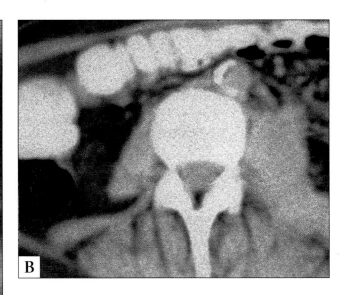

FIGURE 7-14.

Retroperitoneal fistulas. When a sinus tract penetrates posteriorly from the ileum to the retroperitoneum, the resulting phlegmon may entrap the right ureter and compress it against the psoas muscle, resulting in noncalculous hydroureter and hydronephrosis. (*From* Sachar *et al.* [1]; with permission.)

FIGURE 7-15.

A–B, More advanced cases of retroperitoneal fistulization may produce a frank psoas abscess. The computed tomographic scan shows an abscess in the psoas muscle, which is nearly three times its normal thickness and contains an area of central liquefaction. (*From* Sachar *et al.* [1]; with permission.)

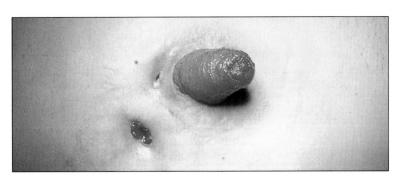

FIGURE 7-16.

Enterocutaneous fistulas. Enterocutaneous fistulas follow the path of least resistance. Therefore, in a patient who has undergone previous surgery, an enterocutaneous fistula invariably emerges through the surgical scar, as shown here. In the absence of earlier surgery, it may dissect along a persistent urachal segment and drain through the relatively thin fascia layer at the umbilicus. Alternatively, it may track along the psoas muscle and present in the groin or extend directly to the anterior abdominal wall in the right lower quadrant. (*Courtesy of* Dr. Adrian Greenstein.)

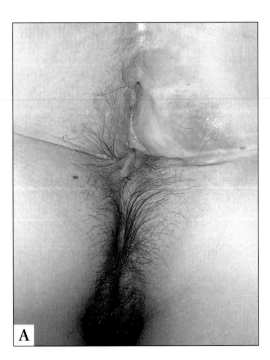

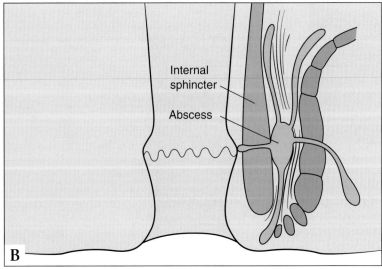

tions are more prevalent in patients with colonic disease, they are also seen in up to one quarter of patients with small-bowel disease alone. **B,** Perianal fistulas develop from the extension of intersphincteric abscesses. The lesions generally follow a course independent of the intra-abdominal disease. (**A,** *Courtesy of* Dr. Daniel Present. **B,** *Adapted from* Wexner [1a].)

FIGURE 7-17.

Perianal fistulas. **A,** Perianal lesions occur in as many as one third of all patients with Crohn's disease. Although perianal complica-

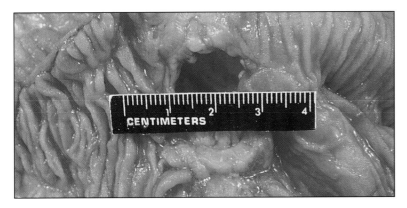

FIGURE 7-18.

There is an increased incidence of gastrointestinal (GI) carcinoma in Crohn's disease. Most of the GI malignancies in Crohn's disease occur in grossly diseased bowel, but as many as one third may arise in clinically uninvolved areas of the GI tract. This figure shows a small ileal carcinoma in an inactive ileum. The predominant risk factor for small-bowel carcinoma in Crohn's disease is a very long duration of disease, usually 20 years or more, applying equally to bypassed loops and to bowel in continuity with the rest of the intestine. In extensive Crohn's disease of the colon, the risk for colorectal cancer is as high as that for ulcerative colitis of comparable extent and duration (*Courtesy of* Dr. Adrian Greenstein).

CLINICAL PATHOLOGIC CORRELATION: DISEASE PATTERNS

Inflammatory pattern

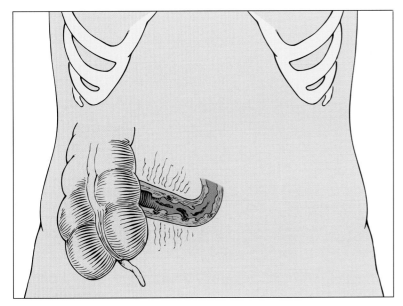

FIGURE 7-19.

Acute inflammatory presentation. The initial presentation of Crohn's disease often mimics acute appendicitis, with right lower quadrant tenderness, fever, and a palpable mass. A careful history, however, will usually uncover a pattern of preceding bowel complaints.

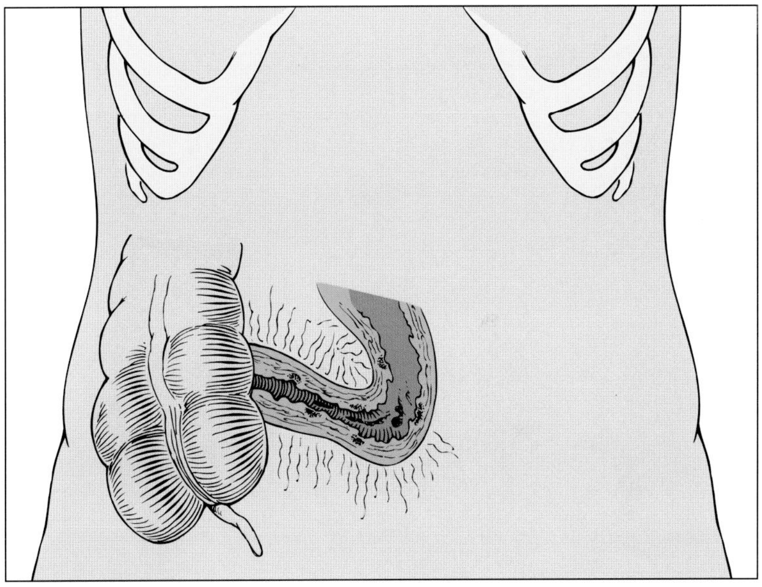

FIGURE 7-20.

Chronic inflammatory presentation. The hallmark of chronic, active Crohn's disease is recurrent episodes of pain and diarrhea. The pain is usually colicky, as intestinal contents pass through edematous and narrowed segments of inflamed bowel. Fever is usually low grade and associated with the inflammatory process.

Stenosing pattern

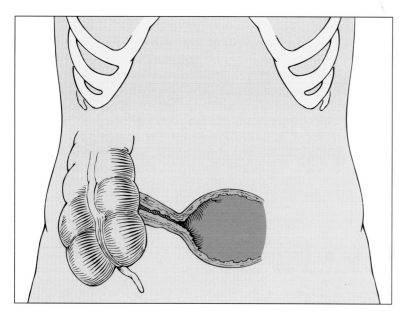

FIGURE 7-21.

As persistent inflammation progresses to scarring and narrowing, diarrhea may gradually give way to constipation and, ultimately, to bowel obstruction. Acute episodes of obstruction in Crohn's disease typically subside spontaneously with simple supportive care, but recurrent episodes signal the need for elective surgery to restore a normal quality of life.

Fistulizing pattern

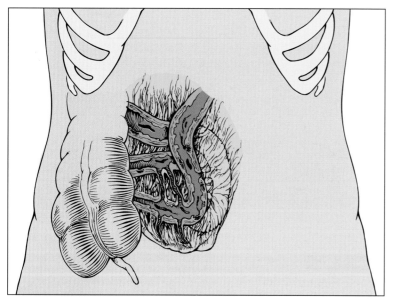

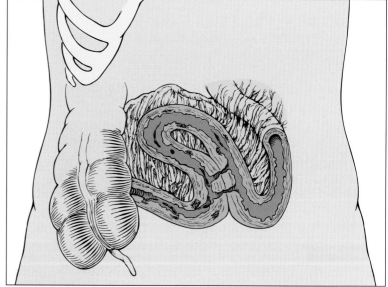

FIGURE 7-22.

Localized phlegmon. The presentation in fistulizing disease may be similar to the acute inflammatory presentation of "acute appendicitis," but with a more persistent palpable mass and more systemic signs of a suppurative process.

FIGURE 7-23.

Enteroenteric fistulas are the most common type encountered in Crohn's disease. They may be relatively asymptomatic, or even salutary, when they represent "nature's way" of bypassing an obstructing stricture.

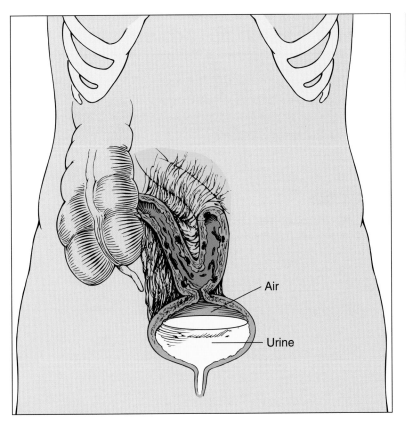

FIGURE 7-24.

Enterovesical fistulas. Enterovesical fistulas typically present with pneumaturia, dysuria, or recurrent bladder infections. Less common is fecaluria.

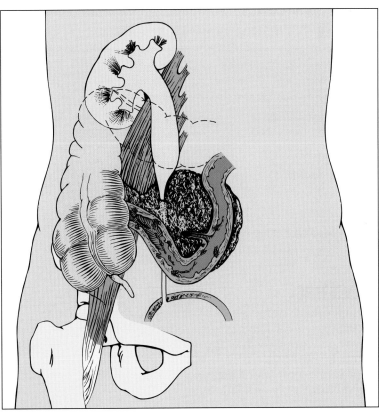

FIGURE 7-25.

Retroperitoneal fistulas. Classic clinical presentation of psoas abscess is pain in the hip, thigh, or knee, accompanied by hip flexion and a limp. Hydroureter and hydronephrosis secondary to ureteral entrapment by phlegmon or abscess do not result in chronic kidney damage. These renal manifestations readily subside once the underlying bowel pathology is corrected.

■ CLINICAL PATHOPHYSIOLOGY RELATED TO SMALL-BOWEL DISEASE

TABLE 7-1. CLINICAL PATHOPHYSIOLOGY RELATED TO SMALL-BOWEL DISEASE

Malabsorption
Renal disease
Gallstones

TABLE 7-1.

Although many systemic complications of Crohn's disease are parallel to those of ulcerative colitis and are related to colonic inflammation, others are directly attributable to pathophysiologic consequences of small-bowel disease, dysfunction, or resection [2].

TABLE 7-2. MALABSORPTION

Inadequate absorptive surface

Extensive disease
Extensive resection
Long bypassed segment
    Fistulous
    Surgical

Bacterial overgrowth

Stenosis → proximal dilation → stagnation → bacterial
    overgrowth (*see* Figs. 7-9, 7-10, 7-11, 7-21, and 7-23)
Bypassed loop
Coloenteric communication
    Fistulous
    Surgical

TABLE 7-2.

Malabsorption is related to inadequate absorptive surface resulting in diminished absorption of bile acids or bacterial overgrowth secondary to stricturing or fistulization.

TABLE 7-3. RENAL COMPLICATIONS

Stones
    Enteric hyperoxaluria → oxalate stones
    Uric acid stones
Infection
Dehydration
Bladder fistulas
Retroperitoneal fistulization → hydroureter and hydronephrosis
Amyloidosis
    Seen somewhat more with colonic than small-bowel Crohn's disease,
    appears to be associated mainly with chronic suppuration

TABLE 7-3.

Calcium oxalate stones are due to increased colonic oxalate absorption (enteric hyperoxaluria) whereas uric acid stones are due to increased metabolism or impaired urinary dilution and alkalinization. Bladder fistula may present with urinary tract infections, pneumaturia, or fecaluria. Retroperitoneal fistulization may result in hydroureter or hydronephrosis.

TABLE 7-4. BILIARY TRACT COMPLICATIONS

Gallstones
Reduction in the size of the bile-salt pool secondary to ileal dysfunction or resection predispose to gallstone formation

Primary sclerosing cholangitis
May be seen in association with colitis

TABLE 7-4.

Alterations in the bile salt pool secondary to ileal dysfunction or ileal resection predispose to gallstone formation by imposing bile salt reabsorption from the terminal ileum.

■ (CLINICAL) NATURAL HISTORY

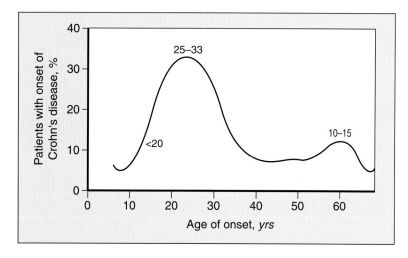

FIGURE 7-26.

Crohn's disease occurs primarily in younger people, with 25% to 33% of patients presenting before age 20. Approximately 10% to 15% of patients experience onset of Crohn's disease after the age of 60. This bimodal distribution, with the "second peak" presenting after the age of 60, may be more apparent than real. Many of those cases with later onset may in fact represent a different entity because the onset of classical ileitis is atypical in the elderly. Most of the cases beginning in older age are colonic, with at least some of them possibly representing variants of ischemic colitis or diverticulitis.

TABLE 7-5. PRESENTATION IN CHILDREN AND ADOLESCENTS

Failure of growth
Fever
Anemia
Arthritis

TABLE 7-5.

In children and adolescents, the typical gastrointestinal manifestations of Crohn's disease may be overshadowed by extraintestinal and systemic symptoms. Growth failure, fever of unknown origin, anemia, and weight loss are particularly prominent in young patients with small-bowel disease. Arthritis and arthralgias are the most common extraintestinal manifestation, occurring in approximately 15% of children and often preceding the first bowel symptoms by months to years.

DIAGNOSIS

TABLE 7-6. HISTORY, PHYSICAL EXAMINATION, RADIOGRAPHIC AND LABORATORY FINDINGS

History
Abdominal pain
Diarrhea
Weight loss or failure of growth
Fever
Family history of inflammatory bowel
    disease
Physical examination
Right lower quadrant tenderness, with or
    without mass

Radiography
Abnormal small-bowel follow-through
    radiographs
Barium enema with ileal reflux showing
    abnormal terminal ileum
Laboratory
Anemia
Elevated erythrocyte sedimentation rate
Hypoalbuminemia
Hypocholesterolemia

TABLE 7-6.

History. The inflammatory pattern of small-bowel Crohn's disease characteristically presents with recurrent episodes of right lower quadrant pain and fever, although a careful history usually uncovers preexisting bowel complaints. Persistent inflammation and scarring may progress to stenosis with repeated bouts of obstruction.

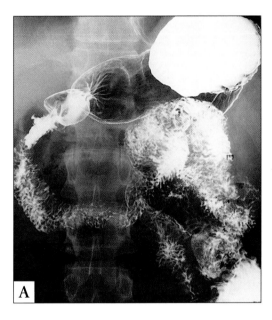
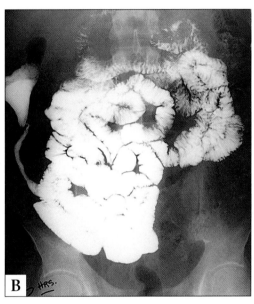

A   B

FIGURE 7-27.

When the history, physical examination, and laboratory testing suggest Crohn's disease, an upper gastrointestinal (**panel A**) and small-bowel series (**panel B**) is generally the best first diagnostic test. If only an upper gastrointestinal series is performed, however, without thorough small-bowel follow-through and visualization of the terminal ileum, even the most obvious diagnosis of Crohn's disease may be completely missed.

DIFFERENTIAL DIAGNOSIS: PROBLEMS OF IDENTITY

TABLE 7-7. DIFFERENTIAL DIAGNOSIS OF CROHN'S DISEASE

DISEASES OF ADJACENT ORGANS

Appendix and cecum
Appendicitis
Appendiceal abscess
Cecal diverticulitis
Cecal carcinoma

Tuboadnexae
Pelvic inflammatory disease
Ovarian cyst or tumor
Endometriosis

INTRINSIC ILEOCECAL DISEASES

Neoplasms
Carcinoid
Lymphoma
Metastatic tumor
Vascular
Oral contraceptives
Systemic vasculitis

Radiation
Infections
    Acute
        Anisakiasis
        Yersinia enterocolitica
    Chronic
        Tuberculosis
        *Mycobacterium
            avium-intracellulare*

Miscellaneous diseases
Chronic nongranulomatous
        ulcerative jejunoileitis
Eosinophilic gastroenteritis
Amyloidosis
Zollinger-Ellison syndrome

TABLE 7-7.

The clinical and radiologic diagnosis of Crohn's disease of the small bowel is rather straightforward. However, not every ileocecal or right lower quadrant lesion represents Crohn's disease. Two major categories of disease that may be confused with regional enteritis are disorders of the adjacent organs and intrinsic disease of the ileum and cecum that mimic the radiographic picture of Crohn's disease.

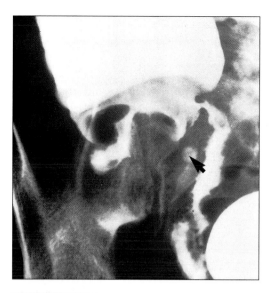

FIGURE 7-28.

Appendiceal abscess. The distal 8 cm of terminal ileum are spastic, irritable, and markedly contracted in association with deformity and narrowing of the cecum. A 1-cm appendicolith is present (*arrow*). In this case, the inflammatory changes in the terminal ileum are secondary to the adjacent appendiceal abscess. (*Courtesy of* Dr. Daniel Maklansky.)

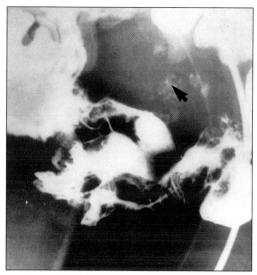

FIGURE 7-29.

Carcinoma of cecum invading the ileocecal valve and terminal ileum. Superficially, this case mimics ileocolitis. The distal 6 cm of terminal ileum are markedly narrowed in association with several short fistulous tracts extending from the ileum to the cecum, which is also markedly contracted. These findings are secondary to an infiltrating mass from a cecal carcinoma. Note the psammoma bodies representing calcifications (*arrow*) in the carcinoma. (*Courtesy of* Dr. Daniel Maklansky.)

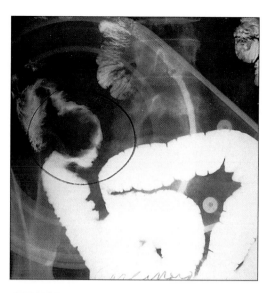

FIGURE 7-30.

Carcinoid. Distal ileum. There is a golf-ball-sized submucosal mass fixing and indenting the distal ileum with minimal pleating of the adjacent folds. (*Courtesy of* Dr. Daniel Maklansky.)

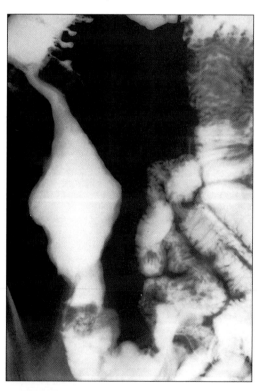

FIGURE 7-31.

Lymphoma dilatation. The distal 15 cm of ileum are dilated in association with scalloped margins indicating mass. These findings represent a large ulcerating neoplasm. The term *aneurysmal* derives from the fact that the ulcerating mass is wider than the normal dimension of the bowel at this site. (*Courtesy of* Dr. Daniel Maklansky.)

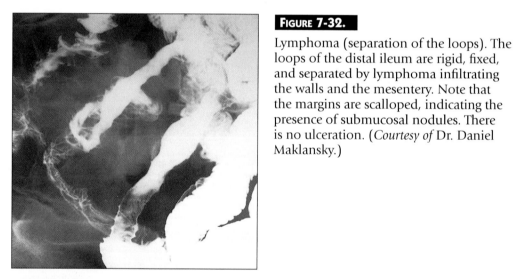

FIGURE 7-32.

Lymphoma (separation of the loops). The loops of the distal ileum are rigid, fixed, and separated by lymphoma infiltrating the walls and the mesentery. Note that the margins are scalloped, indicating the presence of submucosal nodules. There is no ulceration. (*Courtesy of* Dr. Daniel Maklansky.)

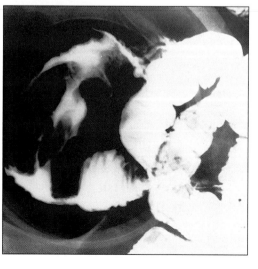

FIGURE 7-33.

Lymphoma. Mid-ileum. There is an irregular ulceration which traverses the center of the mass and divides in two, simulating a fistulous tract. The findings actually represent irregular necrotic changes within the lymphoma mass.

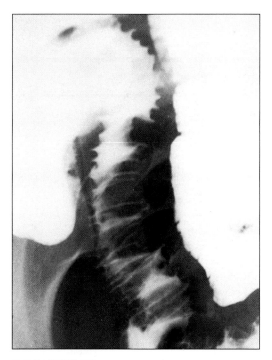

FIGURE 7-34.

Vasculitis and edema of the terminal ileum. The patient is a 29-year-old female on birth control pills presenting with acute right lower quadrant pain. The "stack of coins" appearance indicates edema of the lamina propria and submucosa. (*Courtesy of* Dr. Daniel Maklansky.)

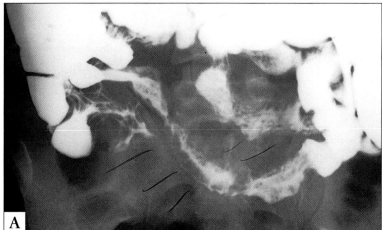

A

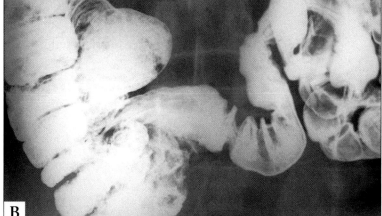

B

FIGURE 7-35.

A, Tuberculosis A. The distal 15 to 20 cm of ileum are involved with an inflammatory mass characterized by extensive linear ulceration, slight transverse ulceration, and separation of the loops. There are no fistulae. From the roentgen findings alone, this cannot be differentiated from Crohn's disease. **B**, Tuberculosis B. Same patient as in **panel A** after 5 months of treatment with appropriate therapy. (*Courtesy of* Dr. Daniel Maklansky.)

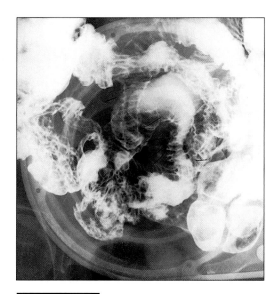

FIGURE 7-36

Radiation enteritis. The loops of the distal ileum are fixed and angulated in position with slight separation. The mucosal folds are thickened, and in some sites, nodular. There are no fistulas or sinus tracts. (*Courtesy of* Dr. Daniel Maklansky.)

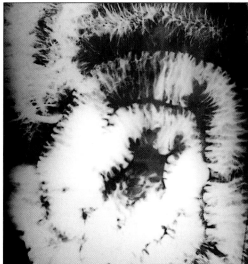

FIGURE 7-37

Amyloid. There is marked thickening and slight rigidity of the valvulae of the jejunum and ileum. Note that the folds in the distal ileum have the appearance of those in the jejunum, termed *jejunization* of the ileum. (*Courtesy of* Dr. Henry Janowitz.)

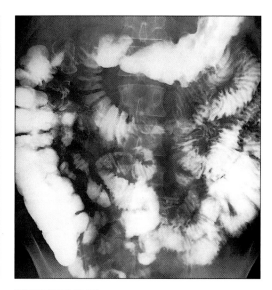

FIGURE 7-38.

Zollinger-Ellison syndrome. There is moderate thickening of the folds of the jejunum and proximal ileum associated with marked increased secretions simulating jejunitis. Markedly thickened gastric folds are also present. (*Courtesy of* Dr. Daniel Maklansky.)

EPIDEMIOLOGY AND RISK FACTORS

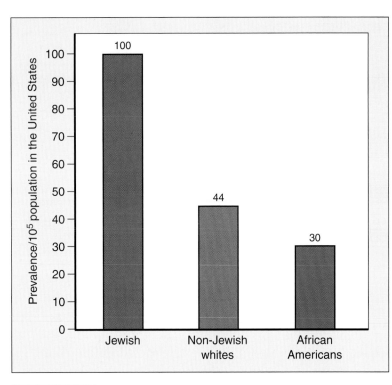

FIGURE 7-39.

Estimates of prevalence from different studies vary by several orders of magnitude. However, several points clearly emerge. Despite recently changing trends, prevalence, even today, is higher in Jewish than non-Jewish whites, and higher in non-Jewish whites than in African-Americans. The differences among these groups are diminishing with the passage of time. Prevalence rates and ethnic specificity vary substantially in different geographic locations. The latter two observations, regarding variations in ethnic-specific prevalence with time and geography, both point to the importance of environmental influences superimposed upon any underlying genetic predispositions [2,3,4,5,6].

TABLE 7-8. POTENTIAL RISK FACTORS

Diet	Nonsteroidal
Infections	anti-inflammatory drugs
Smoking	Oral contraceptives
	Psychosocial factors

TABLE 7-8.

Studies of dietary and infectious exposures in infancy, early childhood, and the years preceding clinical onset of disease have occasionally offered tantalizing clues to the role of infection in the pathogenesis of Crohn's disease, but they have not produced any definitive etiologic conclusions.

Nonsteroidal anti-inflammatory drugs have been associated with asymptomatic mucosal inflammation, strictures, obstruction, perforation, and major hemorrhage. They have also been implicated in flare-ups of established inflammatory bowel disease. Some, but not all, studies have suggested a modest increase in risk for Crohn's disease in patients using oral contraceptives. The possible pathogenesis of any such risk may be related to the thrombogenic properties of oral contraceptives. Although it is unlikely that psychosocial factors are etiologic, Crohn's disease can best be managed with sensitivity to the patient's psychosocial milieu [7,8,9,10,11].

ETIOLOGY

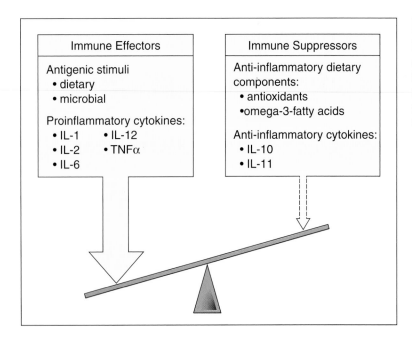

FIGURE 7-40.

Immune dysregulation in Crohn's disease. Just as epidemiologic evidence points to a balance of environmental and genetic factors in the pathogenesis of Crohn's disease, etiologic models suggest that a balance of external stimuli and internal host responses determine the hyperreactivity of the gut immune system that is seen in Crohn's disease [11].

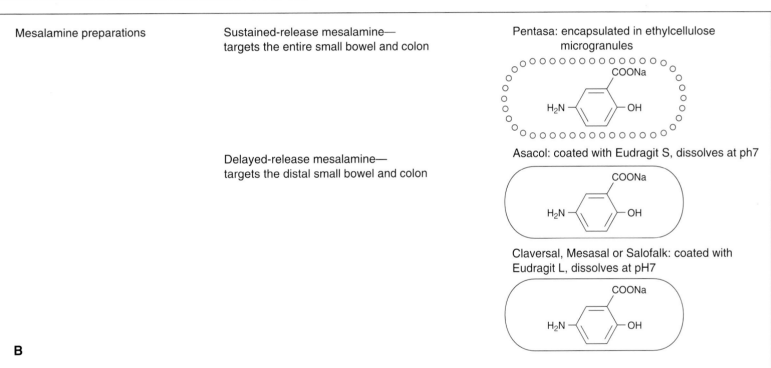

5-Aminosalicylic acid prodrugs

Target the colon and terminal ileum

Sulfasalazine

Azoreductase (colonic bacteria)

5 ASA (mesalamine)　　Sulfapyridine

Olsalazine: 5-aminosalicylate dimer

Azoreductase (colonic bacteria)

(5 ASA) mesalamine

Balsalazide: Aminobenzoylalanine carrier

Azoreductase (colonic bacteria)

aminobenzoylalanine　　(5 ASA) mesalamine

A

Mesalamine preparations

Sustained-release mesalamine— targets the entire small bowel and colon

Delayed-release mesalamine— targets the distal small bowel and colon

Pentasa: encapsulated in ethylcellulose microgranules

Asacol: coated with Eudragit S, dissolves at ph7

Claversal, Mesasal or Salofalk: coated with Eudragit L, dissolves at pH7

B

FIGURE 7-41.

A–B, 5-Aminosalicyclic acid (5-ASA) prodrugs. Because the therapeutically active moiety of 5-ASA is released from the sulfasalazine molecule by colonic bacterial azoreductase, sulfasalazine has less activity in treating small-bowel Crohn's disease and in preventing postoperative recurrence than mesalamine, which can be administered in higher doses, and in some preparations, is released more proximally [12,13].

TABLE 7-9. THE AMINOSALICYLATE (MESALAMINE) PREPARATIONS

Oral	Formulation	Site of delivery	Dose	Treatment	
				Active therapy	**Maintenance therapy**
Azobond preparation					
Azobond Sulfasalazine	5 ASA + Sulfapyridine carrier	Colon	500 mg	4–6 gm divided doses	2–4 gm divided doses
Olsalazine Balsalazide	5 ASA (mesalamine) dimer	Colon	250 mg	?	1.5–3 gm divided doses
	Amino benzoylalanine carrier	Colon	750 mg	2–6 gm	2–6 gm
Mesalamine derivatives: Delayed-release					
Asacol	5 ASA (mesalamine) coated with Eudragit S. Release at pH7	Distal ileum, colon	400 mg	2.4–4.8 gm divided doses	800 mg–4.8 gm in divided doses
Claversal, Mesasal or Salofalk Sustained-release	5 ASA (mesalamine) coated with Eudragit L. Release at pH7	Ileum and colon	250 mg or 500 mg	1.5–3 gm divided doses	750 mg–1.5 gm in divided doses
Pentasa	Mesalamine in enteric-coated Ethylcellulose Microgranules	Stomach (?) ileum colon	250 mg or 500 mg	2–4 gm divided doses	1.5–3 gm in divided doses

TABLE 7-9.

Mesalamine is rapidly absorbed from the upper digestive tract, and therefore requires an enteric delivery system, which delays its rapid absorption. Oral mesalamine preparations have been formulated as either delayed release preparations (Asacol, Claversal, Mesasal, or Salofalk) with a resin (Eudragit) coating, which is degraded at pH 6 or 7, the approximate pH of the ileum and proximal colon, or with sustained release preparations (Pentasa) encapsulated in ethylcellulose microgranules and released throughout the entire small bowel and proximal colon. Like sulfasalazine, those mesalamine preparations with an azo-bond (Olsalazine and Balsalazide) are more active in the colon than in the ileum.

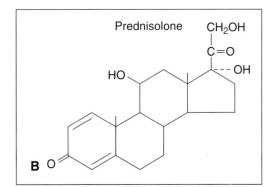

FIGURE 7-42.

Steroids. **A–B,** Glucocorticoids (hydrocortisone, prednisone, prednisolone) are indicated in short-term treatment of severely active Crohn's disease. **C,** Budesonide is a new synthetic corticosteroid that has more topical and less systemic activity [14].

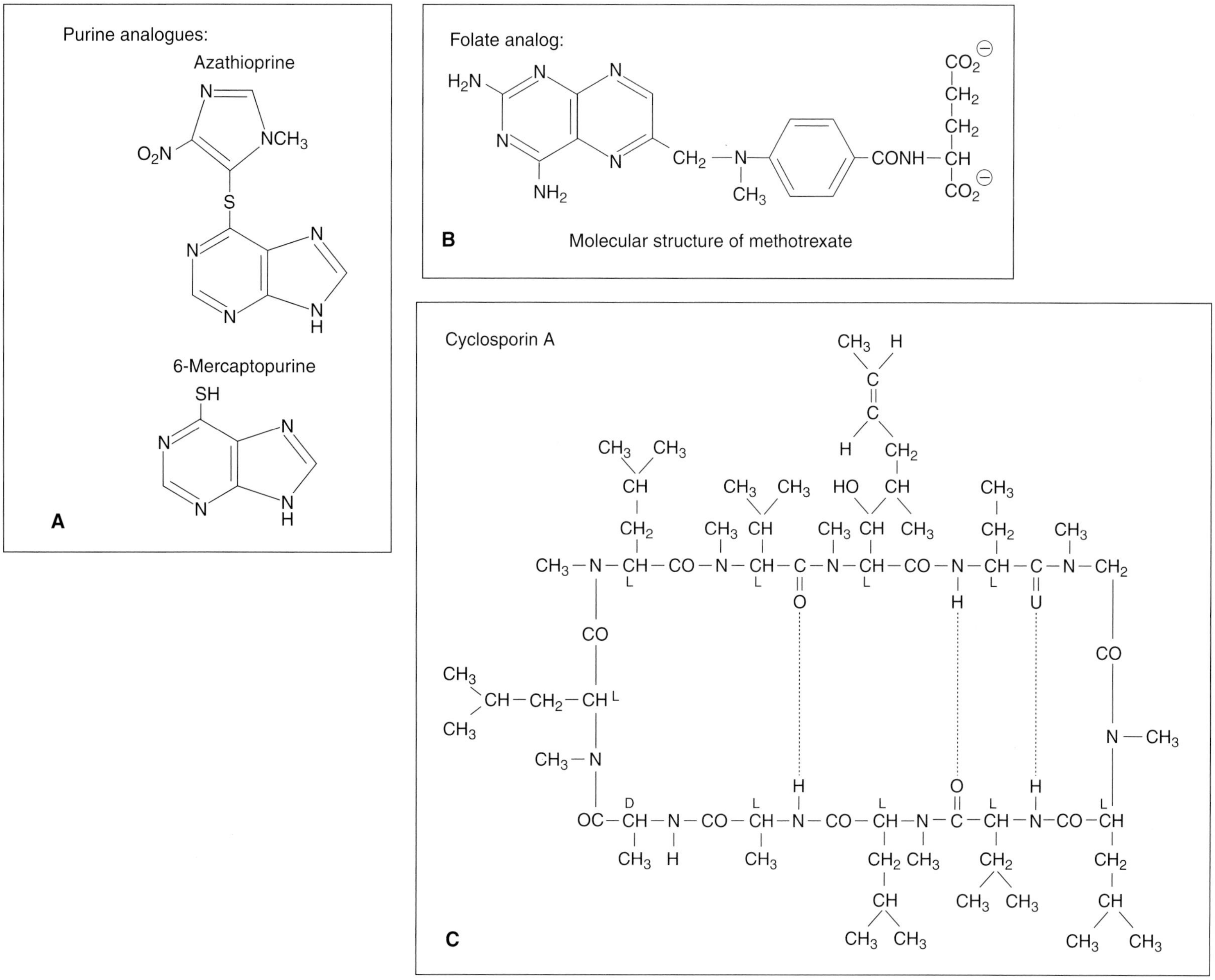

FIGURE 7-43.

Immunomodulators. **A**, Azathioprine is a prodrug that is quickly converted to 6-mercaptopurine (6-MP) in red blood cells. Azathioprine and 6-MP are purine analogues that inhibit nucleotide biosynthesis. These drugs are effective for inducing and maintaining remission of inflammatory and fistulizing Crohn's disease, and especially for reducing corticosteroid requirements, but they require up to 3 to 6 months before the onset of therapeutic action. 6-MP is administered in doses 1.0 to 1.5 mg/kg/day. Azathioprine is administered 1.0 to 3.0 mg/kg/day. Allergic reactions occur in about 5% of patients, including early fever, rash, arthralgias, and acute, reversible pancreatitis, early in the course, or a drug-induced hepatitis later in the course of therapy. Leukopenia is rare, dose related, and reversible. Neither 6-MP or azathioprine has been associated with increased risk of cancer or adverse outcomes of pregnancy, although two cases of CNS lymphoma have been reported in the world experience.

B, Methotrexate is a folate analogue which, like the purine analogues 6-MP and azathioprine, acts as an antimetabolite that inhibits T-lymphocyte function. Indications for treatment include induction of remission in Crohn's disease and reducing corticosteroid requirements. Methotrexate is most effectively administered at a dose of 15 to 25 mg/week, intramuscularly or subcutaneously, for 12 to 18 weeks. Some experts recommend liver biopsy because of the potential for hepatic fibrosis.

C, Cyclosporin A specifically blocks T-helper cell function and proliferation by inhibiting interleukin-2 gene transcription. Although used primarily for inducing remission in severe steroid refractory ulcerative colitis, cyclosporine has also been useful in promoting rapid fistula closure in Crohn's disease and dramatic healing of pyoderma gangrenosum in both Crohn's disease and ulcerative colitis. The usual IV dose is 4 mg/kg/day to achieve levels of 400 to 600 mcg/L using the monoclonal cyclosporine immunoassay.

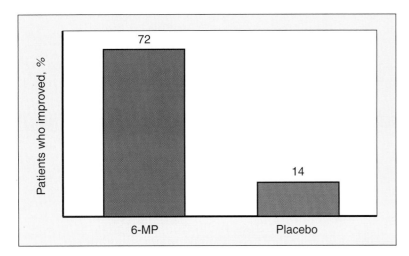

FIGURE 7-44.

6-Mercaptopurine (MP) in the treatment of active Crohn's disease. In a prospective 2-year clinical trial, 83 patients with active Crohn's disease were randomized to receive either 6-MP or placebo. The overall response rate at 12 months was 72% for 6-MP compared to 14% for placebo.

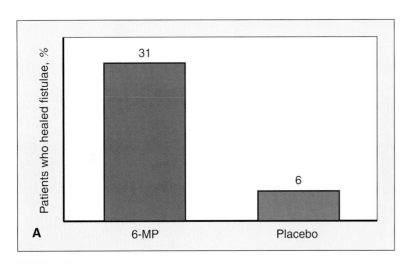

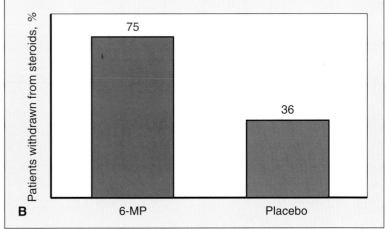

FIGURE 7-45.

A, Healing of fistulas in the 6-mercaptopurine (MP) group with 2-year follow-up occurred in 31% of patients compared with only 6% after treatment with placebo. B, Complete and successful withdrawal from corticosteroids in patients with 6-MP occurred in 75% compared to only 35% of patients receiving placebo.

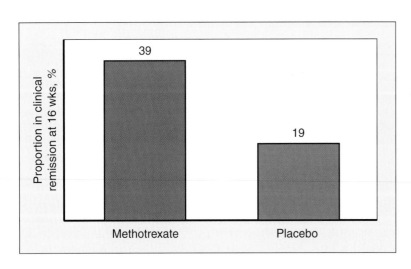

FIGURE 7-46.

Methotrexate. In a 16-week prospective trial, 141 patients with active Crohn's disease were randomized to receive either methotrexate or placebo. The overall response rate was 39% for patients treated with methotrexate compared with 19% for placebo.

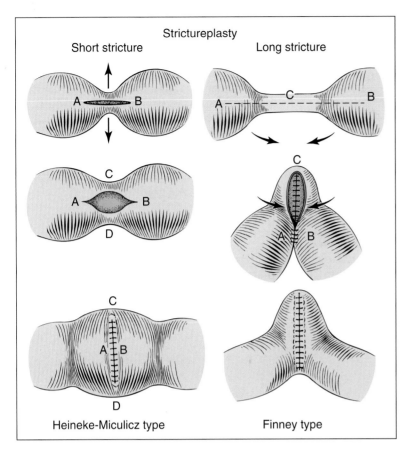

Strictureplasty

Short stricture   Long stricture

Heineke-Miculicz type   Finney type

FIGURE 7-47.

Approximately 70% of patients with Crohn's disease will require surgery at some point in the course of the disease, usually on account of recurrent obstruction, complicated fistulization, abscess formation, or intractability of inflammatory disease. In most instances, the preferred procedure is an ileocolonic resection and anastomosis or ileal resection and ileostomy and proctocolectomy, but when obstructing strictures are too numerous and widespread to allow ileal resection, strictureplasty is available as an alternative procedure.

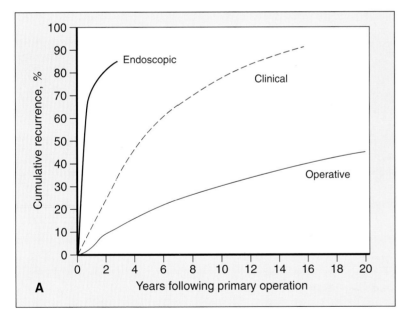

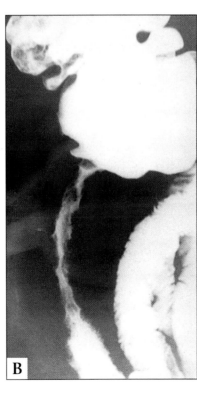

FIGURE 7-48.

Postoperative recurrence of Crohn's disease. **A,** Although surgery is frequently necessary and highly effective in managing complications, achieving rehabilitation, and restoring a healthier quality of life in patients with Crohn's disease, postoperative recurrence is almost inevitable. The magnitude of this problem of postoperative recurrence depends largely on the definition of *recurrence*—whether endoscopic, clinical, or surgical. **B,** Postoperative recurrent ileitis is characterized by edema, ulcerations, and narrowing in the neoterminal ileum.

(*continued on next page*)

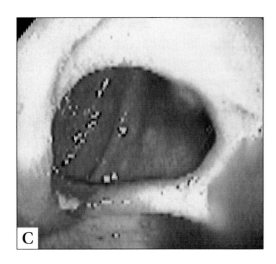

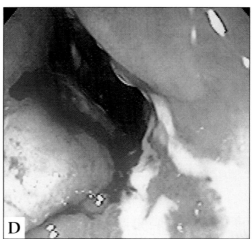

FIGURE 7-48. (*CONTINUED*)

C, Endoscopically, the finding of scattered anastomotic erosions is not uncommon, and does not correlate with symptoms or predict clinical recurrence. **D,** The minority of patients who have anastomotic deep linear ulcerations have a rapid postoperative recurrence and a poor prognosis. No more important challenge faces investigators of Crohn's disease than finding strategies to reduce the incidence of postoperative recurrence [15,16].

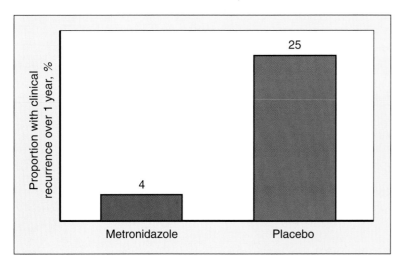

FIGURE 7-49.

Metronidazole for prevention of recurrence in Crohn's disease after ileal resection. Metronidazole treatment for 3 months after ileal resection decreased early recurrence in the neoterminal ileum, as evidenced by endoscopic criteria, and seemed to delay clinical recurrence at least up to 1 year [17].

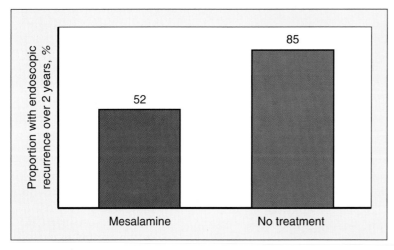

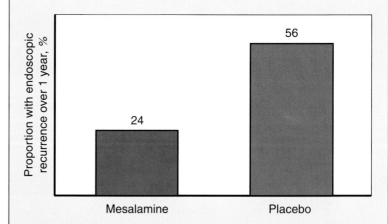

FIGURE 7-50.

Caprilli's study shows that with oral mesalamine (Asacol) treatment, endoscopic recurrence rate at 2 years is reduced from 85% to 52%, reflecting a 39% reduction in recurrence.

FIGURE 7-51.

Another Italian study showed severe endoscopic recurrence 1 year after resection in only 24% of those patients who were taking 3 g mesalamine (Pentasa) compared with 56% on placebo.

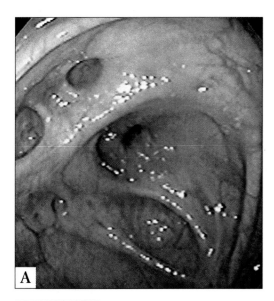 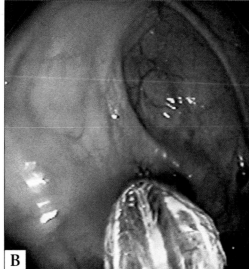 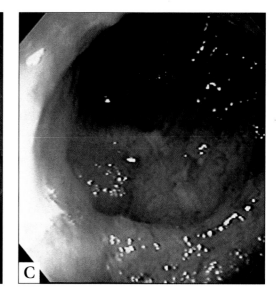

FIGURE 7-52.

A–C, Endoscopic balloon dilation of short postoperative stricture. An alternative strategy for short, inactive ("burnt-out") postoperative strictures is balloon dilation. No controlled trials are currently ongoing to assess this approach, but it offers an intriguing alternative in the management of postoperative recurrence [18,19].

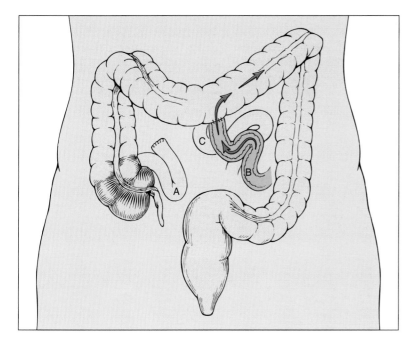

FIGURE 7-53.

The role of the fecal stream in Crohn's Disease. In Crohn's disease, diversion of the fecal stream has been observed to ameliorate the lesion in the bypassed segment, while reestablishment of continuity typically allows recurrent disease to appear at the site of anastomosis. Likewise, postoperative recurrence following anastomotic surgery is much more common than after ileostomy. This figure diagrams the phenomena of (A) quiescence after bypass (a procedure no longer recommended) and (B) recurrence proximal to anastomosis (note that segments adjacent to an anastomosis but not bathed in the fecal stream [C] are generally spared recurrent disease). Thus, the role of the fecal stream may provide a basis for understanding the therapeutic effects of antibiotics, elemental or defined diets, and TPN in the management of Crohn's disease [20].

REFERENCES

1. Sachar D, Peppercorn M, Sweeting J, Burrell M: American Gastroenterological Association Clinical Teaching Project: Inflammatory Bowel Disease. Timonium: Milner-Fenwick 1991

1a. Wexner S: General principles of surgery in ulcerative colitis and Crohn's disease. *Semin Gastrointest Dis* 1991, 2:90–106.

2. Snook J, Jewell D: Management of the extraintestinal manifestation of ulcerative colitis and Crohn's disease. *Semin Gastrointest Dis* 1991, 2:115–125

3. Calkins B: Inflammatory Bowel Diseases. In *Digestive Diseases in the United States*. Edited by Everhart J. U.S. Department of Health and Human Services: National Institutes of Health 1994:511–550.

4. Bayless T, Tokayer A, Polito J, *et al.*: Crohn's disease: Concordance for site and clinical type in affected family members: Potential hereditary influences. *Gastroenterology* 1996, 111:573–579.

5. Sachar D: Crohn's disease: A family affair. *Gastroenterology* 1996, 111:813–815.

6. Ekbom A, Helmick C, Zack M, *et al.*: The epidemiology of inflammatory bowel disease: A large population-based study in Sweden. *Gastroenterology* 1991, 100:350–358.

7. Wurzelmann J, Lyles C, Sandler R: Childhood infections and the risk of inflammatory bowel disease. *Dig Dis Sci* 1994, 39:555–560.

8. Levine J: Exogenous factors in Crohn's disease: A critical review. *J Clin Gastroenterol* 1992, 14:216–226.

9. Lashner B, Kane S, Hanauer S: Lack of association between oral contraceptive use and Crohn's disease: A community-based matched case-control study. *Gastroenterology* 1989, 97:1442–1447.

10. Rhodes J, Thomas G: Smoking: Good or bad for inflammatory bowel disease? *Gastroenterology* 1994, 106:807–810.

11. Kirsner B: Historical Antecedents of Inflammatory Bowel Disease Concepts. In *Inflammatory Bowel Disease*. Edited by Kirsner J, Shorter R. Baltimore: Williams and Wilkins; 1995:3–27.

12. Hanauer S: Drug therapy: Inflammatory bowel disease. *N Engl J Med* 1995, 334:841–847.

13. Meyers S, Sachar D: Medical Therapy of Crohn's Disease. In *Inflammatory Bowel Disease*. Edited by Kirsner J, Shorter R. Baltimore: Williams and Wilkins; 1995:695–714.

14. Sachar DB: New Steroids. In *Management of Inflammatory Bowel Disease*. Edited by Korelitz BI and Sohn N. St. Louis: Mosby Yearbook; 1992:294–288.

15. Greenstein A, Sachar D, Pasternack B, *et al.*: Reoperation and recurrence in Crohn's colitis and ileocolitis: Crude and cumulative rates. *N Engl J Med* 1975, 293:685–690.

16. Rutgeerts P, Geboes K, Vantrappen G, *et al.*: Predictability of postoperative course of Crohn's disease. *Gastroenterology* 1990, 99:956–963.

17. Rutgeerts P, Hiele M, Geboes K, *et al.*: Controlled trial of metronidazole treatment of prevention of Crohn's recurrence after ileal disease. *Gastroenterology* 1995, 108:1617–1621.

18. Caprilli R, Andreoli A, Capuruso L, *et al.*: Oral mesalamine (Asacol) for the prevention of recurrence of postoperative Crohn's disease. *Aliment Pharmacol Ther* 1994, 8:35–43.

19. Brignola C, Cottone M, Pera A, *et al.*: An Italian Cooperative Study Group: Mesalamine in the prevention of endoscopic recurrence after intestinal resection for Crohn's Disease. *Gastroenterology* 1995, 108:345–349.

20. Janowitz H, Croen E: The role of the fecal stream in Crohn's disease: A historical and analytic review. In press.

Chapter
8
Neoplastic Diseases

GORDON D. LUK
HERBERT J. SMITH
EDWARD L. LEE

Despite the markedly greater length and surface area of the small-bowel mucosa (more than 80% of the mucosal surface of the gastrointestinal tract), the small intestine harbors relatively few malignant tumors. This is in contrast to the contiguous "downstream" colon and rectum, which are the most common sites for gastrointestinal malignancies. Several pathogenetic mechanisms have been postulated to explain the relative resistance of the small bowel to malignant transformation, but none has been proven.

The four most common malignant small-bowel tumors are adenocarcinomas, carcinoids, lymphomas, and stromal cell tumors (leiomyosarcomas). Together they account for more than 90% of all malignant small-bowel tumors. Most of this chapter focuses on these four tumor types. Adenocarcinomas are found mostly in the duodenum, and carcinoids are found predominantly in the ileum, especially the terminal ileum. Lymphomas are also more commonly found in the distal small bowel, but leiomyosarcomas are more evenly distributed throughout the gastrointestinal tract.

Except for the duodenum, proximal jejunum, and terminal ileum, most of the small bowel is relatively inaccessible to routine diagnostic procedures and forms a diagnostic blind spot. Even enteroscopy, computed tomography, and MR imaging may not provide definitive reproducible views of the small bowel. Barium examination of the small bowel—conventional small-bowel follow through or enteroclysis—remains the standard mode of preoperative diagnosis. Thus, small-bowel tumors remain diagnostic challenges, and they should be included in the differential diagnosis of intestinal obstruction, abdominal pain, abdominal masses, and gastrointestinal blood loss [1–4].

TABLE 8-1. U.S. GASTROINTESTINAL CANCER STATISTICS, 1995

	ESOPHAGUS	STOMACH	SMALL BOWEL	COLORECTAL
New cases	11,000	24,000	2,500	150,000
Deaths	10,000	14,000	1,000	60,000
5-yr survival rate, %	5	15	60	55

TABLE 8-1.

U.S. gastrointestinal statistics, 1995. (*Adapted from* Parker *et al.* [5] and Luk [6].)

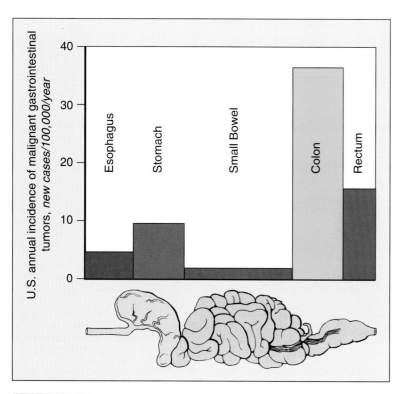

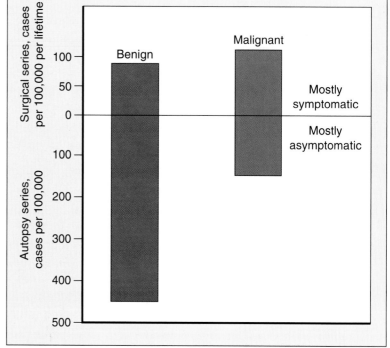

FIGURE 8-1.

Annual incidence of malignant gastrointestinal (GI) tumors in the United States [1,5]. The annual incidence of malignant GI tumors is depicted to show the dramatically lower incidence of small-bowel malignant tumors despite the vastly greater length and surface area of the small-bowel epithelium [1,5].

FIGURE 8-2.

Small-bowel tumors: benign versus malignant (tip of the iceberg). Although it is difficult to directly compare data on the relative frequency of benign versus malignant small-bowel tumors from surgical and autopsy series, it is clear that the vast majority of small-bowel tumors found at autopsy are benign and asymptomatic during life. An attempt has been made to estimate the frequency of clinically detected and surgically excised small-bowel tumors over a lifetime and to compare the estimates with the frequency of tumors found at autopsy. The frequency of malignant tumors from surgical and autopsy data is similar, but the frequency of asymptomatic benign tumors is much greater, suggesting that most small-bowel tumors are benign and asymptomatic [1–4].

TABLE 8-2. PROPOSED PATHOGENETIC MECHANISMS FOR THE LOW FREQUENCY OF SMALL-BOWEL TUMORS

Analogous to colorectal adenocarcinoma

Except

Markedly lower bacterial counts

Rapid transit time

Contents of bowel liquid

Presence of detoxifying enzymes

Abundance of lymphatic tissue and immunoglobin A

Proposed pathogenetic mechanisms for the low frequency of small-bowel malignancies. Despite their being contiguous with one another and being exposed to similar intraluminal contents, and despite their similar cell turnover rate, the small bowel has a dramatically lower frequency of malignant tumors. This has led to several hypotheses of different pathogenetic mechanisms, none of which has been proven; however, the elucidation of the protective mechanisms against malignancies in the small bowel might help in the treatment or prevention of other gastrointestinal malignancies [1,4].

TABLE 8-3. SMALL-BOWEL MALIGNANT TUMORS: RISK FACTORS

Adenocarcinoma

Familial adenomatous polyposis

Crohn's disease (involving small bowel)

Celiac sprue

Ureteroileostomy

Neurofibromatosis

Carcinoid

Multiple endocrine neoplasia syndrome I

Lymphoma

Celiac sprue

Immunosuppression and immunodeficiency

Small-bowel malignant tumors: risk factors. Although small-bowel malignancies are uncommon in the general population, several risk factors predispose to their development in susceptible individuals. For instance, patients with familial adenomatous polyposis have a greater than 50% chance of developing small-bowel (primarily duodenal) adenomas, which often progress to adenocarcinoma. Generally, these risk factors predispose to a specific histologic tumor type. The exception is celiac sprue, which predisposes affected individuals to adenocarcinomas and lymphomas [1–4].

TABLE 8-4. SMALL-BOWEL TUMORS: SIGNS AND SYMPTOMS

ADENOCARCINOMA	CARCINOID	LYMPHOMA	LEIOMYOSARCOMA
Pain	Asymptomatic	Pain	Asymptomatic
Obstruction	Obstruction	Obstruction	Pain
Systemic	Pain	Mass	Gastrointestinal bleeding
(Jaundice with periampullary tumors)		Perforation	Mass
		Gastrointestinal bleeding	Perforation
		Systemic	

Small-bowel tumors: signs and symptoms. Although the majority of small-bowel tumors are asymptomatic or present with mild symptoms only, bulkier tumors can lead to abdominal pain, bowel obstruction, and systemic signs and symptoms. Adenocarcinomas tend to grow circumferentially and lead to pain and obstruction. Jaundice is characteristic of periampullary tumors, which are commonly adenocarcinomas. Carcinoids tend to be smaller than 1 to 2 cm, and are typically asymptomatic, although they may result in obstruction and pain becasue of the occasionally intense desmoplastic tissue reaction and contractures. Lymphomas tend to be bulky and commonly lead to pain, obstruction, a palpable mass, perforation, and bleeding. Although occult gastrointestinal (GI) blood loss may be seen with all small-bowel tumors, gross GI bleeding is seen generally only with lymphomas and leiomyosarcomas. Because leiomyosarcomas tend to be slow growing, they are often asymptomatic until reaching a large size of 5 cm or more, when they may present with pain, GI bleeding, or perforation [1–4,7].

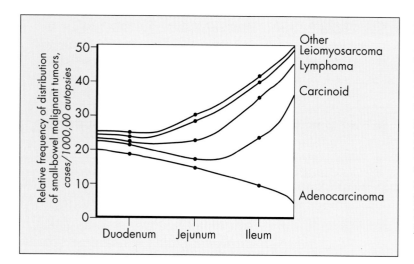

ADENOMAS AND ADENOCARCINOMAS

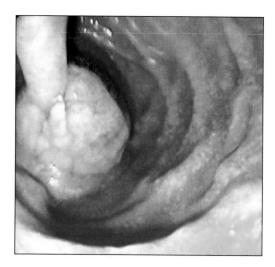

FIGURE 8-4.

Pedunculated adenomatous polyp. This polyp was found in the second portion of the duodenum in a patient with nausea and epigastric discomfort. Although this patient did not carry a diagnosis of familial adenomatous polyposis (FAP), polyps in FAP patients have a similar appearance [10–12].

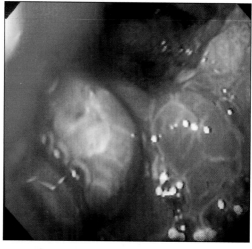

FIGURE 8-5.

Multiple adenomatous polyps. Multiple sessile adenomatous polyps were seen in the second portion of the duodenum in a patient with familial adenomatous polyposis. The surface of the polyps have the slightly lobulated appearance suggestive of adenomas [11,12].

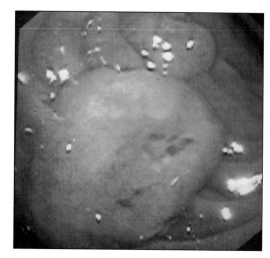

FIGURE 8-6.

Periampullary adenomatous changes. In this patient with familial adenomatous polyposis, the ampulla (foreground) had diffuse involvement with adenomatous changes shown on biopsy. An adenomatous polyp was seen in the background [11,13,14].

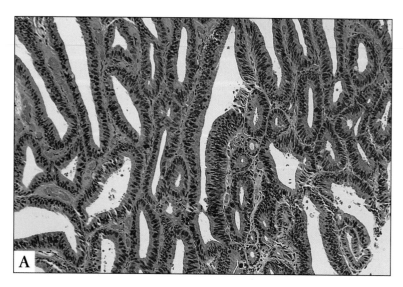

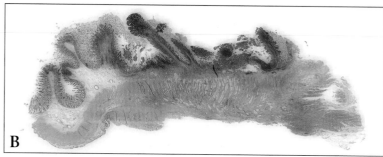

FIGURE 8-7.

Histology of adenomatous polyps. **A,** Adenoma with severe atypia. Note the predominant villous pattern, the tightly packed glands and cells, the elongated hyperchromatic nuclei with loss of basal polarity, and the markedly increased nuclear:cytoplasmic ratio. **B,** Adenoma with mild atypia. Note the well-preserved villus

(continued on next page)

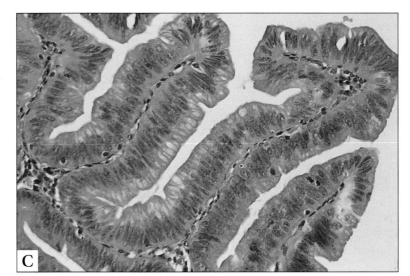

FIGURE 8-7. (CONTINUED)

architecture, with closely packed epithelial glands. The nuclei are hyperchromatic but still retain a predominant basal orientation, with only mildly increased nuclear:cytoplasmic ratio. **C**, Adenocarcinoma. This adenocarcinoma apparently arose from preexisting adenomatous epithelium. Note the transition from relatively normal-appearing mucosa to adenomatous epithelium and to adenocarcinoma.

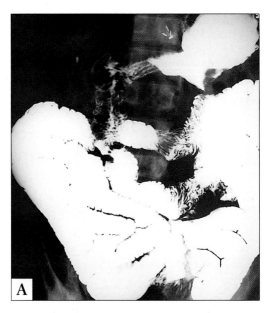

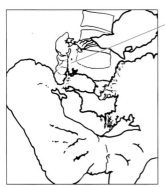

Napkin-ring lesion and displacement of adjacent tissues by mass effect

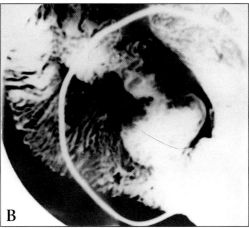

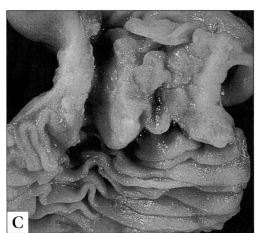

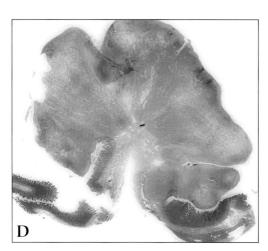

FIGURE 8-8.

Adenocarcinoma. Although many duodenal and proximal jejunal tumors may be seen by endoscopy or enteroscopy, most are beyond the reach of even the longest instruments. Such tumors require either conventional small-bowel follow-through radiograms or enteroclysis for their detection. **A–B**, In this patient, the annular napkin-ringlike lesion was seen to best advantage at enteroclysis. **C**, The marked narrowing of the lumen by the circumferentially growing adenocarcinoma was seen in the resection specimen. **D**, The bulkiness of the tumor was also evident on histologic examination [4,9,10].

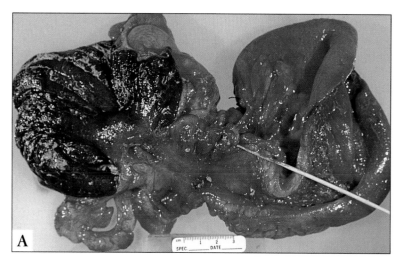

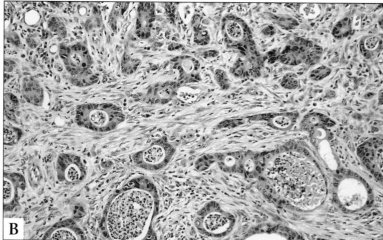

FIGURE 8-9.

Adenocarcinoma in Crohn's disease. The diagnosis of adenocarcinoma in patients with longstanding active Crohn's disease may be extremely difficult. There are strictures, mucosal thickening, and inflammatory changes that may be difficult to differentiate from adenocarcinoma. A high index of suspicion is necessary, and all accessible strictures and masses should undergo biopsy or brushing. This patient with Crohn's disease of 22 years' duration developed worsening abdominal cramping pain and intestinal obstruction. Biopsies of the terminal ileum were highly suspicious for adenocarcinoma. The surgical specimen showed the tumor mass (*white pointer*). **A,** The cecum and proximal colon with melanosis coli are seen on the left side of the specimen. **B,** Histologic examination found moderately well-differentiated adenocarcinoma and active Crohn's disease [4,15].

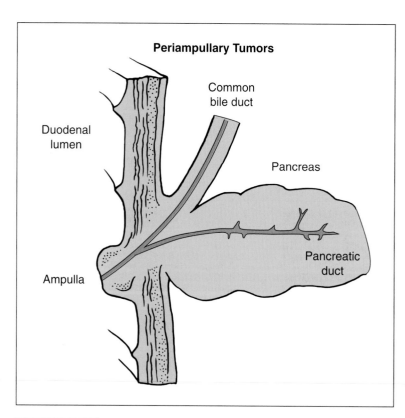

FIGURE 8-10.

Periampullary tumors. Ampullary and periampullary tumors most commonly arise from the pancreatic duct, but may also arise from the ampulla itself or the periampullary duodenal mucosa (commonly in familial adenomatous polyposis), the common bile duct, and even the gallbladder, liver, and other adjacent organs [1,4,14].

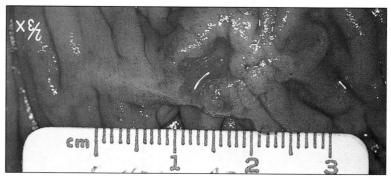

FIGURE 8-11.

Ampullary carcinoma (pancreatic). This ampulla had invasive adenocarcinoma that was found to be pancreatic in origin. The patient underwent a pancreaticoduodenectomy (Whipple's procedure) [14].

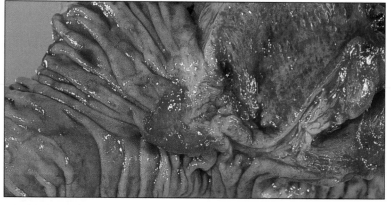

FIGURE 8-12.

Ampullary carcinoma. This ampullary carcinoma was found to arise within the ampulla itself. The common bile duct has been opened lengthwise; no tumor involvement was seen and no evidence of pancreatic involvement was present [14].

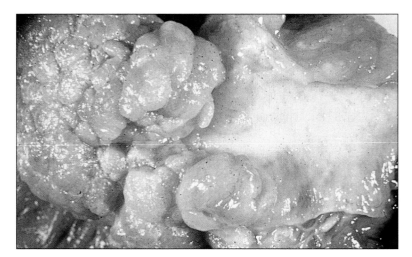

FIGURE 8-13.

Ampullary carcinoma. This was a large tumor mass, virtually obliterating the ampulla. In cases like this, macroscopic dissection to determine the tissue of origin is very difficult. In this case, the tumor histology was highly suggestive of a carcinoma originating from the ampulla [4,14].

CARCINOID TUMORS

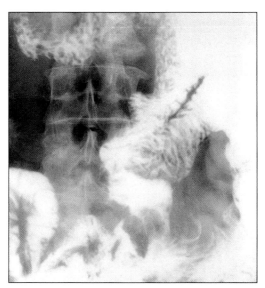

FIGURE 8-14.

Carcinoid. This tumor was visualized as a well-circumscribed intraluminal mass in the midileum by enteroclysis. Without histologic examination, the exact etiology of this polypoid mass cannot be ascertained, although its distal location is suggestive of a carcinoid (*see* Fig. 8-3) [16,17].

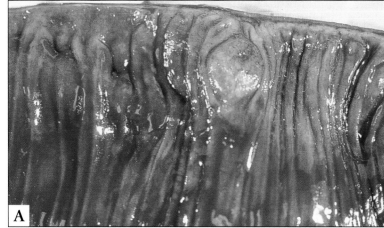

A

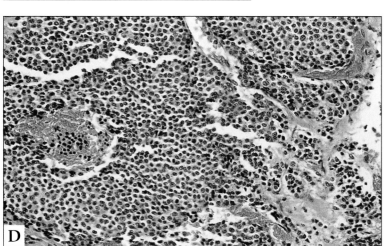

B

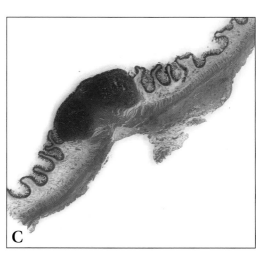

C

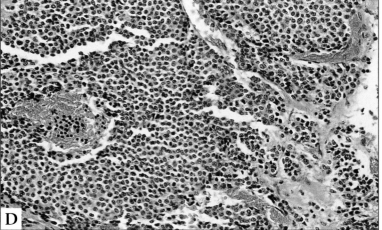

D

FIGURE 8-15.

Carcinoid. **A,** This surgical resection specimen shows a well-circumscribed intraluminal mass with apparently normal overlying mucosa and a central umbilication. **B,** On cut section, the tumor showed a pale-yellow meaty appearance, suggestive of a carcinoid; the muscular layer and serosa have undergone retractile changes that resulted in the formation of a knuckle of bowel, also suggestive of a carcinoid. **C,** The histology shows normal mucosa overlying the submucosal tumor, which consists of a monotonous array of bland tumor cells (**panel D**), which are characteristic of carcinoid [18,19].

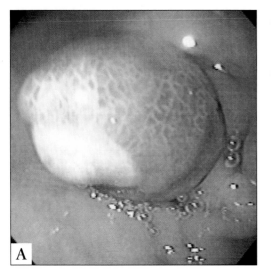
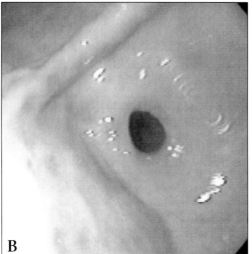

FIGURE 8-16.

Pedunculated duodenal carcinoid. This pedunculated 2-cm duodenal polyp had a long pliable stalk and moved freely through the pylorus into the gastric lumen (**panel A**) and retracted totally into the duodenal bulb (**panel B**) with peristalsis or attempted endoscopic maneuvers.

LYMPHOMA

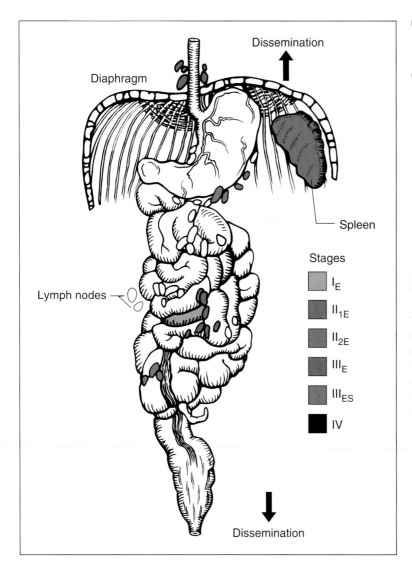

TABLE 8-5. PRIMARY SMALL-BOWEL LYMPHOMA: PROGNOSIS

STAGE	5-YR SURVIVAL RATE, %
I_E	80
II_{1E}	50
II_{2E}	35
III_E	15
III_{ES}	10
IV	5

TABLE 8-5.

Primary small-bowel lymphoma: prognosis. The survival of patients with limited-stage disease (I_E and II_{1E}) who undergo primary excision and radiotherapy or chemotherapy can be very good, with a 5-year survival of 50% to 80% when all gross tumor is resected. With bulky tumors or more advanced-stage disease, management is nonoperative and patients usually receive combination chemotherapy, with the majority of patients dying of their disease within 5 years [1,3,5,20,21]. (*Data from* Lance [1], Jones *et al.* [3], Boring *et al.* [5], Weingrad *et al.* [20], and List *et al.* [21].)

FIGURE 8-17.

Primary small-bowel lymphoma: clinical staging. Primary small-bowel lymphoma is staged by the extent of disease, analogous to other extra-nodal lymphomas. Stage I_{1E} is confined to the small bowel, stage II_{1E} involves adjacent nodes, and stage II_{2E} involves nonadjacent regional nodes. Stage III is more extensive and involves nodes on both sides of the diaphragm, with localized extralymphatic or spleen involvement. Stage IV is metastatic disease with involvement of extralymphatic sites.

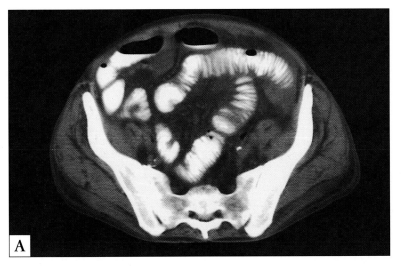

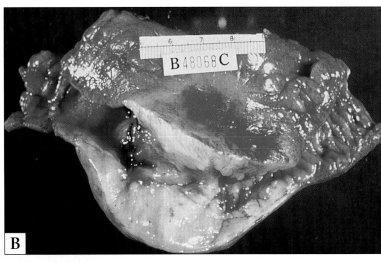

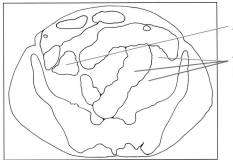

Bowel lumen (contrast)

Thickened bowel well (tissue density)

FIGURE 8-18.

Primary small-bowel lymphoma. Lymphomas may present as diffuse infiltration, ulcerations, circumferential masses, or polypoid masses. **A**, This case of lymphoma with diffuse thickening of the small-bowel wall was visualized by CT scan. **B**, The surgical specimen confirmed the diffuse wall thickening. The cut surface shows the typical fish-flesh appearance [17,20,21].

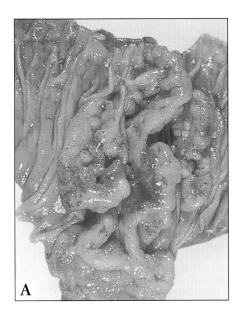

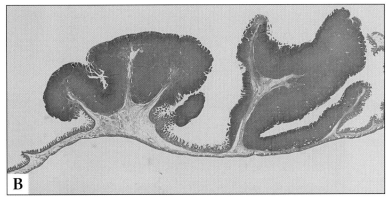

FIGURE 8-19.

Polypoid lymphoma. **A**, This surgical specimen showed the diffuse polypoid involvement of the small-bowel wall by an infiltrative process. **B**, Histology confirmed the diagnosis of lymphoma, with the presence of lymphomatous polyps [20,21].

▌STROMAL TUMORS

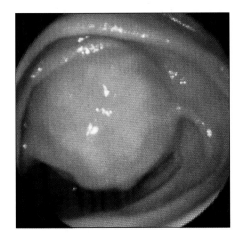

FIGURE 8-20.

Leiomyoma. Leiomyomas and leiomyosarcomas are characteristically spherical submucosal masses with intact overlying mucosa. Large tumors may develop a central ulceration, which can lead to gastro-intestinal bleeding or perforation. Size is an important prognostic factor, and tumors that are 5 cm or larger are generally classified as malignant, although most authors depend on histology (*see* Fig. 8-23). This 3-cm proximal jejunal tumor was visualized by enteroscopy and was histologically a benign leiomyoma. However, surgical resection is almost always indicated and was performed in this patient [22–24].

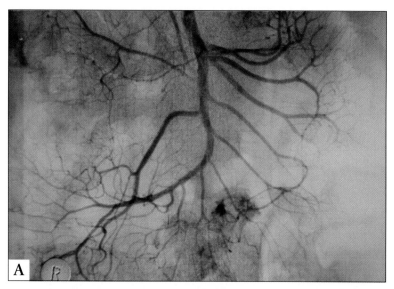

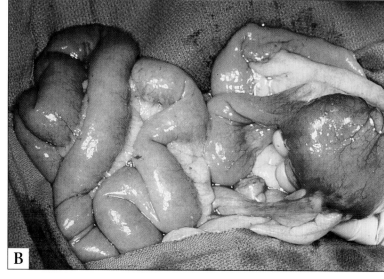

FIGURE 8-21.

Leiomyosarcoma. Most leiomyosarcomas are beyond the reach of even the longest enteroscope. **A,** Arteriography may sometimes be helpful because leiomyosarcomas (and leiomyomas) are hypervascular and have a dense, well-circumscribed blush [25]. **B,** After arteriographic visualization, this patient underwent surgery; the tumor was identified and resected. **C,** The surgical specimen was opened longitudinally and revealed the large bulky hypervascular tumor. This tumor was 6 cm in diameter, and subsequently found to be a leiomyosarcoma by using histology [23,24].

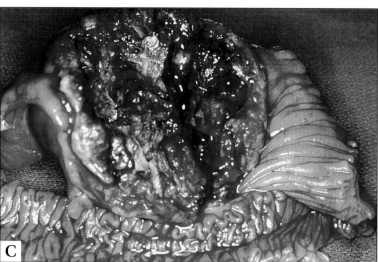

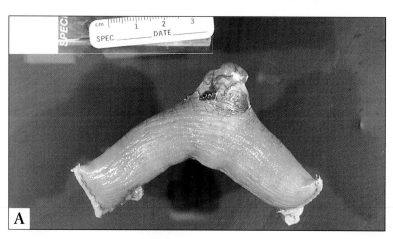

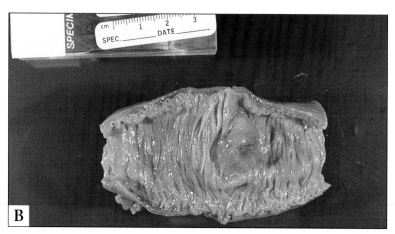

FIGURE 8-22.

Leiomyosarcoma. **A,** This resection specimen revealed a mass eroding through the entire bowel wall. **B,** When the bowel was opened lengthwise, the intraluminal extent of the mass was appreciated. **C,** The cut surface of the mass has a pale, white to tan, whorled appearance with overlying normal-appearing mucosa, suggestive of a stromal cell tumor, leiomyosarcoma, or leiomyoma.

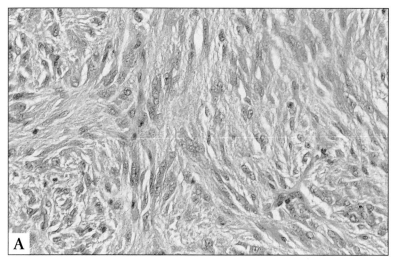

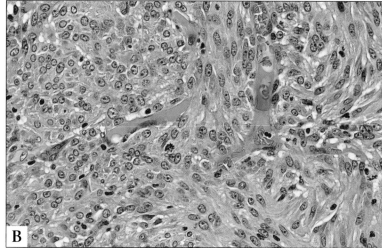

FIGURE 8-23.

Leiomyoma versus leiomyosarcoma. Although size is predictive of the nature of a stromal tumor, with tumors larger than 5 cm tending to be aggressive and malignant, smaller tumors may also be malignant. A reasonable index of malignancy is the level of mitotic activity. Tumors with more than five mitoses per 10 high-power fields tend to be malignant, although even tumors with lower mitotic indices may be or become malignant. Thus, surgical resection is almost always indicated for symptomatic tumors. **A**, No mitoses, a finding suggestive of a benign leiomyoma. **B**, Five mitoses within a single high-power field, a finding strongly suggestive of a malignant leiomyosarcoma [23,24].

■ OTHER TUMORS AND MASSES

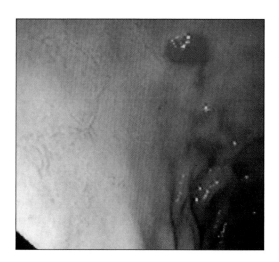

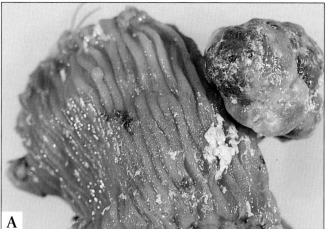

FIGURE 8-25.

Metastatic melanoma. Melanoma is the most common tumor metastatic to the small bowel and is found in about half of patients dying with metastatic melanoma. The metastases may appear as a single mass (**panel A**) or multiple masses (**panel B**). Most melanoma metastases are pigmented. Because tumors tend to be bulky, patients often develop obstruction or intussusception [27].

FIGURE 8-24.

Kaposi's sarcoma. Kaposi's sarcoma in patients with AIDS might be considered a systemic disease, and has been found to arise throughout the entire gastrointestinal tract. In this patient there are multiple flat and raised reddish submucosal lesions, with only a thin layer of overlying mucosa in the distal duodenum. Although patients with AIDS are often found to harbor Kaposi's sarcoma on endoscopic examination, it is unclear whether these small lesions cause symptoms. Biopsy will often yield the diagnosis [26].

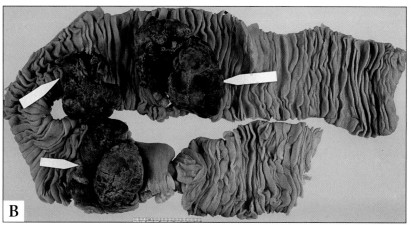

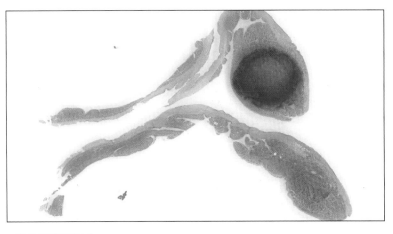

FIGURE 8-26.

Metastatic melanoma. The pigmented nodular lesion is clearly demarcated from the adjacent normal intestinal mucosa, confirming the metastatic nature of the lesion.

FIGURE 8-27.

Metastatic lung carcinoma. This metastatic tumor from a primary squamous cell carcinoma of the lung was ulcerated. Metastatic lung carcinoma to the small intestine has led to perforation. Metastases to the small intestine have been found from primary tumors of the breast, ovary, kidney, and colon, in addition to melanoma and lung carcinomas [4,28].

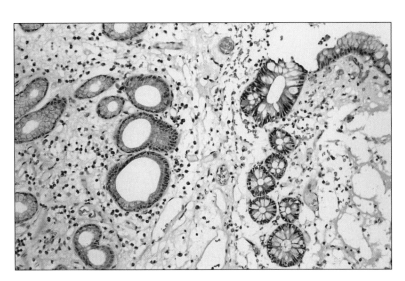

FIGURE 8-28.

Pyloric gland hyperplasia. Biopsy of a small proximal duodenal nodule revealed gastric mucosal elements with pyloric gland hyperplasia underlying normal-appearing duodenal mucosa. This is entirely benign and most likely asymptomatic.

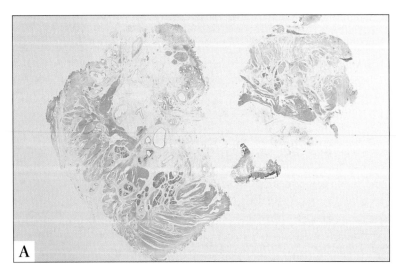

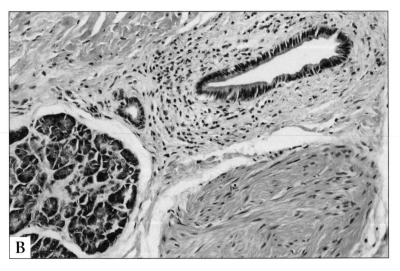

FIGURE 8-29.

Heterotopic pancreas. Biopsy of a small periampullary nodule with intact overlying mucosa (**panel A**) revealed dilated duct-like structures admixed with muscle fibers and acinar tissue (**panel B**), which is diagnostic of heterotopic pancreas. This is entirely benign.

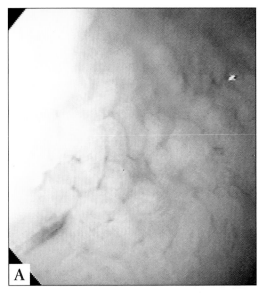

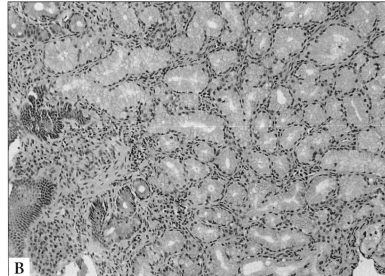

FIGURE 8-30.

Brunner's gland hyperplasia. **A,** This duodenal bulb showed diffuse nodularity with a cobblestone appearance. **B,** Biopsy revealed dilated Brunner's glands with abundant ductal structures. Occasionally, Brunner's gland hyperplastic nodules may enlarge to form polyps, rarely up to 3 cm in diameter. These polyps have been termed *Brunner's gland hamartomas.*

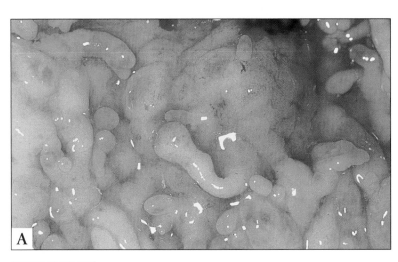

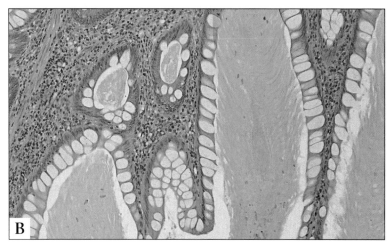

FIGURE 8-31.

Juvenile polyps. These serpentine, translucent polyps were seen in the proximal jejunum of a patient who was complaining of dyspepsia, but who was otherwise healthy. **A,** This surgical specimen shows their characteristic translucent appearance. **B,** Histology revealed the hamartomatous nature of the polyp with distended mucus-filled glands and edematous lamina propria. Except in familial juvenile polyposis syndromes, these juvenile polyps are considered benign [29].

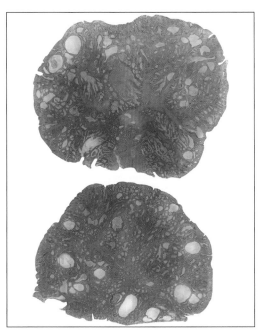

FIGURE 8-32.

Peutz-Jeghers polyp. This 2-cm surgical specimen was found in the midjejunum of a patient with Peutz-Jeghers syndrome who had intermittent intestinal obstruction. The histology reveals the characteristic arborization of smooth muscle and epithelial elements, along with cystic dilation and edematous lamina propria containing abundant vasculature. Although the syndrome has been associated with an increased risk of carcinoma, primarily outside the gastrointestinal tract, the polyps themselves are not considered premalignant [29].

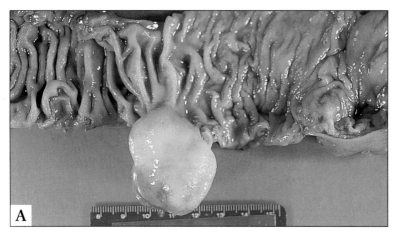

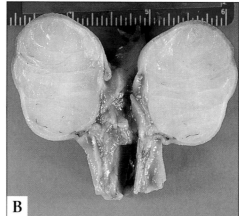

FIGURE 8-33.

Lipoma. This 3-cm polyp was found in the distal ileum of a patient with intermittent intestinal obstruction. **A**, The surgical specimen had the characteristic glistening, yellowish appearance of a lipoma. **B**, The cut surface revealed the characteristic color and texture of fat.

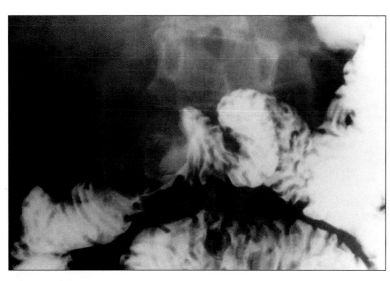

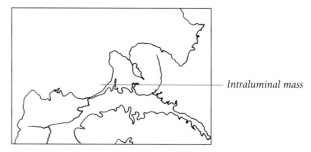

Intraluminal mass

FIGURE 8-34.

Neurofibroma. This large intraluminal mass with a smooth domed surface was visualized by enteroclysis. Subsequently, the mass was found to be a neurofibroma.

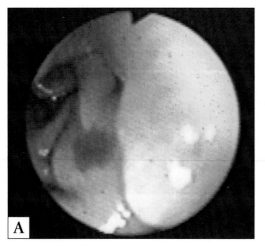

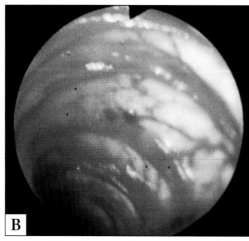

FIGURE 8-35.

Hemangioma. **A**, Hemangiomas of the small intestine may be single, as was the case for this proximal jejunal lesion. **B**, Hemangiomas can also be multiple or diffuse, occasionally with a spider-like appearance, as in this midjejunal hemangioma seen on enteroscopy.

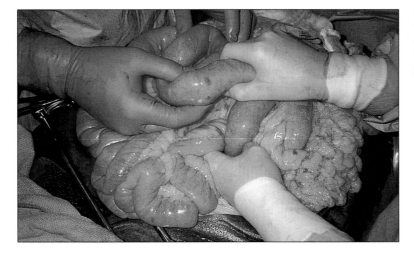

FIGURE 8-36.

Hemangioma. At surgery, this hemangioma was clearly seen through the intact bowel wall, shown here between the surgeon's gloved fingers.

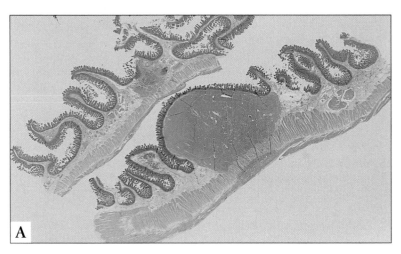

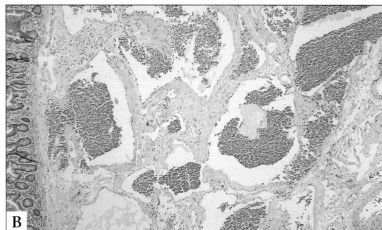

FIGURE 8-37.

Hemangioma. **A,** The low-power view of this hemangioma specimen showed cavernous dilation of the vascular structures. **B,** Higher magnification revealed that almost all vascular structures are dilated.

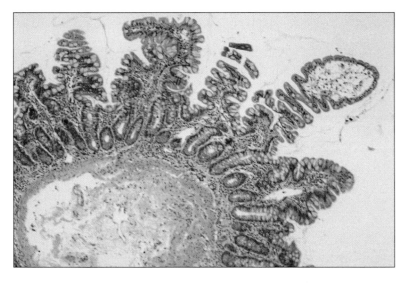

FIGURE 8-38.

Lymphangioma. This small nodule in the proximal jejunum revealed lymphangiectasia, with dilation of the endothelium-lined lymphatic structures (no erythrocytes were seen within the dilated vessels). These lymphangiectatic lesions may become large, but are usually clinically silent. When the lymphangiectasia is diffuse or involves large segments of the small bowel, malabsorption or protein-losing enteropathy may occur [13].

■ REFERENCES

1. Lance P: Tumors and other neoplastic diseases of the small bowel. In *Textbook of Gastroenterology*. Edited by Yamada T. Philadelphia: JB Lippincott; 1995:1696.

2. Moertel CG: Gastrointestinal carcinoid tumors and the malignant carcinoid syndrome. In *Gastrointestinal Disease*, edn 5. Edited by Sleisenger MH, Fordtran JS. Philadelphia: WB Saunders; 1993:1363.

3. Jones DV, Levin B, Salem PA: Primary small intestinal lymphomas. In *Gastrointestinal Disease*, edn 5. Edited by Sleisenger MH, Fordtran JH. Philadelphia: WB Saunders; 1993:1378.

4. Sinar DR: Small bowel neoplasms (other than carcinoid and lymphoma). In *Gastrointestinal Disease*, edn 5. Edited by Sleisenger MH, Fordtran JH. Philadelphia: WB Saunders; 1993:1393.

5. Parker SL, Tong T, Bolden S, Wingo PA: Cancer statistics, 1997. *CA Cancer J Clin* 1997, 47:5.

6. Luk GD: Cancer surveillance strategies. In *Gastrointestinal Disease*, edn 5. Edited by Sleisenger MH, Fordtran JH. Philadelphia: WB Saunders; 1993:115.

7. Donohue JH: Malignant tumours of the small bowel. *Surg Oncol* 1994, 3:61.

8. Weiss NS, Yang C-P: Incidence of histologic types of the small intestine. *J Natl Cancer Inst* 1987, 78:653.

9. Zollinger RM, Sternfeld WC, Schreiber H: Primary neoplasms of the small intestine. *Am J Surg* 1986, 151:654.

10. Galandiuk S, Hermann RES, Jagelman DG, *et al.*: Villous tumors of the duodenum. *Ann Surg* 1988, 207:234.

11. Kurtz RC, Sternberg SJ, Miller HH, DeCosse JJ: Upper gastrointestinal neoplasia in familial polyposis. *Dig Dis Sci* 1987, 32:459.

12. Offerhaus GJA, Giardiello FM, Krush AJ, *et al.*: The risk of upper gastrointestinal cancer in familial adenomatous polyposis. *Gastroenterology* 1992, 102:1980.

13. Hanagiri T, Baba M, Shimabukuro T, *et al.*: Lymphangioma in the small intestine: Report of a case and review of the Japanese literature. *Jpn J Surg* 1992, 22:363.

14. Tarazi RY, Hermann RE, Vogt DP, *et al.*: Results of surgical treatment of periampullary tumors: A thirty-five year experience. *Surgery* 1986, 100:716.

15. Lashner BA: Risk factors for small bowel cancers in Crohn's disease. *Dig Dis Sci* 1992, 37:1179.

16. Maglinte DDT, Hall R, Miller RE, *et al.*: Detection of surgical lesions of the small bowel by enteroclysis. *Am J Surg* 1984, 147:225.

17. Nolan DJ: Radiology of the small intestine. In *Surgery of the Small Intestine*. Edited by Nelson RL, Nyhus LM. Norwalk: Appleton & Lange; 1987:59.

18. Godwin DJ: Carcinoid tumors: An analysis of 2,837 cases. *Cancer* 1975, 36:560.

19. MacGillivray DC, Snyder DA, Drucker W, ReMine SG: Carcinoid tumors: The relationship between clinical presentation and the extent of disease. *Surgery* 1991, 110:68.

20. Weingrad DN, DeCosse JJ, Sherlock P, *et al.*: Primary gastrointestinal lymphoma: A 30-year review. *Cancer* 1982, 49:1258.

21. List AF, Greer JP, Cousar C, *et al.*: Non-Hodgkin's lymphoma of the gastrointestinal tract: An analysis of clinical and pathologic features affecting outcome. *J Clin Oncol* 1988, 7:1125.

22. Lewis BS, Kornbluth A, Waye JD: Small bowel tumours: Yield of enteroscopy. *Gut* 1991, 32:763.

23. Akwari OE, Dozois RR, Weiland LH, Beahrs OH: Leiomyosarcoma of the small and large bowel. *Cancer* 1978, 41:1375.

24. Walker MJ: Sarcomas of the small intestine. In *Surgery of the Small Intestine*. Edited by Nelson RL, Nyhus LM. Norwalk: Appleton & Lange; 1987:243.

25. Allison DJ, Hemingway AP, Cunningham DA: Angiography in gastrointestinal bleeding. *Lancet* 1982, ii:30.

26. Danzig JB, Brandt LJ, Reinus JF, Klein RS: Gastrointestinal malignancy in patients with AIDS. *Am J Gastroenterol* 1991, 86:715.

27. Patel K, Didolkar MS, Pickren JW, Moore RH: Metastatic pattern of malignant melanoma: A study of 216 autopsy cases. *Am J Surg* 1978, 135:807.

28. McNeill PM, Wagman LD, Neifeld JP: Small bowel metastases from primary carcinoma of the lung. *Cancer* 1987, 59:1486.

29. Luk GD: Colonic polyps: Benign and premalignant neoplasms of the colon. In *Textbook of Gastroenterology*. Edited by Yamada T, Alpers DH, Owyang C, *et al.* Philadelphia: JB Lippincott; 1991:1645.

Chapter 9

Small-Bowel Bleeding

Francisco C. Ramirez

The small intestine between the ligament of Treitz and the ileocecal valve is up to 5 m long in the adult. It is not only this considerable length, but also factors that limit the use and interpretation of imaging techniques that have made this portion of the small bowel relatively inaccessible. The need for particularly long instruments has made the small intestine the last frontier in gastrointestinal endoscopy.

Small-bowel lesions located between the second portion of the duodenum and the ileocecal valve account for approximately 3% to 5% of all causes of gastrointestinal hemorrhage. The evolution of enteroscopy through recent years has made it possible to evaluate areas never investigated before and has allowed physicians to make the diagnosis of lesions responsible for gastrointestinal bleeding with unprecedented precision. Enteroscopy may provide specific diagnosis for the 38% of patients with iron-deficiency anemia in whom routine upper and lower gastrointestinal investigation failed to identify the source of bleeding. The parallel development of endoscopic therapeutic techniques also has allowed endoscopists to provide successful treatment for small-bowel bleeding.

▐ CLINICAL PRESENTATION AND EVALUATION OF SMALL-BOWEL HEMORRHAGE

Patients with small-bowel hemorrhage present with either overt or occult bleeding that can be acute, recurrent, or chronic. Most of these patients present with bleeding of obscure origin, in which routine endoscopic and radiographic evaluation of both the upper and lower gastrointestinal tracts does not yield a diagnosis.

The initial work-up of acute gastrointestinal bleeding depends on the clinical presentation. In patients with hematemesis, coffee-grounds emesis, or melena, upper gastrointestinal endoscopy usually is the first diagnostic modality employed. Colonoscopy after bowel preparation, on the other hand, is indicated initially if hematochezia or maroon stools are the mode of presentation. In the presence of clinically severe, active bleeding, a negative endoscopic investigation of the upper gastrointestinal tract and colon should be followed by selective angiographic examination. Alternatively, if the bleeding has slowed down or stopped, scintigraphy ("bleeding scan") is often recommended prior to angiography, but this approach may not be defensible. If the cause of acute hemorrhage remains obscure, laparotomy with intraoperative enteroscopy is the final step. For patients with chronic gastrointestinal blood loss manifested by guaiac-positive stools or iron-deficiency anemia, routine colonoscopy and upper gastrointestinal endoscopic examination are in order to identify the source of bleeding. When this is not diagnostic, enteroscopy, enteroclysis, or even exploratory laparotomy with intraoperative enteroscopy should be considered.

CAUSES OF SMALL-BOWEL HEMORRHAGE

Vascular anomalies, smooth muscle tumors, and Meckel's diverticulum account for the majority of lesions responsible for small-bowel bleeding, and hemorrhage is the most common mode of presentation for these lesions. Other pathologic conditions reported to cause small-bowel bleeding include aortoenteric fistula, hemobilia, hemosuccus pancreaticus, vasculitis, small-bowel diverticula, duodenal reduplication, small-bowel varices, and ulcers.

MANAGEMENT OF SMALL-BOWEL HEMORRHAGE

Depending on the mode of presentation, the diagnostic method used to identify the bleeding site, and the patient's overall clinical status (including surgical risk), the management of a patient with small-bowel bleeding may involve endoscopic therapy (thermal and injection therapy methods), intravenous or intra-arterial vasopressin injection, selective embolization of the bleeding vessel, or surgical resection.

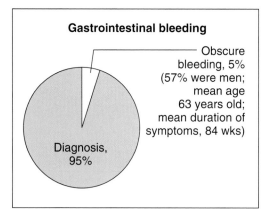

FIGURE 9-1.

Gastrointestinal bleeding of obscure origin. The patient population affected by gastrointestinal bleeding of obscure origin characteristically suffers from a chronic and debilitating course, requiring multiple blood transfusions. Of 852 patients with gastrointestinal hemorrhage of obscure origin in whom data were available [1–7], 484 (56.8%) were men and 368 (43.2%) were women; their mean age was 63 years (range, 2 years to 95 years). The mean duration of symptoms in this collected group of patients was 84 weeks (range, 1 day to 25 years), and the mean number of units of blood transfused was 14 (range, 0 to >100).

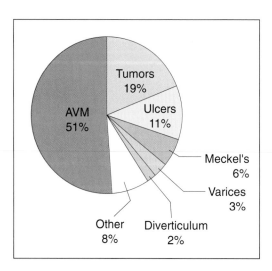

FIGURE 9-2.

Etiology of small-bowel bleeding. Based on 519 patients in whom a lesion thought to be responsible for small-bowel bleeding was identified [1–17], mucosal vascular anomalies (AVMs) were the most frequently found (51%), followed by small-bowel tumors (19%). Of these neoplasms, primary smooth muscle tumors represented 34% (79% benign, 21% malignant). Other malignant solid tumors (primary or metastatic) represented 25% of tumors, lymphoma 15%, nonspecified neoplasms 12%, and others 13% (carcinoid, leukemia, endometrioma, polyps). Small-bowel ulcerations, excluding those induced by nonsteroidal anti-inflammatory drugs (NSAIDs), were responsible for gastrointestinal bleeding in 11% of cases. Meckel's diverticulum was the source of bleeding in 6% of cases, whereas varices and diverticula accounted for 3% and 2%, respectively. Other diagnoses (erosions, aortoenteric fistula, NSAID-associated ulcers, and bleeding without an identified source) were responsible for the remaining 8% of cases.

TABLE 9-1. DIAGNOSTIC TECHNIQUES AVAILABLE FOR EVALUATION OF SMALL-BOWEL BLEEDING

Barium Contrast Radiologic Studies
Small-bowel series
Enteroclysis
Nuclear Medicine Studies
^{99m}Technetium sulfur colloid scintigraphy
^{99m}Technetium-labeled erythrocyte scintigraphy
^{99m}Technetium sodium pertechnetate scan (Meckel's scan)
Enteroscopy
Push enteroscopy (jejunoscopy)
Sonde enteroscopy
Arteriography
Exploratory Laparotomy
Alone
With intraoperative angiography
With intraoperative scintigraphy
With intraoperative enteroscopy

TABLE 9-1.

A list of the diagnostic techniques available for the work-up of patients with suspected small-bowel bleeding is arranged from the least to the most invasive. Typically, patients with small-bowel bleeding not only have multiple, but also repeated tests during the course of their evaluation. Some of these techniques are also capable of delivering therapy, such as electrocoagulation with jejunoscopy, vasopressin infusion or embolization with arteriography, and resection with exploratory laparotomy. The choice of the diagnostic tool to be used depends on the severity of gastrointestinal bleeding, its mode of presentation, and the patient's overall clinical condition.

TABLE 9-2. BARIUM STUDIES IN THE EVALUATION OF SMALL-BOWEL BLEEDING

DIAGNOSTIC YIELD	SMALL-BOWEL SERIES, %	ENTEROCLYSIS, %
Overall (all indications)	6.6–7.1	37
Bleeding	0–5.6	10 (Increased to 20% if done only after negative UGI/LGI work up)

ADVANTAGES	DISADVANTAGES
Noninvasive	Time-consuming
Low complication rate, safe	Operator dependent
	Low diagnostic yield
Relatively easy to perform	Requires duodenal intubation (enteroclysis)
	Should not be used in the presence of acute bleeding
Lower cost than other options	Fails to identify mucosal vascular abnormalities
	Incidental findings may be misleading (seen in 15%)
Widely available	May identify a lesion, but not necessarily the source of bleeding

TABLE 9-2.

The yield of barium studies for the evaluation of small-bowel bleeding depends on the technique used [8,18–20]. Enteroclysis is reported to have a higher diagnostic yield (10%) than small-bowel series (5.6%). This yield can be increased even further (up to 20%) if enteroclysis is performed after negative routine upper and lower gastrointestinal work-up. The advantages and disadvantages of these techniques are listed in this table. UGI—upper gastrointestinal; LGI—lower gastrointestinal.

TABLE 9-3. TYPES OF NUCLEAR MEDICINE STUDIES FOR THE EVALUATION OF SMALL-BOWEL BLEEDING

^{99m}Tc SULFUR COLLOID	^{99m}Tc-LABELED RBC
By 12–15 minutes, most activity is cleared from the intravascular space	Remains in intravascular space for up to 24 hours
Useful for the acute ongoing bleeding	Useful for intermittent bleeding

ADVANTAGES	DISADVANTAGES
Detects slow bleeding rates (0.1 mL/min)	Background activity in esophagus, stomach, duodenum, spleen, and liver
Readily available techniques	Limited use in the upper gastrointestinal tract
Lower complication rate	Delayed films may be misleading for correct anatomic location
Relative low cost	Poor positive and negative predictive value
Noninvasive	Regarded as screening procedure only
Safe	

TABLE 9-3.
Radionuclide studies play an important role in the diagnostic evaluation of gastrointestinal bleeding of obscure origin. There are basically two types of radionuclide substrates that can be used for scintigraphic evaluation of gastrointestinal bleeding. Whereas the disadvantages and some of the advantages are common to these two substrates, some of the advantages also depend on the substrate to be used [21–26].

TABLE 9-4. DIAGNOSTIC YIELD OF NUCLEAR MEDICINE STUDIES FOR SMALL-BOWEL BLEEDING

Overall yield for all gastrointestinal bleedings [22–28] (patients with positive scan/total patients)	25%–64%
Overall correct localization confirmed by other means [22–28] (positive scans in which confirmation attempted)	41%–95%
Yield for small-bowel Bleeding [1,2,5,11,12,14]	55% (0%–100%)
Correct localization of small-bowel bleeding site [1,5,11,12,14]	47% (10%–100%)

TABLE 9-4.
Even in the setting of acute, massive bleeding, 45% of patients with known small-bowel bleeding lesions identified by other means undergo a negative radionuclide study [22–29]. The overall yield of scintigraphic studies for all types of gastrointestinal bleeding (including upper and lower gastrointestinal sources) varies from 25% to 64% [22–29]. A similar yield is seen in those patients being evaluated for small-bowel bleeding (55%) [1,2,5,11,12,14]. The correct localization of the small-bowel bleeding site was only 47% in the collected series presented here [1,5,11,12,14]. Failure to accurately locate the source anatomically may mislead the surgeon and lead to the performance of an incorrect surgical procedure. In at least one study [25], the high rate of incorrect anatomic location in patients with lower gastrointestinal bleeding would have led to a surgical error 42% of the time. Despite evidence from at least one study [26] that a positive scan does not predict a positive subsequent arteriography, some have considered this technique as a screening tool that should be done routinely before angiography. The poor positive predictive value of scintigraphy makes this approach debatable.

TABLE 9-5. DIAGNOSTIC VALUE OF MECKEL'S SCAN IN THE ADULT POPULATION

SENSITIVITY	SPECIFICITY	ACCURACY	PPV
62.5%	9%	46%	60%

PPV=positive predictive value

Causes of false-negative scans

Absent/insufficient (> 1.8 cm^2 required [35]) or necrotic ectopic gastric mucosa

Bad technique or failure in interpretation

Dye washout (rapid bleeding)

Vascular compromise

Yield of Meckel's Scan in the bleeding patient: 55%

Causes of false-positive scans

Ectopic gastric mucosa in absence of diverticulum

Inflammatory reactions

Neoplastic conditions

Renal abnormalities

Vascular lesions

TABLE 9-5.

^{99m}Tc sodium pertechnetate scan (Meckel's scan) [30–38]. Although only 16% of all Meckel's diverticula contain ectopic gastric mucosa, such gastric mucosa and ulceration are present in most Meckel's diverticula complicated by bleeding [30–32]. This provides the rationale for radioisotope scanning because Meckel's diverticulum containing gastric secretory mucosa will take up ^{99m}Tc sodium pertechnetate [33]. Pretreatment with a histamine-$_2$ receptor antagonist, such as cimetidine, enhances the radionuclide uptake, prevents its secretion into the gastric lumen, and decreases interference with interpretation [38]. In the setting of acute bleeding, 300 mg of cimetidine is administered intravenously over 20 minutes, and imaging is started 1 hour later [38].

TABLE 9-6. ARTERIOGRAPHY IN THE DIAGNOSIS OF SMALL-BOWEL BLEEDING

Advantages

Accurately identifies the anatomic location of bleeding

May allow hemostatic therapy

Disadvantages and complications

Invasive

High cost

Requires invasive radiologist and special equipment

Major complications (< 2%):

Formation of false aneurysm

Occlusion of the artery at the site of catheter insertion

Contrast-related allergic reactions; acute renal failure

Complications specific to therapeutic methods used

Reasons for false-negative results (overall)

Bleeding stopped

Insufficient contrast

Short period of observation

Very slow active bleeding (< 0.5–1 mL/min)

Failure to include the bleeding site on the film

Early termination because of patient's clinical deterioration

The bleeding vessel may be overlooked or not selectively opacified

Unfavorable anatomy (stenosis, anomalies, aneurysms, tortuous arteries)

May be difficult to differentiate from normal mucosal blush if bleeding is diffuse

Dilution of contrast in the venous phase may prevent visualization from varices

TABLE 9-6.

Arteriography in the diagnosis of small-bowel bleeding. Arteriography may provide an accurate anatomical location of the bleeding site. Therapeutic intervention at the moment of such procedure may prove to be life-saving for a particular patient. The technique, however, may yield false-negative results, and has important disadvantages that preclude its routine use in the setting of small-bowel bleeding. The advantages and factors associated with false-negative results, as well as the disadvantages and complications of arteriographic studies, are listed in this table.

TABLE 9-7. ARTERIOGRAPHY IN GASTROINTESTINAL BLEEDING

Overall diagnostic yield: 57.6%
Yield for small-bowel bleeding: 61.3%

	SENSITIVITY, %	SPECIFICITY, %	PPV, %	NPV, %
Chronic occult bleeding	40	100	100	75
Recurrent acute bleeding	30	100	100	46
Acute bleeding	47	100	100	11
Overall	37.5	100	100	47

Based on 58 patients with gastrointestinal bleeding undergoing 62 arteriographic examinations [48]

TABLE 9-7.

Arteriography in gastrointestinal bleeding. The overall yield of arteriography for gastrointestinal bleeding is 57.6% [1,10,12,22, 24,26,39–50]. Based on 58 patients with gastrointestinal bleeding who underwent 62 arteriographic examinations, the overall sensitivity was 37.5%, specificity was 100%, positive predictive value was 100%, and negative predictive value was 47% [48]. The sensitivities and negative predictive values varied depending on the bleeding setting, as illustrated in this table. The reported yield for small-bowel bleeding in different series analyzed was 61% [1,2,6,10,11,14,49].

TABLE 9-8. ENTEROSCOPY IN THE DIAGNOSIS AND MANAGEMENT OF SMALL-BOWEL HEMORRHAGE

	PUSH ENTEROSCOPY (JEJUNOSCOPY)	SONDE ENTEROSCOPY
Instruments	Adult or Pediatric Colonoscope or Prototypes (*ie,* Olympus XSIF-10.5, SIF-100 [Olympus America, Inc., Lake Success, NY])	Different Prototypes (Olympus SIF-VI KAI, SSIF-VI KAI, XSIF-VI KAI3, SIF-SW, SSIF-VII, Pentax ESI-2000 [Pentax Precision Instruments Corp., Orangeburg, NY])
Maximum depth of insertion	Jejunum	Terminal ileum
Special operator skills	Not needed	Desirable
Procedure time	Short	Long
Therapeutic capability	Yes	No
Complete mucosal visualization possible	Yes	No

TABLE 9-8.

Enteroscopy has revolutionized the approach of patients with suspected small-bowel bleeding and nonbleeding lesions. There are two types of enteroscopic examinations: push and sonde-type enteroscopy. The former involves the use of either an adult or pediatric colonoscope, or a specially designed enteroscope that allows the endoscopist to visualize an average of 30 and 80 cm beyond the ligament of Treitz. This type of evaluation should be more appropriately called *jejunoscopy*. The same type of endoscope can be used to evaluate longer portions of the small intestine and even in its entire length during the course of an exploratory laparotomy (intraoperative enteroscopy). To overcome the length limitation of push enteroscopy, a sonde-type endoscope is available. This is thinner, measures 250 cm in length, and is the only endoscope that allows visualization of the entire small intestine without surgery. It lacks therapeutic capability, requires an expert endoscopist and still does not permit complete mucosal visualization.

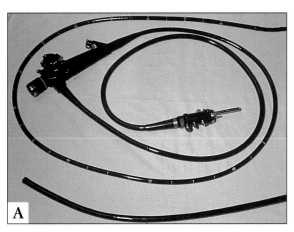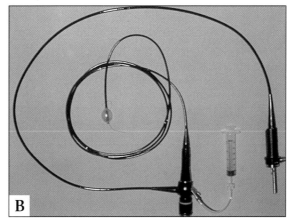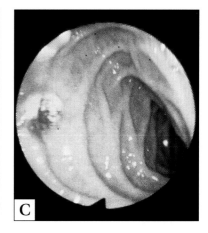

FIGURE 9-3.

A, Push enteroscope with overtube (Olympus SIF-10L [Olympus America, Inc, Lake Success, NY]). B, Sonde-type enteroscope (Olympus SIF-SW). C, SIF-SW sonde-type enteroscope with its inflated balloon tip is seen advancing in the small bowel.

TABLE 9-9. PUSH ENTEROSCOPY (JEJUNOSCOPY) FOR GASTROINTESTINAL BLEEDING OF OBSCURE ORIGIN

	TOTAL PATIENTS	OVERALL POSITIVE STUDY (%)	POSITIVE STUDIES WITHIN REACH OF EGD (% POSITIVE)	POSITIVE STUDY BEYOND LT (% OF SMALL-BOWEL EXAMINATIONS THAT WERE POSITIVE WHEN EGD WAS NEGATIVE)
Foutch et al. [2] Instrument **Colonoscope** Insertion: 45–60 cm beyond LT Mean procedure time: 50 min Complications: None	39	16 (41)	1/39 (2.5)	15/38 (39)
Chong et al. [15] Instrument: **SIF 10.5L/SIF 3000** Insertion: 90–113 cm beyond LT Mean procedure time: 60 min Complications: 1 pharyngoesophageal tear Needs overtube	55	35 (64)	21/55 (38)	14/34 (41)
Barkin et al. [17] Instrument: **SIF 100** Insertion: 108 cm beyond LT Complications: None Needs overtube	20	16 (80)	10/20 (50)	6/10 (60)
Berner et al. [7] **Instrument**: Pediatric colonoscope Complications: None	553	105 (19)	11/553 (2)	94/542 (17)

EGD indicates esophagogastroduodenoscopy (standard endoscopy).
LT—Ligament of Trietz.

TABLE 9-9.

Push enteroscopy (jejunoscopy) for gastrointestinal bleeding of obscure origin. The rate of positive endoscopic identification for the source of gastrointestinal bleeding of obscure origin is depicted in this table. The overall yield varied from 19% to 80%, but it must be noted the rates of positive identification within the reach of routine upper endoscopy (in up to 50% in one of the series) may be significant. Different instruments were used in the 4 different studies.

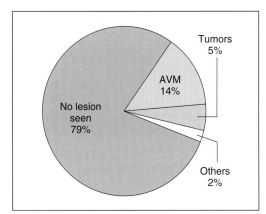

Figure 9-4.

Yield of jejunoscopy for small-bowel bleeding (excludes patients with lesions found within reach of esophagogastroduodenoscopy). Based on a series of 624 patients [2,7,15,17] undergoing jejunoscopy for evaluation of gastrointestinal bleeding of obscure origin mucosal vascular anomalies, such as arteriovenous malformations (AVMs), were the most common small-bowel lesions found (66% of lesions), followed by small-bowel tumors (22%). Other lesions found included diverticula, small-bowel erosions and ulcers, varices and prominent vessels, and aortoenteric fistulas. Endoscopic therapy (bipolar cauterization) was delivered to 14 patients (13 with AVMs and 1 with prominent vessels).

TABLE 9-10. SONDE ENTEROSCOPY

	Total Patients	Overall Positive Study (%)	Positive Studies within Reach of EGD (% positive)	Positive Study Beyond LT (% of small-bowel examinations that were positive when EGD was negative)
Dabezies *et al.* [51] Instrument: **EPM 3000** Video Insertion: LT: 1 Jejunum: 2 Ileum: 4 Mean procedure time: 4.5 h Complications: None	7	1 (14)	0	1/1 (100)
Gostout *et al.* [3] Instrument: **SIF VI KAI** Non-video Insertion: Complete: 5 Mid-distal ileum: 24 Jejunum: 5 Mean procedure time: 4.3 h Complications: None	35	9 (26)	0	9/9 (100)
Morris *et al.* [52] Instrument: **SIF SW** Non-video Insertion: 140 cm small bowel Mean procedure time: 6 h Complications: Two perforations	65	25 (38)	0	25/25 (100)
Gostout *et al.* [53] Instument: **SSIF-VI KAI/XSIF-VI KAI3** Non-Video Complications: None	24	13 (54)	0	13/13 (100)
Berner *et al.* [7] Instrument: **SIF SW** Non-video Insertion: Ileocecal valve: 57 Distal ileum: 221 Distal jejunum: 110 Proximal jejunum: 27	553	144 (26)	15/553 (2.7)	129/538= (24)

EGD—esophagogastroduodenoscopy (standard endoscopy).
LT—Ligament of Trietz.

Table 9-10.

Sonde endoscopy. The yield of sonde enteroscopy for identifying the source of bleeding of obscure origin is shown in this table, and ranged from 14% to 54%. In contrast to push enteroscopy studies, lesions thought to be responsible for obscure gastrointestinal bleeding were less frequently found within the reach of routine upper endoscopy (0–2.7%). Different instruments were used in the different series analyzed.

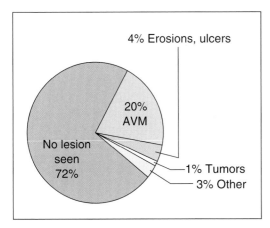

FIGURE 9-5.

Sonde endoscopy. Of 684 patients undergoing sonde enteroscopy [3,7,51–53] for investigation of gastrointestinal bleeding, arteriovenous malformations (AVMs) were the most commonly found lesions (71% of lesions), followed by small-bowel erosions and ulcers (12.5%) and tumors (5%). Other lesions found and thought to be responsible for gastrointestinal hemorrhage included active bleeding without visible lesions, polyps, phlebectasia, diverticula, and various others representing 11% of small-bowel lesions.

TABLE 9-11. INTRAOPERATIVE ENTEROSCOPY

Indications

To use as the ultimate test in the diagnostic work-up of bleeding of obscure origin

To confirm the source(s) of bleeding detected preoperatively or by gross examination at laparotomy

To determine the limits of intestinal pathology

To identify other potential sources of bleeding

To help in the guidance of surgical therapy (*eg*, local versus segmental resection, oversewing) or endoscopic therapy (*eg*, electrocoagulation)

To identify nonpalpable intestinal lesions

To use as a diagnostic tool in an emergency situation when no other localizing diagnostic tests are possible

Limitations

Dense adhesions

Short mesentery

Massive ongoing hemorrhage precluding appropriate mucosal visualization

May be associated with severe mucosal trauma, including perforation and ischemia

TABLE 9-11.

Intraoperative enteroscopy. Intraoperative enteroscopy is considered the gold standard test for gastrointestinal bleeding of obscure origin; however, it should be reserved only for those in whom other imaging and endoscopic techniques failed to reveal the source of bleeding. The indications and limitations of intraoperative enteroscopy are depicted in this table.

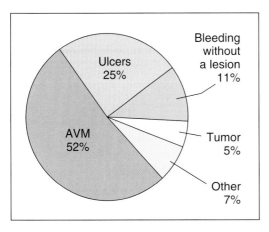

FIGURE 9-6.

Small-bowel lesions found during intraoperative enteroscopy for gastrointestinal hemorrhage of obscure origin. Of a total of 118 patients [4,5,11,14,16,50,54–61] undergoing intraoperative enteroscopy for evaluation of gastrointestinal bleeding, vascular lesions (AVMs) were the most commonly found (52%), followed by small-bowel ulcers (25%), active bleeding without a discernible lesion (11%), and tumors (5%). Other lesions (7%) found included Crohn's, aortoenteric fistulas, polyarteritis nodosa, diverticula, and nonspecific changes.

TABLE 9-12A. CLASSIFICATION OF VASCULAR MALFORMATIONS THAT CAUSE GASTROINTESTINAL HEMORRHAGE

Arteriovenous malformations (AVMs): Dilation of existing vascular structures

Type I AVM (angiodysplasia, vascular ectasia of the colon, vascular dysplasia of the colon)

Dilatation and ectasia of veins, venules, and capillaries in colonic mucosa and submucosa

Important cause of lower gastrointestinal bleeding

Majority of patients are older than 60 years of age

20%–25% have aortic stenosis

Usually are multiple and occur mainly in the right colon

Difficult to identify

Type II AVM

Rare, probably congenital

Bleeding usually occurs before the age of 50

Small bowel is the most common location but may occur anywhere

Larger than type I AVMs

May be visible at laparotomy

Type III AVM (hereditary hemorrhagic telangiectasia, Osler-Weber-Rendu syndrome)

Rare

Autosomal dominant

Throughout the gastrointestinal tract

Repeated bleeding episodes from nasopharynx and gastrointestinal tract

Most have a positive family history

Lesions readily visible on face, oral, and nasopharyngeal mucosa

TABLE 9-12B. VASCULAR ANOMALIES WITH ASSOCIATED SKIN LESIONS

Usually multiple and widespread

Hereditary hemorrhagic telangiectasia (Osler-Weber-Rendu syndrome)

Blue rubber bleb nevus syndrome

Calcinosis cutis, Raynaud's phenomenon, sclerodactyly, and telangectasia

TABLE 9-12C. VASCULAR ANOMALIES NOT ASSOCIATED WITH SKIN LESIONS

Angiodysplasia (vascular ectasia)

Most common

Affects older patients

Mostly in cecum and ascending colon

Also in small bowel and stomach, especially in those with underlying renal disease. In these, estrogen-progesterone therapy may be of use

Etiology unknown

Arteriography: Vascular tuft with early filling veings in the arterial phase. In the venous phase: Densely opacified dilated and slowly emptying draining veins.

Endoscopy: flat, bright red and "fern-like"

True Arteriovenous Malformations

Most likely congenital

Affects younger patients

Most common in the upper gastrointestinal tract

Consist of dilated, thick-walled arteries and nondilated, thick-walled veins that communicate with each other

Dieulafoy's Syndrome

Submucosal artery aneurysm eroding through an otherwise normal epithelium

Most common in gastric fundus, but also described in the small bowel

TABLE 9-12.

A–C, Different classifications of vascular malformations, of which arteriovenous malformations are the most common cause of gastrointestinal bleeding from the small bowel [62,63].

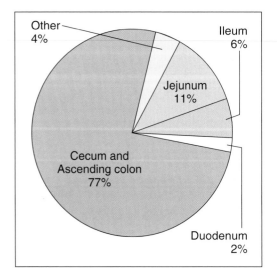

FIGURE 9-7.

Arteriovenous malformations (AVMs) in the gastrointestinal tract. In a revised series of 218 patients with confirmed AVMs [64], cecum with or without involvement of the ascending colon (77.5%) was the most frequent anatomic location for these lesions. AVMs were also found in the jejunum (10.5%), ileum (5.5%) and duodenum (2.3%).

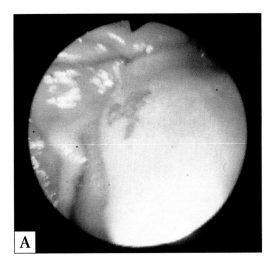

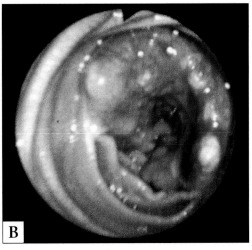

FIGURE 9-8.

Endoscopic views of small-bowel arteriovenous malformations found during enteroscopic evaluations in two patients with gastrointestinal hemorrhage of obscure origin. **A,** A lesion is found in the proximal jejunum using the push-type enteroscope. **B,** A similar lesion is found in the midjejunum by using the sonde-type enteroscope.

TABLE 9-13. CHARACTERISTICS OF PATIENTS WITH ARTERIOVENOUS MALFORMATIONS AS THE CAUSE OF GASTROINTESTINAL BLEEDING

Number of patients: 173

Sex ratio: men:women = 1.4:1 (102/71)

Mean age = 72.3 years (range 19–91)

Mean duration of symptoms = 26.5 months

Mean number of blood transfusions required = 23.2 units per patient

Associated Medical Conditions:

Valvular heart disease: 76

End-stage renal disease: 25

Cirrhosis: 15

von Willebrand's disease: 5

Previous radiation therapy: 4

Osler-Weber-Rendu disease: 1

TABLE 9-13.

Characteristics of patients with small-bowel arteriovenous malformations as the cause of gastrointestinal bleeding [7]. This table shows that the patient population with small-bowel arteriovenous malformations as the cause of gastrointestinal bleeding is older and has a chronic clinical course requiring multiple blood transfusions.

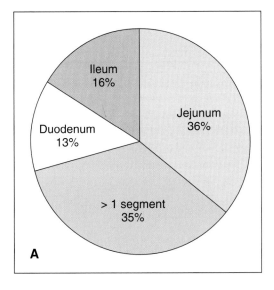

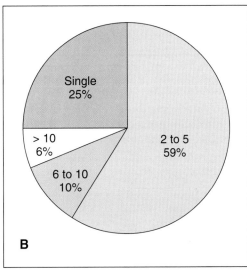

FIGURE 9-9.

Anatomic location of small-bowel arteriovenous malformations (AVMs) responsible for gastrointestinal bleeding [7]. **A,** In 173 patients diagnosed by enteroscopy with AVMs as the cause of gastrointestinal hemorrhage, lesions were found in one anatomic segment alone in 65% (111) of the patients. AVMs located in more than one anatomic segment were seen in 35% (62). **B,** Distribution by number of lesions found in these patients: single lesions were found in 44 patients (25%), 2 to 5 lesions in 100 (59%), 6 to 10 lesions in 18 patients (10%), and more than 10 lesions in 11 patients (6%).

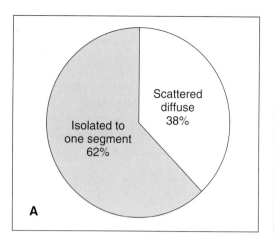

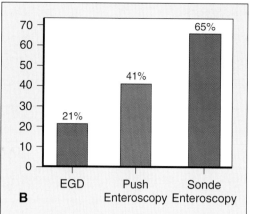

FIGURE 9-10.

Small-bowel arteriovenous malformations as the cause of gastrointestinal hemorrhage: distribution by anatomic segment (**panel A**) and yield of different endoscopic methods (**panel B**) [7].

TABLE 9-14. SMALL-BOWEL TUMORS AS THE CAUSE OF GASTROINTESTINAL HEMORRHAGE

General Concepts of Small-Bowel Tumors:

Represents only 1%–2% of gastrointestinal malignancies

Except for adenocarcinoma, small-bowel tumors are more common distally

Bleeding (overt or occult) is a prominent feature, being more common with benign than with malignant lesions.

Among malignant tumors, leiomyosarcoma is most commonly associated with bleeding. Bleeding with adenocarcinoma is less frequent, and rarely occurs with carcinoid tumors.

Sensitivity of barium studies depends on whether the calculation is made for any abnormality or only for the actual tumor. Thus, for malignant tumors the sensitivity for small-bowel follow-through when using the former criteria varies from 53% to 83% whereas it drops to 30% to 44% for visualization of the actual tumor. Enteroclysis, however, may increase these sensitivities up to 90% and 95%, respectively.

TABLE 9-14.

Small-bowel tumors as the cause of gastrointestinal hemorrhage [65–70]. This table shows some general concepts linked to small-bowel tumors as a cause of gastrointestinal bleeding, stressing the fact that benign tumors are more common than malignant tumors and that enteroclysis is a sensitive, noninvasive technique to detect them.

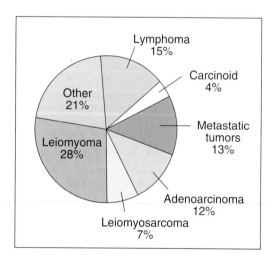

FIGURE 9-11.

Gastrointestinal hemorrhage of obscure origin arising from small-bowel tumors. Small-bowel tumors are found in 19% of patients evaluated for gastrointestinal hemorrhage of obscure origin when standard upper gastrointestinal tract endoscopy and colonoscopy are negative. Among 99 tumors reported as a cause of obscure gastrointestinal hemorrhage [1,2,4,6–10,12,13,15] primary smooth muscle tumors were the most common (35%); 28% were benign (leiomyomas) and 7% were malignant (leiomyosarcomas). Adenocarcinoma was found in 12% and metastatic tumors in 13%. Lymphoma of the small bowel was another common cause of gastrointestinal hemorrhage of obscure origin (15%), but carcinoid tumors represented only 4%. Other tumors, including those reported only as "neoplasms," represented 21% of the total. Small-bowel tumors are the most common cause of bleeding detected through enteroscopy in patients younger than 50 years of age [71].

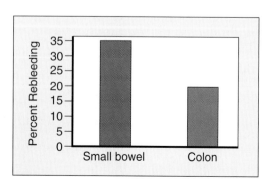

FIGURE 9-12.

Surgical treatment of arteriovenous malformations. Of a total of 65 patients [1,5,14,16, 34,54,61,72–74] undergoing resection for small-bowel arteriovenous malformations thought to be the source of bleeding, 23 (35%) rebled. The range of follow-up was 1 week to 54 months. For comparison, the rebleeding rate in a series of 102 patients with colonic angiodysplasias undergoing corrective surgery in whom postoperative data were available was 20% [64].

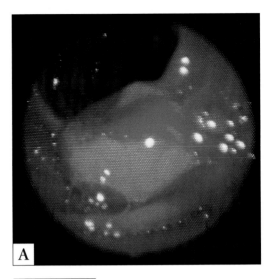 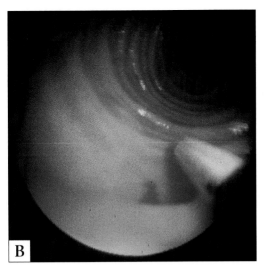 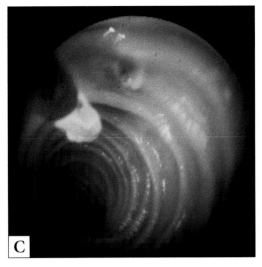

FIGURE 9-13.

Endoscopic views of a malignant-appearing tumor (**panel A**), a bleeding leiomyoma (**panel B**), and villous adenoma with adenocarcinoma (**panel C**) in three patients presenting with gastrointestinal bleeding of obscure origin. These diagnoses were made possible by enteroscopy.

TABLE 9-15. TREATMENT OPTIONS FOR SMALL-BOWEL BLEEDING LESIONS

OPTIONS	USEFUL IN THESE CIRCUMSTANCES	APPLICATIONS	LIMITATIONS
Medical Iron Supplementation Blood Transfusion Estrogen/Progesterone	1. Chronic slow bleeding 2. Patient unfit for invasive diagnostic work-up 3. Patient unfit for surgery 4. After rebleeding despite other therapies	Diffuse arteriovenous malformations (AVMs) Metastatic disease	Temporary Bleeding recurs if therapy stops
Endoscopic Heater Probe Electrocoagulation Laser	1. Active bleeding discovered during endoscopy 2. When multiple lesions are diffuse and therefore not suitable for surgical therapy	AVMs Ulcers	Endoscopic skills needed Persistent/recurrent bleeding
Radiographic Vasopressin Embolization	1. Active bleeding discovered during angiography 2. Patient unfit for surgery 3. Widespread metastasis	Ulcers Tumors AVMs	Temporary Recurrence Invasive
Surgical Excision Local Resection Segmental Resection	1. Bleeding uncontrolled by other modalities 2. Isolated bleeding lesion 3. Suspected malignancy	Tumors Meckel's diverticulum Isolated AVMs	Invasive Persistent/recurrent bleeding

TABLE 9-15.

Treatment options for small-bowel bleeding lesions. The four major therapeutic options for bleeding small-bowel lesions include medical, which is primarily directed to achieve secondary goals, and include iron supplementation, blood transfusion, or use of estrogen/progesterone preparations (*eg*, diffuse arteriovenous malformations, metastatic disease); endoscopic, directed to achieve primary goals, such as to arrest active bleeding, and remove or ablate the source of bleeding (*eg*, arteriovenous malformations, ulcers); radiographic, which include the use of vasopressin or direct embolization (*eg*, ulcers, tumors, arteriovenous malformations); and surgical, in which excision and local or segmental resection attempts to achieve primary goals (*eg*, tumors, Meckel's diverticulum, isolated arteriovenous malformations). Each option has utility in certain circumstances. Each modality has its own limitations. Thus, recurrent bleeding occurs frequently if medical therapy is stopped, therefore providing only temporary relief of the problem. Some techniques (all surgical and some radiographic) are considered invasive and may not be suitable for the fragile, unfit patient. Recurrent or persistent bleeding may also occur with endoscopic and surgical techniques, especially with multiple diffuse lesions. Special endoscopic skill is needed for performing enteroscopy with or without therapy.

TABLE 9-16. GOALS OF TREATMENT OF SMALL-BOWEL BLEEDING LESIONS

Primary

To remove or ablate the source of bleeding (*ie*, resection, endoscopic cauterization)

To stop active hemorrhage (*ie*, resection, endoscopic therapy, vasopressin infusion, or embolization)

Secondary

To keep normal or adequate hemoglobin levels, prevent rebleeding, and stop or reduce blood transfusion requirements (*ie*, blood transfusion, chronic iron supplementation, resection endoscopic cauterization, estrogen-progesterone preparations)

TABLE 9-16.

Goals of treatment of small-bowel bleeding lesions. Once the source of bleeding is identified, efforts must be made to treat these lesions to halt the chronic process the patient has been subjected to, and thus to improve his or her quality of life. Alternatively, whether the source has been or has not been identified, secondary goals, such as maintenance of normal hemoglobin levels and reduction in the number of blood transfusions, become important.

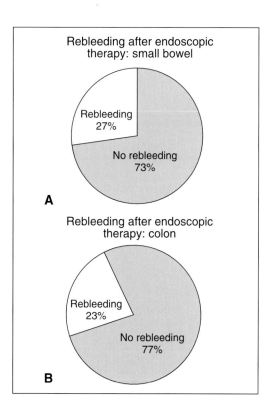

A — Rebleeding after endoscopic therapy: small bowel
Rebleeding 27%
No rebleeding 73%

B — Rebleeding after endoscopic therapy: colon
Rebleeding 23%
No rebleeding 77%

FIGURE 9-14.

Endoscopic therapy of angiodysplasias. Of 11 patients reported to have had bipolar (BICAP) electrocoagulation as the primary therapy of small-bowel angiodysplasias, the rebleeding rate was 27% [2] (**A**). In comparison (**B**), the rebleeding rate of 151 patients undergoing cauterization of large-bowel lesions (68 with BICAP [75], and 83 with Nd-YAG laser [76]) was 23%. The blood transfusion requirement after endoscopic electrocoagulation of small-bowel angiodysplasias (0.35±0.96 U/mo) was significantly decreased when compared with the transfusion requirement before therapy (2.34±3.0 U/mo) ($P < 0.0001$) [77].

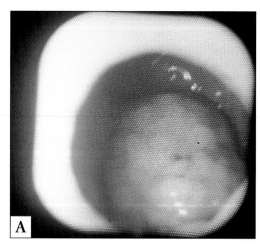
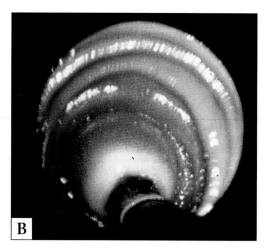

A **B**

FIGURE 9-15.

Endoscopic therapy of a bleeding small-bowel arteriovenous malformation. The malformation was found in the proximal jejunum with an enteroscope in a patient with recurrent bleeding and negative routine upper and lower endoscopy and a negative enteroclysis. **A**, A bipolar coagulation (BICAP) probe was passed through the working channel of the enteroscope and advanced toward the lesion. **B**, After a few gentle pulses against the vascular anomaly, successful electrocoagulation was achieved.

TABLE 9-17. HORMONAL THERAPY OF SMALL-BOWEL ANGIODYSPLASIAS

Author	Study Design	Patients (N)	Drug(s)	Results
Bronner *et al.* [78]	Uncontrolled	7	Mestranol 0.075–0.15 mg + norethisterone 1 mg	Arrested bleeding in all patients
Van Cutsem *et al.* [79]	Placebo-controlled	10	Norethindrone 1 mg + ethinylestradiol 0.05 mg	Significant reduction of bleeding in treated group ($P<0.002$)
Lewis *et al.* [80]	Cohort	64	Norethynodrel 5–10 mg + mestranol 0.075–0.15 mg or conjugated estrogens 0.625 mg	No difference in transfusion requirements

TABLE 9-17.

Hormonal therapy of small-bowel angiodysplasias. The mechanism of action of hormonal therapy in the setting of bleeding angiodysplasias (both acquired and inherited) remains unknown. Improvement in the endothelial integrity in patients with Osler-Weber-Rendu disease [81], blood stasis within mesenteric microcirculation in animals [82], shortened bleeding time in dialysis patients [83], and effects on the endothelium such as reduction in prostacyclin production [84] have been some of the phenomena observed in response to estrogen therapy.

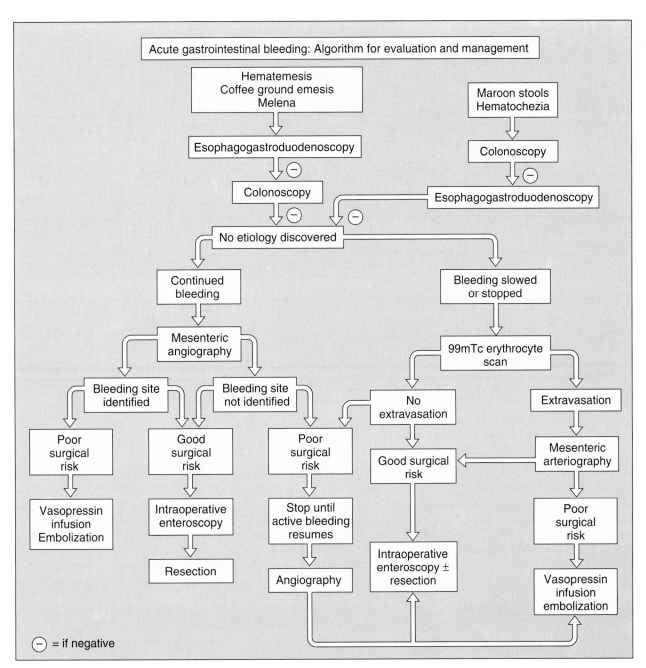

FIGURE 9-16.

This figure depicts a proposed algorithm for the evaluation and management of acute hemorrhage, whether it is from the upper or lower gastrointestinal tract.

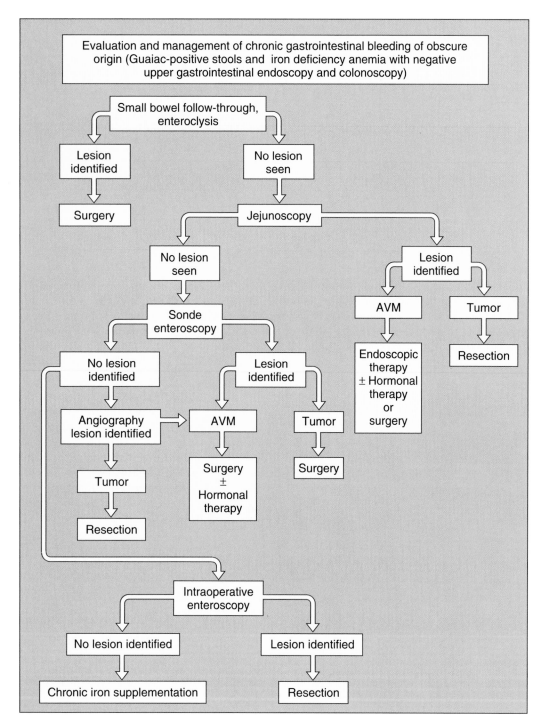

FIGURE 9-17.

Evaluation and management of chronic gastrointestinal bleeding of obscure origin (guaiac-positive stools and iron deficiency anemia with negative upper gastrointestinal endoscopy and colonoscopy).

■ REFERENCES

1. Thompson JN, Salem RR, Hemingway AP, *et al.*: Specialist investigation of obscure gastrointestinal bleeding. *Gut* 1987, 28:47–51.

2. Foutch PG, Sawyer R, Sanowski RA: Push enteroscopy for diagnosis of patients with gastrointestinal bleeding of obscure origin. *Gastrointest Endosc* 1990, 36:337–341.

3. Gostout CJ, Schroeder KW, Burton DD: Small bowel enteroscopy: An early experience in gastrointestinal bleeding of unknown origin. *Gastrointest Endosc* 1991, 37:5–8.

4. Ress AM, Benacci JC, Sarr MG: Efficacy of intraoperative enteroscopy in diagnosis and prevention of recurrent, occult gastrointestinal bleeding. *Am J Surg* 1992, 163:94–99.

5. O'Connell H, Martin CJ: Intraoperative enteroscopy in the management of bleeding small bowel lesions. *Aust N Z J Surg* 1992, 62:394–396.

6. Lau WY, Yuen WK, Chu KW, *et al.*: Obscure bleeding in the gastrointestinal tract originating in the small intestine. *Surg Gynecol Obstet* 1992, 174:119–124.

7. Berner JS, Mauer K, Lewis BS: Push and sonde enteroscopy for the diagnosis of obscure gastrointestinal bleeding. *Am J Gastroenterol* 1994, 89:2139–2142.

8. Retzlaff JA, Hagedorn AB, Bartholomew LG: Abdominal exploration for gastrointestinal bleeding of obscure origin. *JAMA* 1961, 177:104–107.

9. Briley CA Jr, Jackson DC, Joshrude IS, Mills SR: Acute gastrointestinal hemorrhage of small bowel origin. *Radiology* 1980, 136:317–319.

10. Tillotson CL, Geller SC, Kantrowitz L, *et al.*: Small bowel hemorrhage: Angiographic localization and intervention. *Gastrointest Radiol* 1988, 13:207–211.

11. Apelgren KN, Vargish T, Al-Kawas F: Principles for use of intraoperative enteroscopy for hemorrhage from the small bowel. *Am Surg* 1988, 54:85–88.

12. Fiorito JJ, Brandt LJ, Kozicky O, *et al.*: The diagnostic yield of superior mesenteric angiography: Correlation with the pattern of gastrointestinal bleeding. *Am J Gastroenterol* 1989, 84:878–881.

13. Rex DK, Lappas JC, Maglinte DDT, *et al.*: Enteroclysis in the evaluation of suspected small intestinal bleeding. *Gastroenterology* 1989, 97:58–60.

14. Desa LA, Ohri SK, Hutton KAR, *et al.*: Role of intraoperative enteroscopy in obscure gastrointestinal bleeding of small bowel origin. *Br J Surg* 1991, 78:192–195.

15. Chong J, Tagle M, Barkin JS, Reiner DK: Small bowel push-type fiberoptic enteroscopy for patients with occult gastrointestinal bleeding or suspected small bowel pathology. *Am J Gastroenterol* 1994, 89:2143–2146.

16. Hoffman JS, Cave DR, Birkett D: Intra-operative enteroscopy with a sonde intestinal fiberscope. *Gastrointest Endosc* 1994, 40:229–230.

17. Barkin JS, Chong J, Reiner DK: First-generation video enteroscope: Fourth-generation push-type small bowel enteroscopy utilizing an overtube. *Gastrointest Endosc* 1994, 40:743–747.

18. Rabe FE, Becker GJ, Besozzi MJ, Miller RE: Efficacy study of the small-bowel examination. *Radiology* 1981, 140:47–50.

19. Fried AM, Poulos A, Hatfield DR: The effectiveness of the incidental small bowel series. *Radiology* 1981, 140:45–46.

20. Sanders DE, Ho CS: The small bowel enema: Experience with 150 examinations. *AJR Am J Roentgenol* 1976, 127:743–751.

21. Alavi A, Dann RW, Baum S, Biery DN: Scintigraphic detection of acute gastrointestinal bleeding. *Radiology* 1977, 124:753–756.

22. Alavi A, Ring EJ: Localization of gastrointestinal bleeding: Superiority of ^{99m}Tc sulfur colloid compared with angiography. *AJR Am J Roentgenol* 1980, 137:741–748.

23. McKusick KA, Froelich J, Callahan RJ, *et al.*: ^{99m}Tc red blood cells for detection of gastrointestinal bleeding: Experience with 80 patients. *AJR Am J Roentgenol* 1981, 137:1113—1118.

24. Markisz JA, Front D, Royal HD, *et al.*: An evaluation of ^{99m}Tc-labeled red blood cell scintigraphy for the detection and localization of gastrointestinal bleeding sites. *Gastroenterology* 1982, 83:394–398.

25. Hunter JM, Pezim ME: Limited value of technetium 99m-labeled red cell scintigraphy in localization of lower gastrointestinal bleeding. *Am J Surg* 1990, 159:504–506.

26. Bentley DE, Richardson JD: The role of tagged red blood cell imaging in the localization of gastrointestinal bleeding. *Arch Surg* 1991, 126:821–824.

27. Gupta S, Luna E, Kingsley S, *et al.*: Detection of gastrointestinal bleeding by radionuclide scintigraphy. *Am J Gastroenterol* 1984, 79:26–31.

28. Bunker SR, Lull RJ, Tanesescu DE, *et al.*: Scintigraphy of gastrointestinal hemorrhage: Superiority of ^{99m}Tc red blood cells over ^{99m}Tc sulfur colloid. *AJR Am J Roentgenol* 1984, 143:543–548.

29. Sos TA, Lee JG, Wixson D, Sniderman KW: Intermittent bleeding from minute to minute in acute massive gastrointestinal hemorrhage: Arteriographic demonstration. *AJR Am J Roentgenol* 1978, 131:1015–1017.

30. Berquist TH, Nolan NG, Adson MA, *et al.*: Diagnosis of Meckel's diverticulum by radioisotope scanning. *Mayo Clin Proc* 1973, 48:98–102.

31. Diamond T, Russell CF: Meckel's diverticulum in the adult. *Br J Surg* 1985, 72:480–482

32. Mackey WC, Dineen P: A fifty year experience with Meckel's diverticulum. *Surg Gynecol Obstet* 1983, 156:56–64.

33. Sagar VV, Piccone JM: The effects of cimetidine on blood clearance, gastric uptake and secretion of ^{99m}Tc-pertechnetate in dogs. *Radiology* 1981, 139:729–731.

34. Schwartz MJ, Lewis JH: Meckel's diverticulum: Pitfalls in scintigraphic detection in the adult. *Am J Gastroenterol* 1984, 79:611–618.

35. Priebe CJ, Marsden DS, Lazarevic B: The use of 99m Tc pertechnetate to detect transplanted gastric mucosa in the dog. *J Pediatr Surg* 1974, 9:605–613.

36. Eisenberg D, Sherwood CE: Bleeding diverticulum diagnosed by arteriography and radioisotope imaging. *Dig Dis Sci* 1975, 20:573–576.

37. Farr CM, Iqbal R, Bezmalinovic Z, *et al.*: Bleeding Meckel's diverticulum in an adult. *J Clin Gastroenterol* 1989, 11:208–210.

38. Baum S: Pertechnetate imaging following cimetidine administration in Meckel's diverticulum of the ileum. *Am J Gastroenterol* 1981, 76:464–465.

39. Casarella WJ, Galloway SJ, Taxin RN, *et al.*: Lower gastrointestinal tract hemorrhage: New concepts based on arteriography. *AJR Am J Roentgenol* 1974, 121:357–368.

40. Moore JD, Thompson W, Appelman HD, Foley D: Arteriovenous malformations of the gastrointestinal tract. *Arch Surg* 1976, 111:381–389.

41. Welch C, Athanasoulis C, Galdabini J: Hemorrhage from the large bowel with special reference to angiodysplasia and diverticular disease. *World J Surg* 1978, 2:73–83.

42. Johnsrude IS, Jackson DC: The role of the radiologist in acute gastrointestinal bleeding. *Gastrointest Radiol* 1978, 3:357–368.

43. Boley S, DiBiase A, Brandt L, Sammartano R: Lower intestinal bleeding in the elderly. *Am J Surg* 1979, 137:57–64.

44. Wright H, Pellicia O, Higgins E, *et al.*: Controlled semi-elective segmental resection for massive colonic hemorrhage. *Am J Surg* 1980, 139:535–538.

45. Nath R, Sequeira J, Weitzman F, *et al.*: Lower gastrointestinal bleeding: Diagnostic approach and management conclusions. *Am J Surg* 1981, 141:478–481.

46. Bowden TA, Hooks VH III, Mansberger AR Jr: Intestinal vascular ectasias: A new look at an old disease. *South Med J* 1982, 75:1310–1317.

47. Britt L, Warren L, Moore O: Selective management of lower gastrointestinal bleeding. *Am Surg* 1983, 49:121–125.

48. Browder W, Cerise E, Litwin MS: Impact of emergency angiography in massive lower gastrointestinal bleeding. *Ann Surg* 1986, 204:530–536.

49. Spiller RC, Parkins RA: Recurrent gastrointestinal bleeding of obscure origin: Report of 17 cases and a guide to logical management. *Br J Surg* 1983, 70:489–493.

50. Flickinger EG, Stanforth AC, Sinar DR, *et al.*: Intraoperative video panendoscopy for diagnosing sites of chronic intestinal bleeding. *Am J Surg* 1989, 157:137–144.

51. Dabezies MA, Fisher RS, Krevsky B: Video small bowel enteroscopy: Early experience with a prototype instrument. *Gastrointest Endosc* 1991, 37:60–62.

52. Morris AJ, Wasson LA, MacKenzie JF: Small bowel enteroscopy in undiagnosed gastrointestinal blood loss. *Gut* 1992, 33:887–889.

53. Gostout CJ: Improving the withdrawal phase of sonde enteroscopy with the "push away" method. *Gastrointest Endosc* 1993, 39:69–72.

54. Greenberg GR, Phillips MJ, Tover EB, Jeejeebhoy KN: Fiberoptic endoscopy during laparotomy in the diagnosis of small intestinal bleeding. *Gastroenterology* 1976, 71:133–135.

55. Bowden TA Jr, Hooks VH III, Mansberger AR Jr: Intraoperative gastrointestinal endoscopy. *Ann Surg* 1980, 191:680–687.

56. Bowden TA Jr, Hooks VH III, Teeslink CR, *et al.*: Occult gastrointestinal bleeding: Locating the cause. *Am Surg* 1980, 46:80–87.

57. Yamamoto Y, Sano K, Shigemoto H: Detection of the bleeding source from small intestine: Intraoperative endoscopy and preoperative abdominal scintigraphy by technetium 99m pertechnetate. *Am Surg* 1985, 51:658–660.

58. Mathus-Vliegen EMH, Tytgat GNJ: Intraoperative endoscopy: Technique, indications and results. *Gastroenterology* 1986, 32:381–384.

59. Schwartz RW, Hagihara PF, Griffen WO Jr: Intraoperative endoscopy for recurrent gastrointestinal bleeding. *South Med J* 1988, 81:1106–1108.

60. Lau WY: Intraoperative enteroscopy—Indications and limitations. *Gastrointest Endosc* 1990, 36:268–271.

61. Lewis BS, Wenger JS, Waye JD: Small bowel enteroscopy and intraoperative enteroscopy for obscure gastrointestinal bleeding. *Am J Gastroenterol* 1991, 86:171–174.

62. Spechler SJ, Schimmel EM: Gastrointestinal tract bleeding of unknown origin. *Arch Intern Med* 1982, 142:236–240.

63. Peterson WL: Obscure gastrointestinal bleeding. *Med Clin North Am* 1988, 72:1169–1176.

64. Meyer CT, Troncale FJ, Galloway S, Sheahan DG: Arteriovenous malformations of the bowel: An analysis of 22 cases and a review of the literature. *Medicine* 1981, 60:36–48.

65. Zollinger RM, Stemfeld WC, Schreiber H: Primary neoplasms of the small intestine. *Am J Surg* 1986, 151:654–658.

66. Ashley SW, Wells SA Jr: Tumors of the small intestine. *Semin Oncol* 1988, 15:116–128.

67. Gourtsoyiannis NC, Bays D, Papaioannou N, *et al.*: Benign tumors of the small intestine: Preoperative evaluation with a barium infusion technique. *Eur J Radiol* 1993, 16:115–125.

68. Vuori JVA, Vuorio MK: Radiological findings in primary malignant tumors of the small intestine. *Ann Clin Res* 1971, 3:16–21.

69. Ekberg O, Ekholm S: Radiography in primary tumors of the small bowel. *Acta Radiol* 1980, 21:79–84.

70. Bessette JR, Maglinte DD, Kelvin FM, Chernish SM: Primary malignant tumors in the small bowel: A comparison of the small bowel enema and conventional follow-through examination. *AJR Am J Roentgenol* 1989, 153:741–744.

71. Lewis BS, Kornbluth A, Waye JD: Small bowel tumours: Yield of enteroscopy. *Gut* 1991, 32:763–765.

72. Iacconi P, Aldi R, Ricci E, *et al.*: Small bowel angiodysplasia: Usefulness of perioperative enteroscopy. *Ital J Gastroenterol* 1993, 25:68–71.

73. Biener A, Palestro C, Lewis BS: Intraoperative scintigraphy for active gastrointestinal bleeding. *Surg Gynecol Obstet* 1990, 171:388–392.

74. Kanter IE, Schwartz AJ, Fleming RJ: Localization of bleeding point in chronic and acute gastrointestinal hemorrhage by means of selective visceral arteriography. *AJR Am J Roentgenol* 1968, 103:386–399.

75. Gostaut CJ, Bowyer BA, Ahlquist DA: Mucosal vascular malformation of the gastrointestinal tract: Clinical observations and results of endoscopic neodynium:ytrium-aluminum-garnet laser therapy. *Mayo Clin Proc* 1988, 63:993–1003.

76. Jensen DM, Machicado GA, Kovacs TOG: Bleeding colonic angiomata: Diagnosis, treatment and outcome [abstract]. Gastrointest Endosc 1989, 35:173.

77. Askin M, Lewis B: Long term success of endoscopic cauterization of small intestinal angiodysplasia [abstract]. Gastrointest Endosc 1994, 40:P15.

78. Bronner MH, Pate MB, Cunningham JT, *et al.*: Estrogen-progesterone therapy for bleeding gastrointestinal telangiectasias in chronic renal failure. *Ann Intern Med* 1986, 105:371–374.

79. Van Cutsem E, Rutgeerts P, Vantrappen G: Treatment of bleeding gastrointestinal vascular malformations with oestrogen-progesterone. *Lancet* 1990, 335:953–955.

80. Lewis BS, Salomon P, Rivera-MacMurray S, *et al.*: Does hormonal therapy have any benefit for bleeding angiodysplasia? *J Clin Gastroenterol* 1992, 15:99–103.

81. Richtmeier W, Weaver G, Stretch W, et al.: Estrogen and progesterone therapy receptors in hereditary hemorrhagic telangiectasia. Otolaryngol Head Neck Surg 1984, 92:564–570.

82. Nagamine Y, Komatsu S, Suzuki J: New embolization method using estrogen: Effect of estrogen on microcirculation. Surg Neurol 1983, 20:269–275.

83. Livio M, Mannucci P, Vigano G: Conjugated estrogens for the management of bleeding associated with renal failure. N Engl J Med 1986, 315:731–735.

84. Hull R, Hasbargen J, Fall S, O'Barr T: Conjugated estrogens reduce endothelial prostacyclin production and fail to reduce postbypass blood loss. Chest 1991, 99:1116–1119.

Chapter 10

Mesenteric Vascular Insufficiency

ARVEY I. ROGERS
CHARLES M. ROSEN

The term *ischemia of the small intestine* covers a wide range of disorders that has as its unifying characteristic hypoxic injury caused by alterations in blood flow. A contributing factor is reperfusion injury occurring as a consequence of the production of toxic oxygen metabolites accumulating after blood flow has been reestablished [1].

Clinical presentations depend on anatomic factors such as the mechanism of ischemia (occlusive or nonocclusive), the degree of collateral circulation, the duration of the injury (acute or chronic), the site of ischemic insult, and the type of vessel involved (artery or vein) [1].

Advances in this area include a better understanding of the complex anatomic and physiologic factors regulating splanchnic circulation, refinements in interventional techniques for diagnosis and treatment, and improved intensive care unit support [1].

Mesenteric ischemic syndromes are common and often fatal. Although the improvements mentioned have reduced the previously high rates of morbidity and mortality, the clinician must have a very high index of suspicion and move rapidly to diagnose these syndromes if patients are to survive and their small intestines are to be salvaged [2].

■ PATHOPHYSIOLOGY

Arterial blood is supplied to the splanchnic viscera by the celiac, superior mesenteric, and inferior mesenteric arteries. The small intestine is at risk of sustaining ischemic injury when it is deprived of oxygen and nutrients necessary to maintain normal cellular metabolism and integrity. Decreased blood flow may be a consequence of poor systemic circulation or may result from local alterations in the splanchnic vasculature and flow dynamics. Stenosis of mesenteric vessels, embolic phenomena, vasculitis, primary thrombosis, or vasospasm can all cause inadequate perfusion at a cellular level. Whatever the cause, the end results of intestinal ischemia are the same: a broad spectrum of injury ranging from reversible functional abnormalities to transmural hemorrhagic necrosis of segments or all of the small bowel [3].

CLINICAL ASPECTS

Various clinical factors predispose patients to the occurrence of acute intestinal ischemia. Thrombosis of the superior mesenteric artery can occur in the setting of known vascular disease (severe atherosclerosis or vasculitis) or hypercoagulable states. Embolism occurs in the setting of atrial fibrillation (with or without atrial thrombus), valvular heart disease, or recent myocardial infarction. Mesenteric venous thrombosis should be considered in patients with known hypercoagulable states, such as polycythemia vera, pancreatitis, cirrhosis, carcinomatosis, or deficiency of antithrombin III, protein C, or protein S. Nonocclusive ischemia can result from shock, congestive heart failure resulting in poor cardiac output, or treatment with digitalis compounds, α-adrenergic agonists, β-adrenergic antagonists, or vasopressin [2].

PRESENTATION AND TREATMENT

Most patients with acute mesenteric ischemia have some degree of abdominal pain. Initially, it may be moderate, but can become severe; it is often accompanied by ileus, bloody diarrhea, and vomiting. The results of an abdominal examination may be entirely normal in the presence of severe pain.

Abdominal pain out of proportion to the physical findings should raise the suspicion of acute mesenteric ischemia in the proper clinical setting [2].

No pathognomonic abdominal findings exist early in the course of intestinal ischemia. Rebound tenderness and guarding occur late in the course, when they strongly indicate the likelihood of infarcted bowel. Leukocytosis and metabolic acidosis should heighten the suspicion that infarction and cell death have occurred.

Plain abdominal radiographic films are usually normal before infarction occurs. With time, dilated small-bowel loops, mucosal thumbprinting, pneumatosis intestinalis, or free air may be seen. Selective mesenteric angiography is the mainstay of diagnosis and provides the opportunity for initial treatment of both occlusive and nonocclusive forms of acute mesenteric ischemia [2].

The clinical picture of mesenteric venous thrombosis tends to evolve more slowly than that of arterial occlusion. Abdominal pain may be mild and is ultimately associated with diarrhea, which is frequently bloody, and with vomiting. Rapid referral for abdominal venography or contrast-enhanced computed tomographic scan is paramount.

Chronic mesenteric ischemia, also called *intestinal angina*, is the result of severe diffuse arteriosclerotic disease of the celiac, superior mesenteric, and inferior mesenteric arteries with total occlusion of two or more of these vessels, one of which must be the superior mesenteric artery. Clinical features include diffuse postprandial abdominal pain, chronic weight loss, and fear of eating. Diagnosis is by abdominal arteriography. Current treatment of this syndrome is primarily surgical [2].

ANATOMY

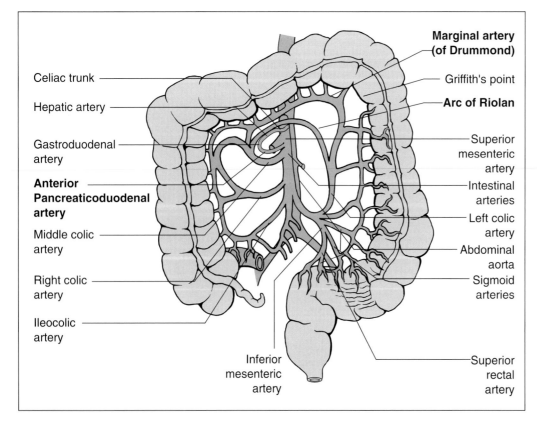

FIGURE 10-1.

Mesenteric arterial anatomy. Three unpaired arterial branches of the aorta provide the small and large intestines with arterial blood. Direct arterial flow to the small intestine depends on patent celiac and superior mesenteric arteries (SMA). Potential exists for the development of collateral (anastomotic) channels between celiac arteries and SMA, as well as between superior and inferior mesenteric arteries when gradual occlusion of the primary vascular trunks occurs. These collateral channels are represented schematically in Figure 10-4.

In most instances, veins parallel arteries in the mesenteric circulation. The superior mesenteric vein joins the splenic vein to form the portal vein, which enters the liver at its hilum. The inferior mesenteric vein anastomoses with the splenic vein near the point at which the superior mesenteric and splenic veins join to form the portal vein [1]. (*Adapted from* Rogers and David [1].)

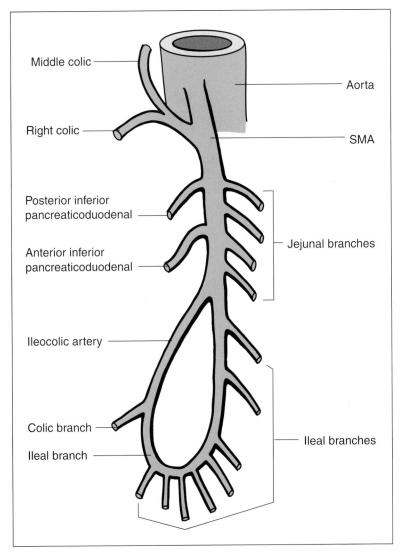

Middle colic

Right colic

Aorta

SMA

Posterior inferior
pancreaticoduodenal

Anterior inferior
pancreaticoduodenal

Jejunal branches

Ileocolic artery

Colic branch

Ileal branch

Ileal branches

FIGURE 10-2.

Anatomy of the superior mesenteric artery (SMA) [1]. The SMA originates posterior to the body of the pancreas and the splenic vein at the level of L-1. It arises just beneath the origin of the celiac axis, then proceeds downward and forward over the uncinate process of the pancreas and anterior to the third portion of the duodenum. The SMA perfuses the entire small bowel, cecum, and large bowel to the level of the mid-transverse colon as well as portions of the duodenum and pancreas. Its four major branches are the inferior pancreaticoduodenal, middle colic, right colic, and ileocolic arteries. There are also up to 20 jejunal and ileal branches. The main trunk of the SMA ends in the ileocolic artery, which supplies the terminal ileum, cecum, and right colon [1].

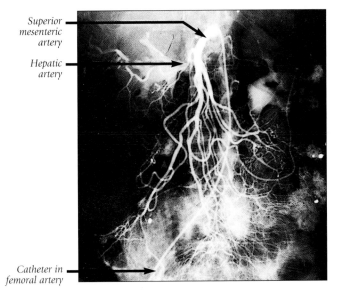

Superior
mesenteric
artery

Hepatic
artery

Catheter in
femoral artery

FIGURE 10-3.

Superior mesenteric artery anatomy seen arteriographically. This arteriogram was performed by selective injection of the superior mesenteric artery (SMA). The catheter is shown ascending from its entrance site in the right femoral artery, traversing the abdominal aorta, with the catheter tip in the SMA (obscured by the contrast medium). The hepatic artery is the first major branch, as seen in this patient; an anatomic variant occurs in approximately 25% of normal individuals [4]. (*From* American Gastroenterological Association [4]; with permission.)

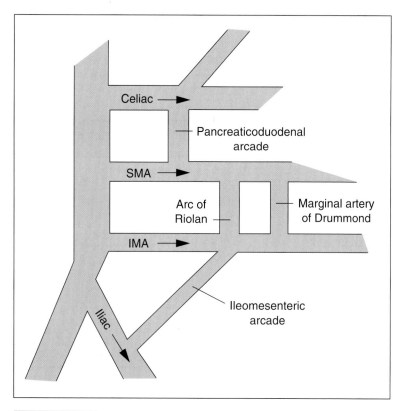

FIGURE 10-4.

Schematic representation of collateral channels among the three major mesenteric arteries. There are several major collateral channels between the three principal mesenteric arteries. Any one of the three major mesenteric vessels can supply all of the intra-abdominal viscera if adequate time has allowed development of alternative anastomoses and, therefore, collateral flow [1]. The major anas-

tomoses between the celiac artery (CA) and the superior mesenteric artery (SMA) are via the anterior and posterior branches of the superior pancreaticoduodenal artery that encircle the head of the pancreas and anastomose with the anterior and posterior branches of the inferior pancreaticoduodenal artery, a branch of the SMA [5,6]. This network is referred to as the *pancreaticoduodenal arcade*.

There are two key anastomotic connections between the SMA and inferior mesenteric artery (IMA). The most important is the one between the left branch of the middle colic artery (from the SMA) and the left colic artery (from the IMA). This tortuous artery is usually situated in an avascular area of the mesocolic mesentery, and is referred to as the *meandering mesenteric artery* or the *Arc of Riolan*. When present, the meandering artery indicates with certainty that either the SMA or the IMA has been occluded. The other important anastomotic connection is between the arterial arcades running along the mesenteric border of the colon. This arterial connection provides a continuous channel of collateral blood flow via the vasa recta to the small and large bowel [7]. This anastomosis is known as the *marginal artery of Drummond*. An important anastomosis between the mesenteric and systemic circulation exists via the superior hemorrhoidal artery (from the IMA) and the inferior hemorrhoidal artery (from the hypogastric artery, a branch of the iliac artery). These collateral channels help to maintain blood supply to the rectum [1].

Regions of the colon and rectum that are located at a point of arterial anastomoses may be fed by arteries of narrow caliber. As a result, they may be relatively underperfused during episodes of systemic hypotension. These "weak" points relate to the occasional absence of anastomosing arcades close to the gut wall. These gaps are often noted between the inferior pancreaticoduodenal artery and the first or second jejunal artery, as well as an absent or tenuous anastomosis at the splenic flexure. These areas, including the splenic flexure (SMA-IMA) and the rectosigmoid junction (IMA-hypogastric artery), are known as *watersheds* [1]. (*Adapted from* Rogers and David [1]; with permission.)

FIGURE 10-5.

Intramural vascular anatomy. The smallest branches of the mesenteric arterial arcades (*ie*, the vasa recta) arborize as they traverse the serosa, penetrate the muscularis, and terminate in the submucosal plexuses. It is estimated that the submucosa and serosa receive 75% of total intestinal arterial flow. The network of serosal arteries and branches of the submucosal plexus provide arterial flow to the muscular layers. Arteries to the mucosa separate into those entering the villi at their bases to branch into a dense capillary network and those penetrating the muscularis mucosae to perfuse the glands lining the crypts. The basic intramural vascular anatomy consists of the arteriole, the capillaries, and the venule. The viscosity of blood presented to the capillary network, the length of the vessel through which it must flow, and the vascular resistance encountered at the precapillary level influence flow characteristics across the capillaries through which exchange occurs [1]. (*Adapted from* Rogers and David [1].)

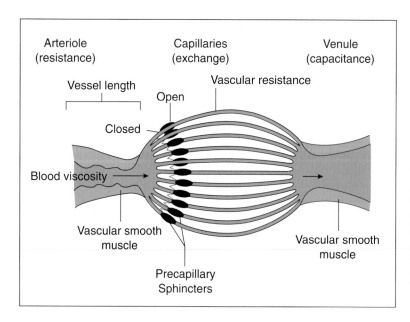

TABLE 10-1. VASCULAR RESISTANCE AND AUTOREGULATION

Extrinsic factors	Intrinsic factors
Neural	*Neural*
Sympathetic Nervous System	Enteric nervous system
Humoral	Myenteric plexus
Endocrine System	Submucosal plexus
Angiotensin II	*Humoral*
Catecholamines	Paracrine system
Gastrointestinal hormones	Serotonin
Secretin	Histamine
Cholecystokinin	Bradykinin
Gastrin	Prostaglandin
	Metabolic factors
	H^+, K^+, CO_2, lactate, osmolarity

TABLE 10-1.

Vascular resistance and autoregulation. Important factors influence the amount of extractable oxygen available to the mucosa, submucosa, and muscular layers delivered through the capillary network. Resistance is related to the fourth power of the vessel radius so that small changes in vessel diameter, can cause a marked reduction in intestinal blood flow. Extrinsic compression or luminal occlusion of arterial channels are the factors reducing arterial diameter. When arterial flow is compromised, the arteriolar capillary bed can enlarge (dilate) to maintain resting blood flow, but additional demands for arterial flow, such as meal stimulation, cannot be met. The ability to maintain constant blood flow is termed *autoregulation*. The process of autoregulation depends almost entirely on the arterial smooth muscle tone, which is responsive to local (intrinsic) and systemic (extrinsic) factors.

Neural (sympathetic nervous system) and humoral (angiotensin II, catecholamines, gastrointestinal peptide hormones) factors contribute to the extrinsic regulation of flow. Intrinsic regulation derives from the intrinsic nervous system of the gut (*ie*, the myenteric and submucosal plexuses), humoral and paracrine secretions, and metabolites produced as a consequence of both normal and compromised arterial flow [1].

TABLE 10-2. CAUSES OF VASCULAR INSUFFICIENCY

Nonocclusive factors (low flow)	Venous
Impaired cardiac output	Thrombosis
Reduced systemic arterial flow	Intrinsic
Vasoconstriciton (drugs)	Extrinsic
Occlusive vascular disease	Trauma
Arterial	Neoplasm
Thrombosis	Hypertension (*ie*, Portal)
Embolism	

TABLE 10-2.

Causes of vascular insufficiency. Occlusive or nonocclusive arterial disease leads to insufficiency of blood flow and may result in ischemia or infarction. Decreased cardiac output and systemic blood flow occur in hypotension resulting from hypovolemia, sepsis or hemorrhage, congestive heart failure, aortic stenosis, myocardial infarction, and arrhythmias. Examples of locally vasoconstrictive drugs include norepinephrine, vasopressin, and digitalis.

Arterial occlusion can be caused by a thrombus (usually on or into an atheromatous plaque), embolus, vasculitis, trauma, or neoplasm. Venous occlusion is secondary to thrombus (from a variety of hypercoagulable states), trauma, or neoplasm [4]. (*Adapted from* American Gastroenterological Association [4].)

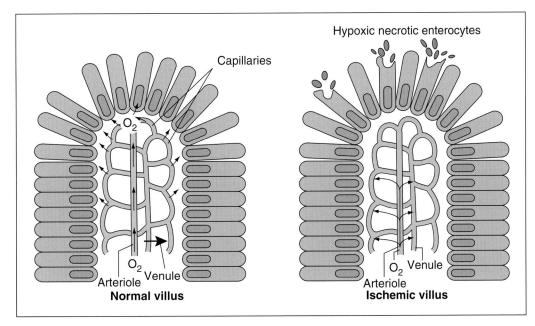

FIGURE 10-6.

Effect of ischemia on oxygenation of villus tip enterocytes. In the normal villus, most plasma oxygen is delivered to the villus tip by the arteriole and then flows into the capillaries before diffusing out to the enterocytes lining the villus. In the ischemic villus, an oxygen countercurrent exchanger extracts much of the plasma oxygen before it reaches the villus tip, thereby aggravating ischemia and killing the enterocytes. (*Adapted from* Levine and Jacobson [8]; with permission.)

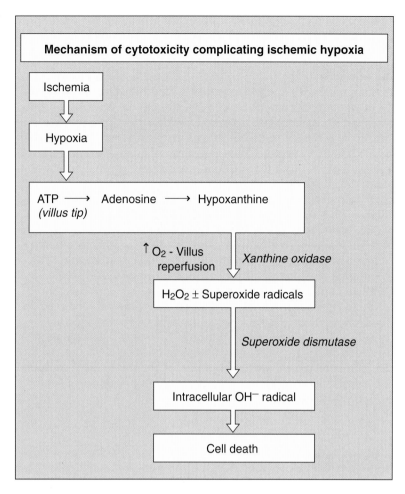

FIGURE 10-7.

Ischemic hypoxia of the gut: mechanism of cytotoxicity. One proposed mechanism of ischemic injury is that during a reduced blood flow state with resulting hypoxia, cellular metabolism shifts toward anaerobic conditions with conversion of adenosine triphosphate (ATP) to hypoxanthine. The most metabolically active cells in intestinal ischemia are the enterocytes of the villus tip. These cells contain a large amount of xanthine oxidase. During reperfusion of the cell with oxygen-rich blood, xanthine oxidase converts hypoxanthine into superoxide radicals (O^-_2), hydrogen peroxide (H_2O_2), and hydroxyl radicals (OH^-) within the cell. These final products are toxic to vital enzyme systems [4]. These active oxidants damage cells by causing disulfide formation in membrane proteins and by peroxidizing membrane lipids. These changes in membrane macromolecules increase cellular permeability to extracellular calcium and water. Active oxidants also inhibit cytoprotective agents, like nitrous oxide, and cause vasoconstriction, which intensifies local ischemia. In addition, active oxidants stimulate intracellular proteases, which exacerbate membrane leakiness. (*Adapted from* Levine and Jacobson [8]; with permission.)

■ CLASSIFICATION AND ETIOLOGY

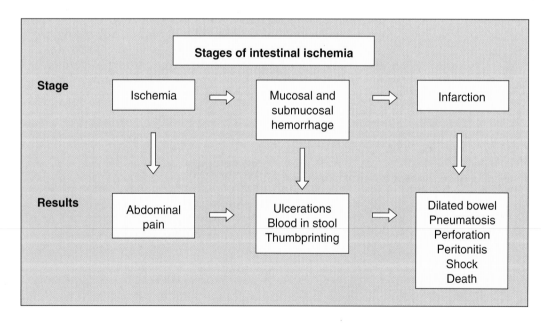

FIGURE 10-8.

Stages of intestinal ischemia. The clinical presentations of intestinal ischemia depend on the completeness and duration of impaired gut blood flow. In mild and potentially reversible ischemia, the only clinical feature is abdominal pain. Blood tests, stool studies, and radiographs are normal. If the ischemia progresses or is more severe initially, necrosis of the surface epithelium occurs with mucosal sloughing and submucosal hemorrhage. Complete infarction, which is irreversible, manifests itself as an "acute abdomen" with features of peritonitis. (*Adapted from* American Gastroenterological Association [4]; with permission.)

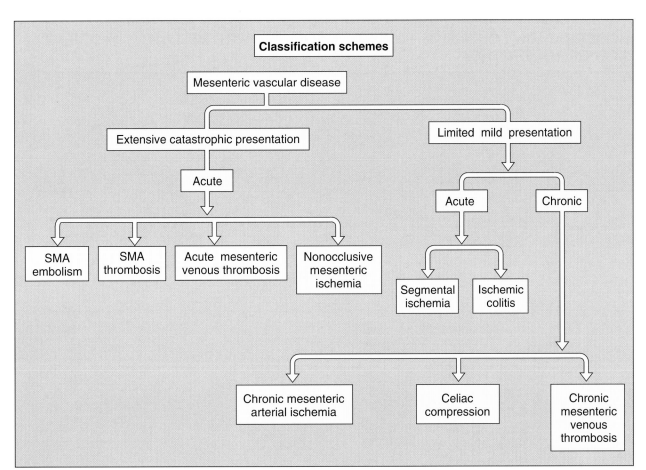

FIGURE 10-9.

Classification of mesenteric vascular disease based on the extent of ischemia. Previous classification schemes have been based on time (acute versus chronic), location (arterial versus venous and mesenteric versus colonic), and the character of the obstruction (occlusive versus nonocclusive). The classification scheme proposed by Williams, which separates disease entities into extensive ischemia and limited ischemia, may facilitate evaluation, diagnosis, and treatment of mesenteric vascular disorders [1]. (*Adapted from* Williams [9].)

TABLE 10-3. CLASSIFICATION OF SMALL INTESTINAL ISCHEMIC DISORDERS

MAJOR PATHOLOGICAL PROCESS	EXAMPLES OF DISEASE ENTITIES
SMA occlusion	SMA thrombosis or embolus
SMA low flow state without occlusion (SMA vasospasm)	Nonocclusive intestinal ischemia as in heart failure, aortic surgery, or circulatory shock
Miscellaneous processes	
Bacterial invasion in susceptible mucosa	Necrotizing enterocolitis
Mesenteric venous occlusion	Extension of a portal thrombus, compression of a mesenteric vein (strangulated hernia, hepatic tumor, ileus, volvulus, adhesions)
Arterial wall connective tissue inflammation	Periarteritis nodosa

TABLE 10-3.

Classification of small intestinal ischemic disorders according to the pathologic process. This organization is based on the predominant pathogenetic process and emphasizes the most common severe intestinal ischemic states. (*Adapted from* Levine and Jacobson [8]; with permission.)

TABLE 10-4. CONDITIONS THAT MAY CONTRIBUTE TO OR BE ASSOCIATED WITH MESENTERIC VASCULAR OCCLUSION OR INSUFFICIENCY

Embolic occlusion
  Cardiac diseases
    Rhythm
      Arrhythmia
      Atrial fibrillation
    Valvular disease
      Rheumatic heart disease
      Prosthetic heart valve
      Endocarditis
      Valvular stenosis
    Heart chamber disease
      Myocardial infarction
      Mural thrombus
      Atrial myxoma
  Vascular diseases
    Invasive radiologic procedures,
      angiographic manipulation
    Arterial plaques
    Vascular aneurysms
    Vascular dissections
    Trauma

Thrombotic occlusion
  Atherosclerosis
  Hypercoagulable state
    Sickle-cell disease
    Polycythemia vera
    Thrombocytosis
    Factor V Leiden mutation
    Antithrombin III deficiency
    Protein C or S deficiency
    Neoplasms (especially
      intra-abdominal)
    Pregnancy
    Migratory thrombophlebitis
  Vascular diseases
    Invasive radiologic procedures,
      angiographic manipulation
    Arterial plaques
    Vascular aneurysms
    Vascular dissections
    Trauma
Nonocclusive mesenteric ischemia
  Hypoperfusion
    Cardiac failure
    Hypovolemia
    Sepsis
    Vasoconstricting drugs

Mesenteric vein thrombosis
  Hypercoagulable states
    Sickle-cell disease
    Polycythemia vera
    Thrombocytosis
    Factor V Leiden mutation
    Antithrombin III deficiency
    Protein C or S deficiency
    Neoplasms (especially intra-abdominal)
    Pregnancy
    Migratory thrombophlebitis
  Local venous stasis
    Portal hypertension
      Cirrhosis
      Congestive splenomegaly
      After sclerotherapy of esophageal varices
    Compression of portal venous radicles by tumor
Portal hypertension
Intra-abdominal inflammation and sepsis
  Abscess (pelvic, intra-abdominal)
  Peritonitis
  Inflammatory bowel disease
  Diverticulitis
  Pancreatitis
Postoperative states
Trauma

TABLE 10-4.

Conditions that may contribute to or be associated with mesenteric vascular occlusion or insufficiency. Whatever the cause, the end result of extensive mesenteric ischemia can be similar and range from mild completely reversible intestinal injury to irreversible, transmural, hemorrhagic necrosis. The degree of ischemia and the length of bowel involved are factors that determine the clinical picture [1]. (*Adapted from* Rogers and David [1].)

■ CLINICAL SYNDROMES

Embolism

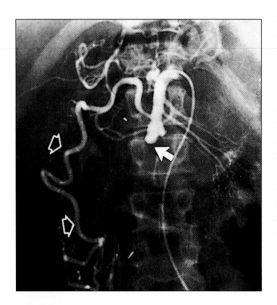

FIGURE 10-10.

Embolic occlusion of the superior mesenteric artery (SMA). The usual origin of a mesenteric arterial embolus is a mural thrombus from the left atrium or ventricle. Predisposing conditions include atrial fibrillation, rheumatic heart disease, prosthetic heart valves, myocardial infarction, ventricular aneurysms, and invasive angiographic procedures. The clinician should be alert to the possibility of embolism to a major mesenteric artery when severe periumbilical abdominal pain, vomiting, diarrhea, and leukocytosis arise acutely in the appropriate clinical setting. Emboli to the SMA most often lodge in the middle colic branch, but can affect any of its four branches. Emboli tend to lodge within 3 to 8 cm of the origin of the SMA, usually where the vessel narrows. This angiogram reveals occlusion of the SMA by a thrombus. The solid arrow points to complete occlusion distal to the origin of the middle colic artery. The open arrows reveal some collateral flow through the middle colic–right colic anastomosis [1]. (*From* Rogers and David [1]; *courtesy of* Stanley Baum, MD, University of Pennsylvania, Philadelphia, PA.)

Pneumatosis intestinalis

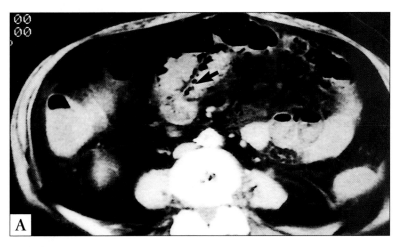 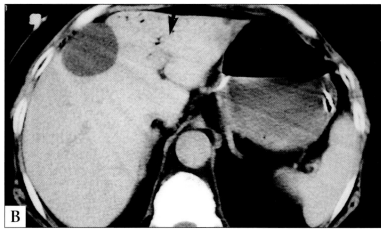

FIGURE 10-11.

Pneumatosis intestinalis with hepatic portal venous gas demonstrated by computed tomography. **A,** Gas collections within the intestinal wall, termed *pneumatosis intestinalis* (PI) in (*arrow*), can be a manifestation of a variety of disorders (*see* Table 10-6). **B,** The additional finding of hepatic portal venous gas (HPVG) (*arrow*) dramatically shortens the list given in Table 10-6. Portal venous gas is virtually always associated with bowel necrosis, bacteremia, or both. It generally represents a grave prognostic sign. Mesenteric vascular occlusion, as in this case, rapidly progresses to intestinal infarction and necrosis of long segments of small bowel, commonly associated with PI. HPVG is often present in this setting [10]. (*Courtesy of* J. Casillas, Miami, FL.)

TABLE 10-5. CAUSES OF PNEUMATOSIS INTESTINALIS

Mesenteric vascular insufficiency	Inflammatory	Miscellaneous
Intrinsic	Neonatal necrotizing enterocolitis	Whipple's disease
Mesenteric vascular	Septic enterocolitis	Leukemia
occlusion	Pseudomembranous enterocolitis	Sprue
Hypoperfusion	Toxic megacolon	Peptic ulcer
Mechanical strangulation	Crohn's disease	Diverticulitis
Volvulus	Inflammatory diarrhea of childhood	Caustic ingestion
Internal hernia	Simple bowel obstruction (any cause)	Trauma
Intussusception	Collagen diseases	Intestinal parasites
	Scleroderma	Idiopathic
	Iatrogenic	Pulmonary
	Endoscopy	Obstructive lung disease
	Umbilical vein catheterization	Pneumothorax
	Hydrogen peroxide enemas	Interstitial emphysema
		Pneumomediastinum

TABLE 10-5.

Causes of pneumatosis intestinalis (PI). PI is an important radiographic manifestation of a number of disorders—it is not a disease. In most clinical conditions PI is asymptomatic, and rapidly disappears once the underlying cause is ameliorated or treated [10]. (*Adapted from* Dodds *et al.* [10].)

Chronic intestinal ischemia

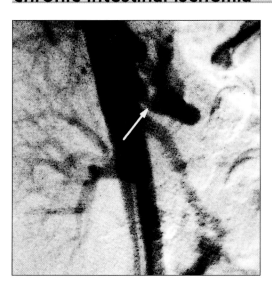

FIGURE 10-12.

Chronic intestinal ischemia. This can be encountered in patients with severe atherosclerotic disease of the splanchnic circulation. These patients present with postprandial abdominal pain, sitophobia (fear of eating), and weight loss. The site of arterial narrowing is often seen near the origin of the feeding artery from the aorta. Shown here is an oblique view of the abdominal aorta during digital subtraction angiography in an individual with chronic upper abdominal pain. There is stenosis of the celiac axis with poststenotic dilation (*arrow*). Although surgical reconstruction may be attempted, the results are often suboptimal. (*From* Pounder *et al.* [11]; with permission.)

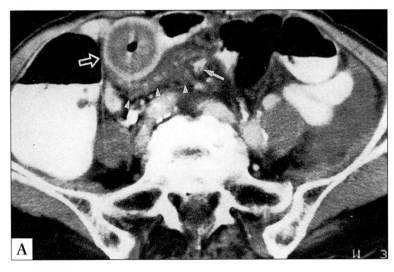

FIGURE 10-13.

Mesenteric venous thrombosis. **A**, Computed tomography with intravenous contrast exhibits marked thickening of the jejunal wall with alternating layers of high and low density and peripheral enhancement. The branches of the superior mesenteric vein have thrombus (*closed arrow*); mesenteric edema is present (*arrowheads*). **B**, The histology of the resected specimen reveals hemorrhage (H), edema (E), and thrombus in submucosal veins (*arrow*). (*From* Kim *et al.* [14]; with permission.)

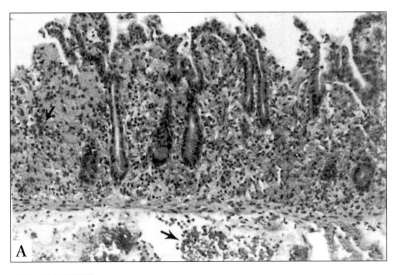

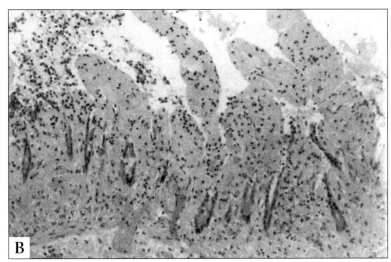

FIGURE 10-14.

Histopathology of ischemia in human small intestinal mucosa. A sequence of destructive changes overcomes the normal architecture of the bowel wall when there is moderate to severe ischemia of longer duration. (Both photomicrographs are x100 magnification with light microscopy). **A**, Moderately severe ileal mucosal injury presents with hemorrhage (*arrow*) in the lamina propria and submucosa, simplification of villi, loss of some villus tips, and partial detachment and injury of surface epithelial cells. **B**, Mucosal infarction produces complete denudation of the surface epithelium, villus ghosts, coagulative necrosis of most of the mucosa, and withered crypt bases. Both sections were obtained from the ileal mucosa of a patient with superior mesenteric venous thrombosis [8]. (*From* Levine and Jacobson [8]; *courtesy of* Dr. George Warren, Director of Pathology, Columbia-Rose Medical Center, Denver, CO.)

Celiac artery compression

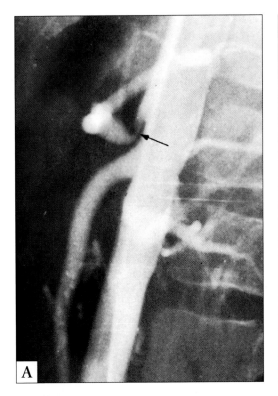

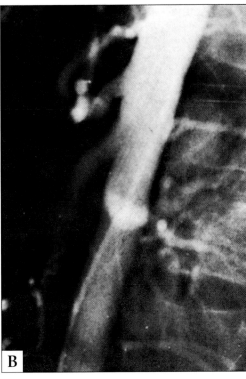

FIGURE 10-15.

Celiac artery compression syndrome. This syndrome presents as chronic recurring upper abdominal pain, which can be attributed to compression of the celiac axis (CA) by surrounding structures. Structures that may contribute to compression of the proximal CA include the inferior portion of the median arcuate ligament of the diaphragmatic crura and the celiac plexus. Patients with this syndrome are generally young and otherwise in good health. They are usually young women with complaints of abdominal discomfort, which is not consistently related to meals and is frequently associated with other symptoms, such as nausea, vomiting, and weight loss. A high- midline systolic bruit that decreases with inspiration may be the only helpful physical finding. The angiogram shown exhibits a smooth tapered compression of the CA in a 12-year-old boy with epigastric pain. A bruit could be heard over the epigastrium. **A,** The lateral abdominal aortogram shows compression of the CA by the median arcuate ligament (*arrow*). **B,** A repeat aortogram after surgical division of the constricting ligament reveals patency of the CA lumen. The child became asymp-tomatic after the surgery. Considerable forethought must be exercised before recommending surgery; this remains a poorly defined syndrome with an unproven pathogenesis [1]. (*From* Rogers and David [1]; *courtesy of* Stanley Baum, MD, University of Pennsylvania, Philadelphia, PA.)

Vasculitis

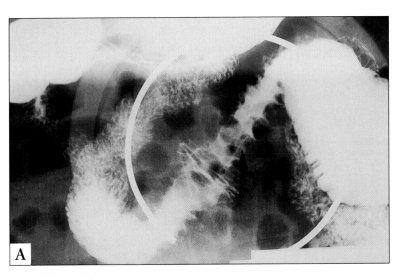

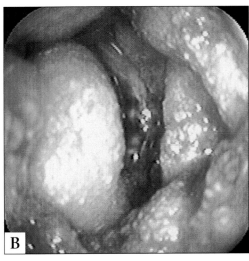

FIGURE 10-16.

Polyarteritis nodosa (PAN). PAN results in a necrotizing vasculitis of medium and small arteries. The presentation of a vasculitis affecting small intestinal arteries can be the first or only manifestation of the patient's disease. The vessel involvement in PAN is classically segmental, as in **panel A**. Note the mucosal effacement and thumbprinting (*arrow*) caused by submucosal edema on this barium contrast study of the upper gastrointestinal tract. **B,** An endoscopic picture of the acute stage of intestinal ischemia characterized by hyperemia and edema [15]. Endoscopy is an important adjunct for the clinician in diagnosis of ischemic diseases of the gastrointestinal tract. It enables a direct inspection of the intestinal mucosa and permits access to perform biopsies, if necessary [16]. (*Courtesy of* Tony DeMondesert, Fort Smith, AR.)

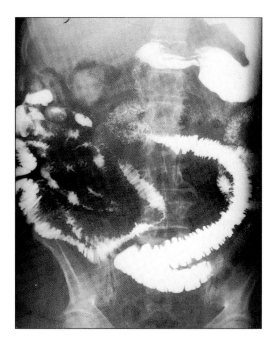

FIGURE 10-17.

Systemic lupus erythematosus (SLE). Vasculitis affecting the mesenteric vasculature is the most serious gastrointestinal complication of SLE. Patients can present with nausea, diarrhea, acute abdominal pain, or gastrointestinal bleeding. Infarction with perforation may also occur, presenting as an "acute abdomen." The prognosis in cases of perforation is poor, with a mortality rate of greater than 66% in most studies. The concomitant use of corticosteroids may mask these signs and symptoms. Histologically, a small vessel arteritis and venulitis are both seen. Thrombotic events leading to intestinal ischemia may also develop in patients with SLE due to the lupus anticoagulant and the antiphospholipid and anticardiolipin antibodies. In this figure the small bowel series in a patient with SLE shows the characteristic appearance of a bowel affected by vasculitis (*ie*, spiculation of the mucosa and separation of the small-bowel loops) secondary to edema of the bowel wall. (*From* Harris and Lewis [15]; with permission.)

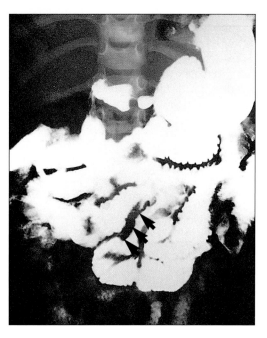

FIGURE 10-18

Henoch-Schönlein purpura. Henoch-Schönlein purpura, a small-vessel vasculitis, frequently involves the gastrointestinal tract. It is characterized by nonthrombocytopenic purpura, renal involvement, and colicky abdominal pain (with or without bloody diarrhea). This disease is most often seen in children between the ages of 4 and 7 years old. Pain may be related to intramural hemorrhage, secondary to the vasculitis. Pain, nausea, and vomiting may also develop if hematoma formation or resultant edema causes intussusception. This upper gastrointestinal series was taken of a 2-year-old child who presented with anemia, abdominal pain, and gastrointestinal bleeding. It reveals narrowing and ulceration of the jejunum and ileum (*arrows*), which are most commonly involved. This appearance can mimic Crohn's disease or lymphoma [15]. (*Courtesy of* Robert Feltman, Miami, FL.)

Volvulus and intussusception

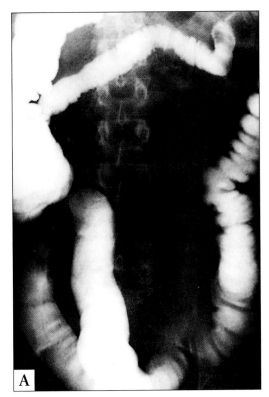

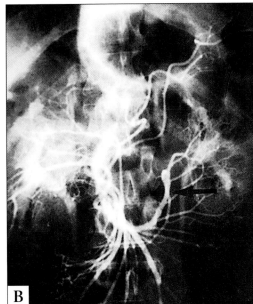

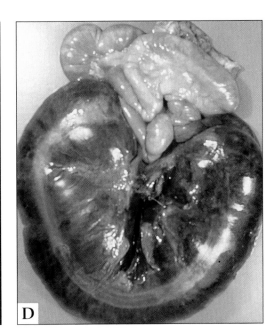

FIGURE 10-19.

Ischemia secondary to midgut volvulus in the adult. Symptomatic intestinal mal-rotation in the adolescent and adult is uncommon. Most cases are silent throughout adulthood and are discovered incidentally, unless there is acute or chronic abdominal pain. The most frequent presentation in the adult is midgut volvulus, usually self-limited and recurrent, but occasionally leading to vascular compromise and infarction. Severity depends on the degree of vessel occlusion and its duration. Surgical treatment of symptomatic patients involves defining the abnormal anatomy first, followed by taking down any adhesions that have formed subsequent to each recurrent volvulus. The intestine is then returned to its normal position. In the event of complete malrotation, the small bowel is placed on the right side. Operative fixation of the intestine is not required, because it will occur naturally through the formation of adhesions.

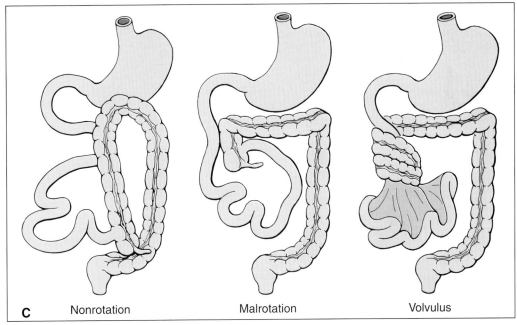

A, View of barium enema of a 46-year-old man with a 2-month history of severe postpran-dial midabdominal pain, bloating, sitophobia, and a 15-lb weight loss. This study reveals the cecum in the right upper quadrant and a long, straight terminal ileum. B, Superior mesenteric arteriography demonstrates the artery curling posteriorly to the left. The jejunal, ileal, and ileocolic vessels were seen higher in the abdomen than normal, and the vessels were abnormally curled toward the left, the so-called "barber-pole sign" (*arrow*). C, Anomalies of rotation and fixation [17]. D, Necrotic surgical specimen of an adult patient with midgut volvulus. (**A–C**, *From* Rowsom *et al.* [17]; with permission. **D**, *Courtesy of* M. Dapena, Miami, FL.)

TABLE 10-6. RADIOLOGIC ABNORMALITIES IN MALROTATION AND VOLVULUS

INVESTIGATION	POSSIBLE FINDINGS
Plain radiographic film of abdomen	Air fluid levels, subhepatic cecum
Upper GI series and small-bowel follow-through	Duodenal obstruction, right-sided duodenojejunal junction; right-sided small bowel, "corkscrew" small bowel, narrow-based mesentery
Barium enema	Mobile subhepatic or left-sided cecum
Angiography	Corkscrew or "barber pole" sign superior mesenteric artery; intestinal varices
Computerized tomography	Whirl-like encircling loops of bowel around superior mesenteric artery; superior mesenteric vein to the left of the superior mesenteric artery
Ultrasonography	Dilatation of distal duodenum (described in infants)

TABLE 10-6.

Radiologic abnormalities in malrotation and volvulus. Arriving at a diagnosis of intestinal malrotation and midgut volvulus in the adult is assisted by an awareness of the condition and recognition of the various radiologic abnormalities. Plain radiographs of the abdomen are frequently normal or may show a partial bowel obstruction. Suspicion may be raised if the cecum is malpositioned [17]. Abnormal rotation of the cecocolic segment may be seen on the barium enema. In the complete nonrotation, the entire colon and ileocecal valve may be found to the left of the midline [17]. The small bowel follow-through may reveal the abnormal position of the small bowel on the right side and may also delineate the ileocecal valve and malrotation of the cecocolic segment [17]. Angiography exhibits the aberrant anatomy of the superior artery (SMA). It normally courses down and to the left of the midline, with the vessels to the small intestine not overlapping. If abnormal, the SMA will be twisted like a corkscrew or described as having the "barber pole sign" [18]. Computed tomography and ultrasound (in infants) have been employed, as described. (*Adapted from* Rowsom *et al.* [17]; with permission.)

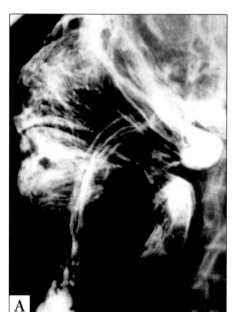

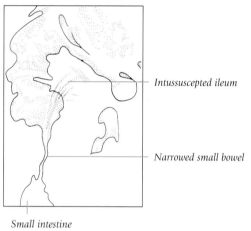

Intussuscepted ileum

Narrowed small bowel

Small intestine

FIGURE 10-20.

Intussusception. Intussusception is the invagination of a portion of the intestine into its contiguous distal segment. Any condition which causes hypermotility may result in an invagination. Examples in children include acute enteritis, allergic reactions, and intestinal spasm. In adults, it may be caused by a pedunculated tumor or polyp, an enlarged Peyer's patch, or a Meckel's diverticulum, which may mark the site at which the wall of the proximal segment turns and intrudes into its distal portion.

Intestinal ischemia may arise when the mesentery of the ensheathed portion of intestine becomes easily compressed, causing the development of edema, peritoneal exudation, vascular strangulation, and finally, intestinal gangrene.

Clinical manifestations include colicky abdominal pain that, as a rule, recurs at intervals of 15 to 20 minutes and is accompanied by signs of acute shock. In approximately 85% of the cases, a movable mass may be palpated in the abdomen.

(*continued on next page*)

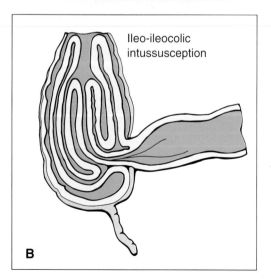

Ileo-ileocolic intussusception

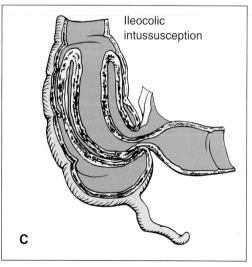

Ileocolic intussusception

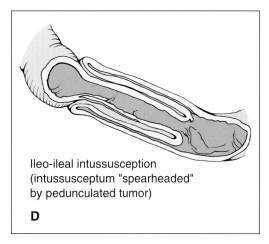

Ileo-ileal intussusception
(intussusceptum "spearheaded"
by pedunculated tumor)

D

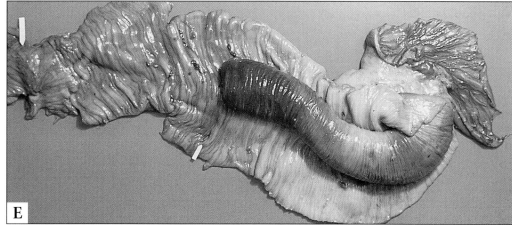

E

FIGURE 10-20 (CONTINUED)

The diagnosis can be established by barium studies (**panel A**); the types of invaginations are shown in **panels B** through **panel D**. Treatment of choice is laparotomy.

Resection is indicated when the lesion is irreducible or when the intestinal loops have been irreversibly compromised (**panel E**). In general, the prognosis of this disease is favorable [19]. (**E**, *Courtesy of* M. Dapena, Miami, Fl).

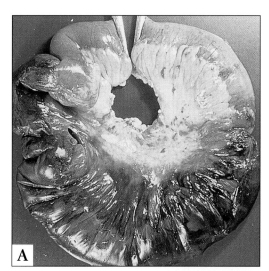

A

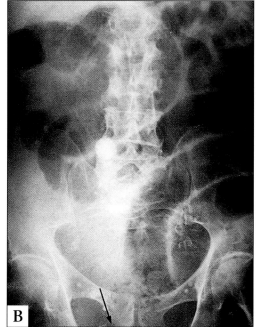

B

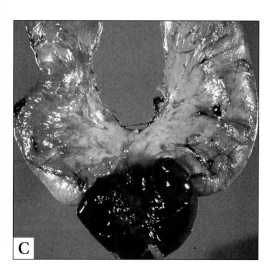

C

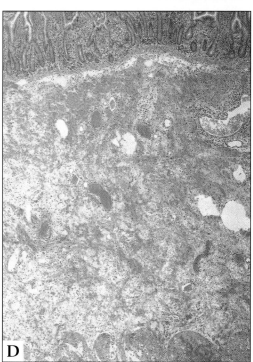

D

FIGURE 10-21.

Strangulated hernia. The diagnosis of strangulation (*ie*, obstruction of the blood supply of a herniated viscus) is usually not difficult. A sharp pain over a tender hernial area is present. Vomiting of gastric contents begins early, but its character changes to bilious shortly thereafter, followed by a feculent quality. Signs and symptoms of shock very quickly develop, requiring urgent surgical intervention. Depending on whether the incarcerated loop is still viable (return of normal color, restoration of elasticity, firmness, and shiny appearance) or has lost its vitality (black, green, or yellowish patches; loss of peritoneal luster; flabby consistency), as in **panel A**, one may either return the loop of bowel into the peritoneal cavity or resect it and perform an end-to-end anastomosis or an exteriorization [19].

B, Dilated, obstructed small bowel loops are seen on this plain abdominal radiograph of another patient; air is noted within the strangulated small bowel loop seen outside the peritoneal cavity (*arrow*) trapped within a hernial sac. C, Resected specimen from a third patient with a strangulated inguinal hernia. Note the gangrenous loop of small bowel. D, Histologic view of the surgical specimen in **panel C**, which reveals mucosal and submucosal edema, congestion, and extravasation of erythrocytes [13]. (**A**, *Courtesy of* M. Dapena, Miami, FL. **B–D**, *From* Pounder *et al.* [11]; with permission.)

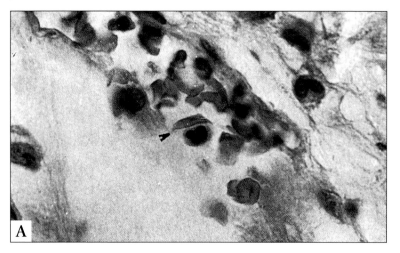
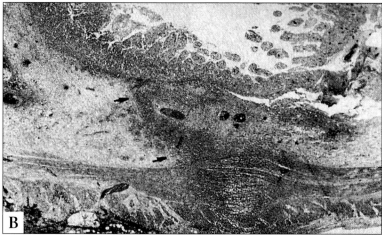

FIGURE 10-22.

Focal small bowel ischemia in the setting of sickle-cell disease. Focal small bowel ischemia can be the result of limited embolism or thrombosis in the setting of a hypercoagulable state, diabetes, collagen-vascular diseases, or, as in this case, sickle-cell disease. **A,** Note the sickled erythrocyte (*arrow*) in a zone of interstitial edema (hematoxylin and eosin stain, original magnification ×268). This microscopic slide was taken from a patient with sickle-cell syndrome with end-stage renal disease who presented with abdominal pain. Complete small-bowel obstruction and diffuse peritonitis necessitated emergency surgery, after which, necrosis of the terminal ileum was found. **B,** Histologically, the bowel wall was edematous with congested blood vessels. Hemorrhagic necrosis involved all layers of the small intestine, and the mucosa was partially ulcerated. Perivascular infiltrates of acute and chronic inflammatory cells were present in the nonviable segment, as well as at the interface between normal and necrotic tissue. Prominent infiltrates of neutrophils were noted at the serosa and within the mesenteric adipose tissue [20].

Because collateral circulation is often adequate to prevent transmural infarction, segmental ischemia is not ordinarily associated with the severe systemic consequences of extensive bowel ischemia. The diagnosis is usually made at laparotomy. Incomplete tissue necrosis can result in complete healing, chronic enteritis, or stricture. The treatment of segmental ischemia is usually surgical, with resection of the diseased segment (as in this case) [1]. (*From* Engelhardt *et al.* [20]; with permission.)

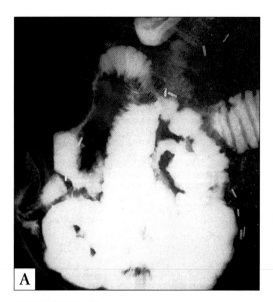
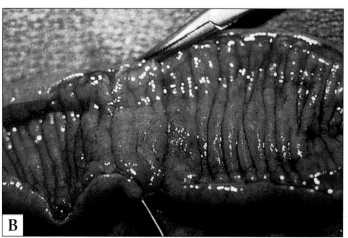

FIGURE 10-23.

Radiation injury to the small intestine. The initial effects of irradiation to the bowel are a direct injury to the intestinal mucosa. Later injury usually appears between 6 and 24 months after radiotherapy, and appears to be secondary to the effects of radiation on the vasculature of the bowel. A progressive vasculitis begins and leads to subendothelial proliferation, medial wall thickening, and interstitial collagen deposition. Ischemia and necrosis occur as small vessels are slowly occluded. Histologically, large foam cells are seen in the subintimal layer with hyaline ring formation around small arteries. Mucosal ulcerations may cause pain or bleeding, and strictures of the bowel wall may develop. Injury seldom occurs with total doses of less than 4000 rads. Concomitant diseases that decrease mesenteric blood flow, such as congestive heart failure, compound the risk of late radiation injury.

A, An upper gastrointestinal series of a 62-year-old white female who 10 years previously had undergone a total abdominal hysterectomy (TAH) and bilateral salpingo-oophorectomy for stage II endometrial carcinoma. She had received 5000 rads to her pelvis 3 weeks before the TAH. She was admitted with crampy abdominal pain, nausea, vomiting, and 3 days of obstipation. This patient had been admitted many times over the previous 2 years for recurrent partial small-bowel obstruction. This radiograph reveals multiple strictures of the distal ileum with an abnormal mucosal pattern. **B,** A localized stricture in the surgical specimen of the distal ileum [21]. (*From* Sher and Bauer [21]; with permission.)

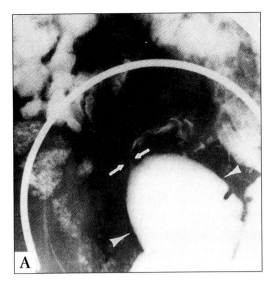
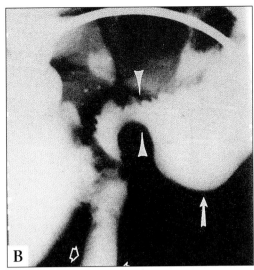
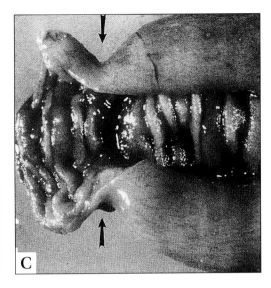

FIGURE 10-24.

Intestinal ischemia related to trauma. The cases shown are from seat-belt injuries sustained in two children after automobile accidents. Both children were readmitted to the hospital with small intestinal obstruction some time after the injury. Barium studies in one case revealed a stricture in the midjejunum in one case (**panel A**) and in the ileum in the other case (**panel B**). The gross specimen of the midjejunum from **panel A** is seen in **panel C**. Note the fibrotic stricture in this longitudinally opened specimen [22,23].

A seat belt may cause blunt trauma to the abdomen with contusion or perforation of the bowel and mesenteric hematoma. Various mechanisms of injury include compression of the intestine between

the vertebrae and the anterior abdominal wall, sudden increase in intraluminal pressure, and tangential tears at fixed points along the bowel. Most patients who have these injuries are symptomatic immediately following the accident. As in these cases, however, signs and symptoms caused by an intestinal stricture can arise a few weeks later [23].

Injury to the mesentery may lead to bowel ischemia with subsequent infarction of the affected segment, which then heals by fibrosis resulting in luminal narrowing. Hematoma or perforation of the bowel may also compromise blood supply and consequent stricture formation [23]. (*From* Shalaby-Rana *et al.* [23]; with permission.)

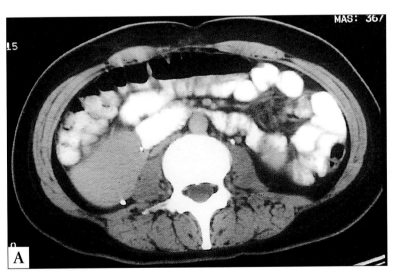
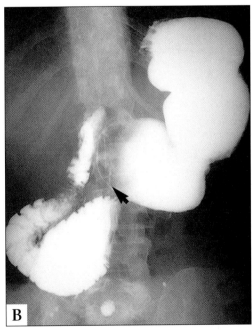

FIGURE 10-25.

Superior mesenteric artery (SMA) syndrome. The SMA branches off from the aorta at an acute angle and, coursing in the root of the mesentery, crosses over the duodenum, usually just to the right of the midline. Rarely, the SMA may pinch the duodenum as it crosses over it (as seen in the computed tomographic scan in **panel A**), possibly because of a more acute angle than normal, between the aorta and the SMA. This may be caused by substantial weight loss, reducing the size of the fat pad separating the SMA from the second and third portions of the

duodenum. Clinical features include epigastric fullness and bloating after meals, bilious vomiting, and midabdominal, crampy pain that may be alleviated by assuming a prone or knee-chest position. The upper gastrointestinal series in **panel B** reveals the stomach and proximal duodenum to be dilated, with a sharp duodenal cut-off just to the right of the midline (*arrow*). Acute treatment involves nasogastric tube decompression with intravenous fluid and electrolyte replacement [24]. (*Courtesy of* Al Weinfield and Martin Tagle, Miami, FL).

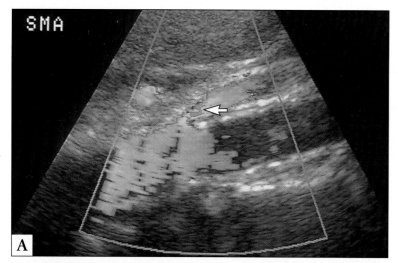

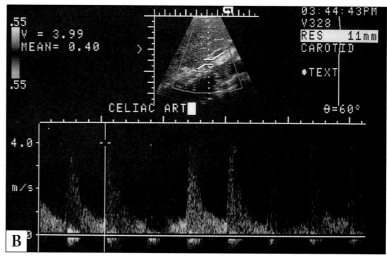

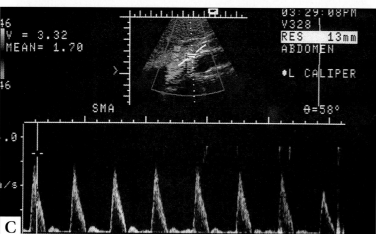

FIGURE 10-26.

Doppler duplex scanning in chronic arterial ischemia. In the study by Moneta *et al.* 100 patients were studied prospectively and findings at Doppler duplex scanning were compared with a lateral aortogram taken within 2 weeks. Fasting peak systolic velocity of greater than 200 cm/sec or no flow in the celiac axis (CA) and a velocity over 275 cm/sec or absence of flow in the superior mesenteric artery (SMA) predicted a 70% or greater stenosis.

The color Doppler in **panel A** is from a patient with chronic abdominal pain and weight loss. It reveals a narrowing of the origin of the SMA (*arrow*) with "aliasing" (*ie,* a change in the color map to blue, indicating an elevated velocity) (Montalvo B, personal communication, June 1995).

In **panel B** and **panel C**, which display spectral wave forms, the peak systolic velocity in the celiac axis (**panel B**) is 400 cm/sec and in the SMA (**panel C**) is 332 cm/sec. Both values are well above their respective upper limit of normal and predict at least a 70% stenosis of both vessels (Montalvo B, personal communication, June 1995). (*Courtesy of* Berta Montalvo, Miami, FL.)

TABLE 10-7. ROUTINE TESTS FOR PATIENTS WITH SUSPECTED INTESTINAL ISCHEMIA

TESTS	FINDINGS WITH ISCHEMIA	NONVASCULAR CAUSES OF FINDING
Routine Laboratory	Anion gap acidosis	Any abdominal catastrophe
	Leukocytosis/bandemia	Any acute inflammation or sepsis
	Hyperamylasemia	Pancreatitis, bowel perforation, penetrating ulcer
Flat and upright radiographs of the abdomen	Thickened bowel wall	Other inflammatory bowel diseases [IBD] (acute dysentery)
	Free intraperitoneal gas	Perforation (diverticulitis, appendicitis, IBD, ulcer)
	Gas in portal venous system or linear pneumatosis	Any cause of bowel infarction

TABLE 10-7.

Routine tests for suspected intestinal ischemia. If ischemia is considered likely in a patient with acute abdominal pain, the laboratory and radiologic studies undertaken may offer supporting evidence and assist in establishing a diagnosis far more rapidly. These tests are insensitive, however, and are usually positive only when infarction has already occurred (*eg,* acidosis). In addition, these tests are nonspecific with similar results (*eg,* hyperamylasemia) present in other disease processes. On the contrary, routine abdominal radiographs or computed tomographic scans revealing intraperitoneal free air or gas in the portal venous system in this setting offer compelling evidence of intestinal infarction and should lead to immediate surgical intervention. (*Adapted from* Levine and Jacobson [8]; with permission.)

TABLE 10-8. SENSITIVITY, SPECIFICITY, POSITIVE PREDICTIVE VALUE, AND NEGATIVE PREDICTIVE VALUE OF DOPPLER DUPLEX SCANNING IN DETECTING 70% OR MORE STENOSIS IN THE CELIAC ARTERY OR SUPERIOR MESENTERIC ARTERY

	VISUALIZATION, %	SENSITIVITY, %	SPECIFICITY, %	PPV, %	NPV, %
Celiac artery	83	87	80	63	94
Superior mesenteric artery	93	92	96	80	99

NPV—negative predictive value; PPV—positive predictive value.

TABLE 10-8.

Sensitivity, specificity, positive predictive value, and negative predictive value of Doppler duplex scanning in detecting 70% or greater stenosis in the celiac artery or superior mesenteric artery (SMA). Using the criteria mentioned in Figure 10-26, a high accuracy is achieved in predicting a 70% or greater stenosis, particularly for the SMA. End diastolic velocity is less reliable than peak systolic velocity. Other sonographic and Doppler criteria, such as the enlargement of the inferior mesenteric artery, retrograde and turbulent flow in the hepatic artery, and postprandial effects on flow, may increase the accuracy of these techniques [12,13]. (*Adapted from* Moneta *et al.* [12].)

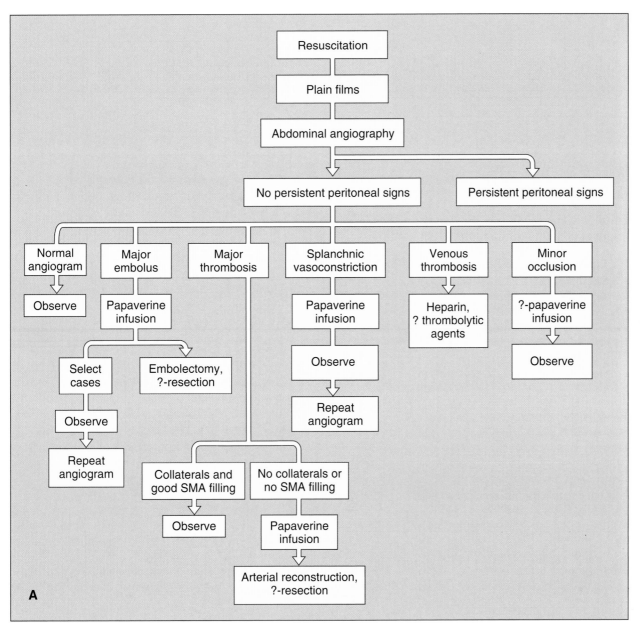

A

FIGURE 10-27.

Algorithm for the management of extensive mesenteric vascular ischemia in the absence (**panel A**) and presence (**panel B**) of persistent peritoneal signs [1]. Factors that increase the risk of mesenteric ischemia include age greater than 50 years old, previous myocardial infarction or embolic events, cardiac arrhythmia, valvular or rheumatic heart disease, low cardiac output, invasive vascular procedures and the use of oral contraception. As described by Boley *et al* [25,26], if a patient with any of these risk factors presents with acute onset of abdominal pain that persists for more than 2 or 3 hours, the diagnosis of extensive mesenteric ischemia must be suspected, and the above protocol for evaluation and treatment should be initiated. The only way to decrease the morbidity and mortality of visceral ischemic injury is by

(*continued on next page*)

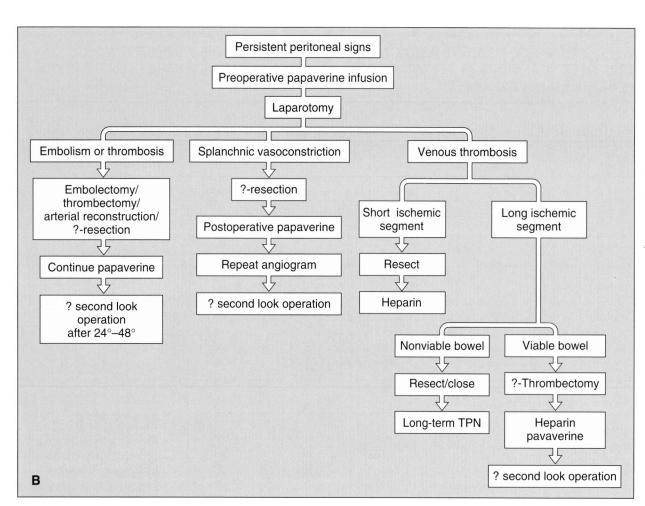

FIGURE 10-27. (*CONTINUED*)

having a high index of suspicion and employing early angiographic examination supplemented by selective mesenteric vasodilation or urgent surgery, when appropriate. If the diagnosis is made after intestinal infarction occurs, the mortality rate is between 70% and 90%. (*Adapted from* Rogers and David [1]; with permission.)

REFERENCES

1. Rogers AI, David S: Intestinal blood flow and diseases of vascular impairment. In *Bockus Gastroenterology*, vol 2, edn 5. Edited by Haubrich WS, Fenton S. Philadelphia: WB Saunders; 1995:1212–1234.

2. Giannella RA: The small intestine. In *Medical Knowledge Self-Assessment Program in the Subspecialty of Gastroenterology and Hepatology.* Edited by Rogers AI. Philadelphia: American College of Physicians; 1993:87–88.

3. Brandt LJ, Boley SJ: Ischemic and vascular lesions of the bowel. In *Gastrointestinal Disease*, vol 2, edn 5. Edited by Sleisenger MH, Fordtran JS. Philadelphia: WB Saunders, 1992:1927–1948.

4. American Gastroenterological Association: *Undergraduate Teaching Project in Gastroenterology and Liver Disease.* Timonium, Maryland: Milner-Fenwick; 1983.

5. Muller RF, Figlu MM: The arteries of the abdomen, pelvis and thigh. *AJR Am J Roentgenol* 1957, 77:296–311.

6. Rogers AI, Cohen JL: Ischemic bowel disease. In *Bockus Gastroenterology*, 4th edition. Edited by Berk JE, Haubrich WS, Kalser MH, et al. Philadelphia: WB Saunders; 1985:1915–1936.

7. Kornblith PL, Boley SJ, Whitehouse BS: Anatomy of the splanchnic circulation. *Surg Clin North Am* 1992, 72:1–30.

8. Levine JS, Jacobson ED: Intestinal ischemic disorders *Dig Dis* 1995, 13:3–24.

9. Williams LF Jr: Mesenteric ischemia. *Surg Clin North Am* 1988, 68:331–353.

10. Dodds WJ, Stewart ET, Goldberg HI: Pneumatosis intestinalis associated with hepatic portal venous gas. *Dig Dis* 1976, 21:992–995.

11. Pounder RE, Allison MC, Dhillon AP: *A Color Atlas of Digestive System* London: Wolfe Publishing Co., 1989:126–127.

12. Moneta GL, Lee RW, Yeager RA, *et al.*: Mesenteric duplex scanning: A blinded prospective study. *J Vasc Surg* 1993, 17:79–86.

13. Shorron P, Lamb G: Radiology of the small intestine. *Curr Opin Gastroenterol* 1994, 10:163–170.

14. Kim JY, Ha HK, Byun JY, *et al.*: Intestinal infarction secondary to mesenteric venous thrombosis: CT-pathologic correlation. *J Comput Assist Tomogr* 1993, 17:382–385.

15. Harris MT, Lewis BS: Systemic diseases affecting the mesenteric circulation. *Surg Clin North Am* 1992, 72:245–259.

16. Kurland B, Brandt LJ, Delany HM: Diagnostic tests for intestinal ischemia. *Surg Clin North Am* 1992, 72:97.

17. Rowsom JT, Sullivan SN, Girvan DP: Midgut volvulus in the adult: A complication of intestinal malrotation. *J Clin Gastroenterol* 1987, 9:212–216.

18. Buranasir SI, Bawm S, Nusbaum M, Turren H: The angiographic diagnosis of midgut malrotation with volvulus in adults. *Radiology* 1973, 109:555–556.

19. Netter F: *The CIBA Collection of Medical Illustrations: The Digestive System*, vol 3. Edited by Oppenheimer E. West Caldwell, New Jersey: CIBA Pharmaceuticals; 1987.

20. Engelhardt T, Pulitzer DR, Etheredge EE: Ischemic intestinal necrosis as a cause of atypical abdominal pain in a sickle cell patient. *J Natl Med Assoc* 1989, 81:1077–1088.

21. Sher ME, Bauer J: Radiation-induced enteropathy. *Am J Gastroenterol* 1990, 85:121–128.

22. Koehler R: Radiology of the small intestine. *Curr Opin Gastroenterol* 1993, 9:224.

23. Shalaby-Rana E, Eichelberger M, Kerzner B, Kapur S: Intestinal stricture due to lap-belt injury. *AJR Am J Roentgenol* 1992, 158:63–64.

24. Lee M, Feldman M: Nausea and vomiting. In *Gastrointestinal Disease* vol 2, edn 5. Edited by Sleisenger MH, Fordtran JS. Philadelphia: WB Saunders; 1992:516–517.

25. Boley SJ, Feinstein FR, Sammartano R, *et al:* New concepts in the management of emboli of the superior mesenteric artery. *Surg Gynecol Obstet* 1981, 153:156–569.

26. Boley SJ, Sprayregan S, Siegelman SS, et al: Initial results from an aggressive roentological and surgical approach to acute mesenteric ischemic. *Surgery* 1977, 82:848–855.

Chapter 11

Small-Bowel Transplantation

JAVIER TABASCO-MINGUILLAN

WILLIAM HUTSON

ATSUSHI SUGITANI

JAMES C. REYNOLDS

Small-bowel transplantation (SBT), the latest achievement in visceral organ transplantation, may soon be a practical therapeutic option for patients with permanent intestinal failure. Successful SBT was first reported in a multivisceral transplantation procedure. Subsequently, in 1990, an isolated intestinal transplant had a reported graft survival exceeding 1 year. The long-term impact of SBT as a therapeutic option for the many disorders that result in dependence on total parenteral nutrition (TPN) is under investigation.

Prolonged use of TPN may lead to chronic liver disease, and even liver failure, particularly in patients with short-bowel syndrome. Therefore, combined liver transplant and SBT would be indicated in patients with short-bowel gut syndrome and liver failure. Other indications for transplantation before the development of end-stage liver disease are also under investigation, including conditions such as Crohn's disease, celiac sprue, vasculitis-induced intestinal dysfunction, and congenital small intestinal disorders, such as visceral myopathy, chronic neuropathic pseudo-obstruction, or microvillus inclusion disease.

Among the group of transplant candidates, two cohorts of patients appear to be ideal: patients with short-bowel gut syndrome who have developed end-stage liver disease, and those patients for whom TPN is an increasingly dangerous and impractical means of providing nutrition (ie, complications from maintaining intravenous lines and from thrombosis of central veins). Patients who are not dependent on TPN are not currently considered for SBT because of the risk of transplantation and need for immunosuppressant drugs. At the same time, patients with severe Crohn's disease, celiac sprue, or vasculitis-induced bowel injury could be among the first to undergo SBT because they already receive immunosuppressant agents (eg, corticosteroids, azathioprine [Imuran], cyclosporine, or tacrolimus [FK506]). Contraindications to SBT include incurable cancer, active infection, including HIV infection, or psychiatric disorders that influence patient compliance.

Improvements in SBT will require advances in the knowledge of the role of preservation solutions to maintain normal neuromuscular function of the gut during cold ischemic injury. In addition, better understanding of factors leading to the long-term survival of patients with small-bowel grafts is needed. Recent observations that the graft and host become chimeric in multiple organs other than the graft may provide one of the keys to graft acceptance. Pharmacologic agents must be developed to limit rejection and excessive immunosuppression. Development of strategies to deal more successfully with bacterial, viral, and fungal infections also is likely to improve patient and graft survival rates.

Small intestinal transplantation has progressed considerably over the past 5 years. Much effort will be required to bring its level of acceptance to that currently enjoyed by more established solid organ transplantation. Recent advances may soon provide a practical solution so that SBT can be made available to patients with intestinal failure who desperately desire a more normal lifestyle.

INDICATIONS AND CONTRAINDICATIONS

TABLE 11-1. INDICATIONS FOR TRANSPLANTATION

IN ADULTS	IN CHILDREN
Short-bowel syndrome resulting from	Short-bowel syndrome resulting from
Ischemic bowel injury	
Mesenteric venous thrombosis	Gastroschisis
Traumatic bowel injury	Malrotation
Gunshot wound	Necrotizing enterocolitis
Motor vehicle accident	Volvulus
Surgical trauma	Intussusception
Polyposis syndromes	Microvillus atrophy
Gardner's syndrome	Pseudo-obstruction
Peutz-Jeghers syndrome	
Desmoid tumor	
Immune-mediated bowel disease	
Advanced Crohn's disease	
Vasculitis-induced injury	
Refractory celiac disease	
Ulcerative jejunitis	

TABLE 11-1.

Indications for transplantation.

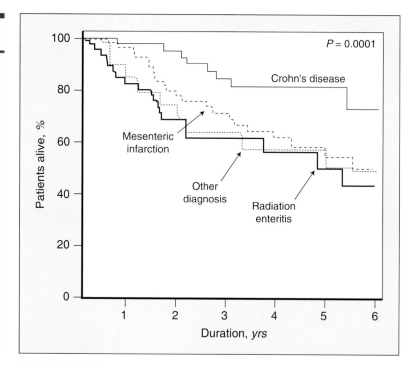

FIGURE 11-1.

Morbidity, mortality, and cost of intestinal failure. The long-term survival rates and costs of small-bowel transplantation must be compared with the currently available therapy for intestinal failure (*ie*, chronic home hyperalimentation). It has been estimated that total parenteral nutrition (TPN) in the home, costs from $75,000 to $150,000 per year. Annual costs are further increased by an average of one to three TPN-related complications requiring hospitalization each year. The survival of patients on home TPN in France is shown in this figure. Similar survival rates were found in a cohort of over 1500 U.S. patients observed for 3 years with 7 selected diagnoses. The 5-year survival rate for patients who do not have cancer or AIDS ranges from 50% to 60%, with 8% to 30% of all deaths directly attributable to TPN. TPN-related deaths occur most commonly because of sepsis, central venous thrombosis, and liver failure. (*Adapted from* Messing [1].)

TABLE 11-2. CONTRAINDICATIONS FOR TRANSPLANTATION

TABLE 11-2.

Contraindications for transplantation.

ABSOLUTE	RELATIVE
Incurable cancer	Patient not dependent on
Uncooperative patient	intravenous feeding
Unable to take medications reliably	Limited central venous access
Active infection	
AIDS	

Gastroschisis

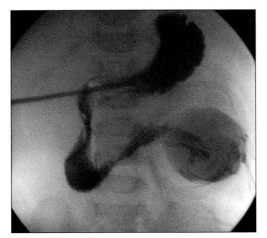

FIGURE 11-2.

Pediatric indications for small-bowel transplantation: gastroschisis. Barium-contrast small-bowel study of a 17-month-old child with short-bowel syndrome since birth caused by complications associated with gastroschisis (congenital extraumbilical abdominal wall defect with extraabdominal intestine). Multiple resections and chronic total parenteral nutrition (TPN) were associated with increasing bilirubin thought to be caused by a TPN-related hepatic injury. This study, performed through a feeding gastrostomy, shows only 10 cm of functioning small intestine remaining. This patient underwent a combined liver and small-bowel transplantation, but the patient succumbed from sepsis on the 29th postoperative day. Sepsis is, by far, the most common complication in small-bowel transplantation.

Short-bowel syndrome

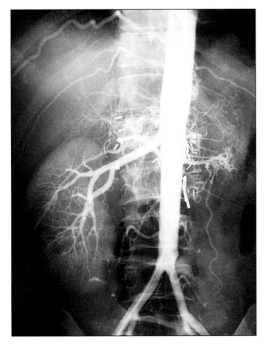

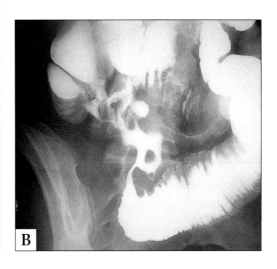

FIGURE 11-3.

Arterial thrombosis causing short-bowel syndrome in an adult. An abdominal aortogram in a 32-year-old man with protein C and protein S deficiency demonstrates absence of the celiac, superior mesenteric, inferior mesenteric, and splenic arteries. The left kidney is atrophic and the right kidney is hypertrophied. Note that the hepatic artery is reconstituted using collaterals. The metallic clips are secondary to the previous resection of necrotic small bowel.

FIGURE 11-4.

Short-bowel syndrome in an adult. Upper gastrointestinal series with small-bowel follow-through in a patient with short-bowel syndrome undergoing evaluation for small-bowel transplantation. The patient was a 41-year-old woman with superior mesenteric artery thrombosis. **A,** Short, dilated upper jejunum with hypertrophy of the valvulae conniventes. **B,** Further passage of the barium into the colon through the ileocecal anastomosis.

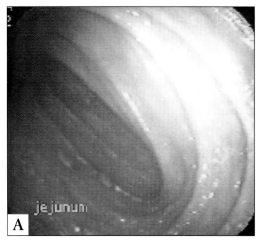 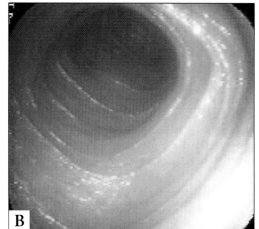

Figure 11-5.

Endoscopic views of short-bowel syndrome. Endoscopic views of the jejunum of a patient with short-bowel syndrome. **A,** The lumen of the jejunum is slightly dilated and the folds are hypertrophied. **B,** Several small ulcerations, probably from use of nonsteroidal anti-inflammatory drugs, can be seen.

Liver injury from total parenteral nutrition

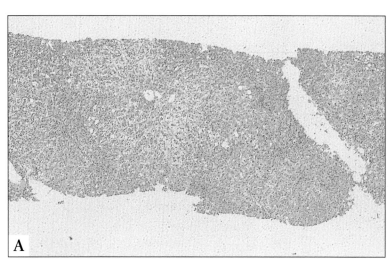 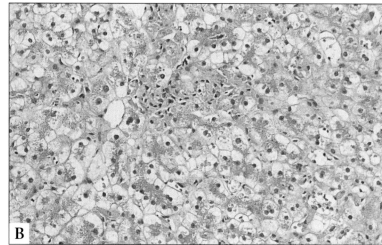

Figure 11-6.

Liver injury caused by total parenteral nutrition (TPN) in a patient with short-bowel syndrome. The patient was placed on TPN for nutritional support. Abnormal liver enzyme elevation with mild jaundice developed after 1 year. A liver biopsy showed preserved hepatic parenchyma (**panel A**) with evidence of steatosis (**panel B**) and cholestasis, but no cirrhosis.

Chronic intestinal pseudo-obstruction

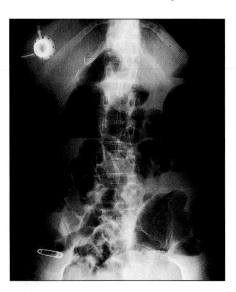

Figure 11-7.

Chronic idiopathic intestinal pseudo-obstruction. This plain abdominal radiograph demonstrates gaseous distention of the bowel with multiple air-fluid levels. It is often difficult to differentiate mechanical obstruction from pseudo-obstruction from these types of radiographic studies. In this patient, however, the abnormalities seen were chronic and long-standing, and the clinical presentation was not consistent with mechanical blockage.

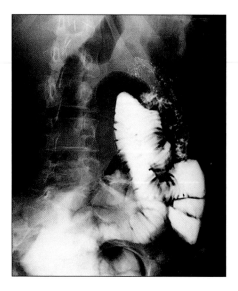

Figure 11-8.

Dilated small intestine caused by chronic idiopathic intestinal pseudo-obstruction. Barium is injected through an existing jejunostomy tube in this patient. There is mild to moderate focal dilatation of the proximal jejunum that increased in dilatation with injection. Interestingly, the subject developed increasing abdominal pain with injection. No mechanical obstruction is present.

■ OPERATIVE PROCEDURE

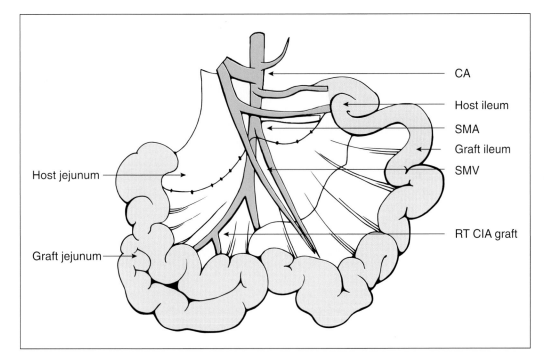

CA

Host ileum

SMA

Graft ileum

SMV

Host jejunum

RT CIA graft

Graft jejunum

FIGURE 11-9.

Schematic representation of the operative procedure. The small intestine is replaced in an orthotopic position. The entire jejunum and ileum from the donor are included. The superior mesenteric artery is implanted in an end-to-side fashion to the aorta. For selected patients, the colon, liver, pancreas, and stomach may also be included in the procedure as a multivisceral transplant.

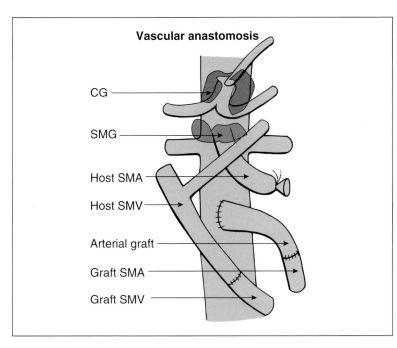

Vascular anastomosis

CG

SMG

Host SMA

Host SMV

Arterial graft

Graft SMA

Graft SMV

FIGURE 11-10.

Vascular anastomosis of the superior mesenteric artery. A critical technical aspect for successful transplantation is vascular anastomosis. The superior mesenteric artery is implanted in an end-to-side fashion to the aorta. The superior mesenteric veins of the donor and recipient are anastomosed in an end-to-end fashion. CG—celiac ganglion; SMG—superior mesenteric artery; SMV—Superior mesenteric vein.

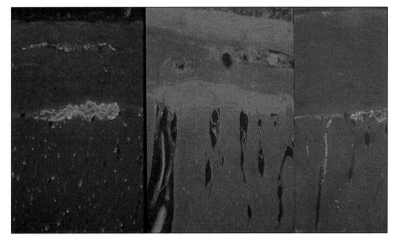

FIGURE 11-11.

Extrinsic reinnervation of the small intestine. All extrinsic neurons to the small intestine are severed during the transplantation process. This deprives the intestine of the normal modulating effects of the central nervous system that reach the small intestine through the sympathetic and parasympathetic nervous systems. It is unknown whether these neurons are able to reinnervate the small intestine in humans. Early examinations of rejected grafts suggest that little to no reinnervation by sympathetic neurons can be detected up to 2 years following the transplantation.

To further address this important issue, we have studied the timing of the reappearance of tyrosine hydroxylase-like immunoreactive (TH-LI) neurons in autotransplanted dogs. **A**, In normal small intestine, numerous brightly staining TH-LI fibers are seen in the myenteric plexus and in both the longitudinal and circular muscle layers in a sham-operated animal. **B**, No TH-LI–positive neurons can be seen 3 months following autotransplantation. **C**, By 12 months, however, some animals began to show scant but convincing evidence of regrowth of TH-LI neurons. This reinnervation of sympathetic neurons occurs more frequently, however, in experimental situations when an end-to-end anastomosis is used, compared with an end-to-side technique, which is used in small-bowel transplantation in humans.

■ COMPLICATIONS

TABLE 11-3.

Complications of small-bowel transplantation.

TABLE 11-3. COMPLICATIONS OF SMALL-BOWEL TRANSPLANTATION

COMPLICATIONS WITH SMALL-BOWEL AND LIVER TRANSPLANTATION	COMPLICATIONS WITH SMALL-BOWEL TRANSPLANTATION BUT NOT WITH LIVER TRANSPLANTATION
Preharvest injury (warm ischemia)	Visceral anastamotic leaks
Harvest injury and cold ischemia	Visceral anastamotic strictures
Reperfusion injury	Bacterial translocation
Acute rejection	Gastroparesis
Chronic rejection	Paralytic ileus or pseudo-obstruction
Vascular anastamotic leaks and strictures	Graft-versus-host disease
Opportunistic infections	
Drug toxicity	
Post-transplantation lymphoproliferative disease (PTLD)	

Acute rejection

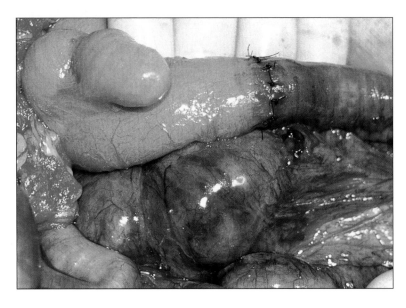

FIGURE 11-12.

Intraoperative view of acute rejection. A marked, obvious difference in color can be easily seen between the host jejunum on the left compared with the blackened graft jejunum to the right and below the anastomosis in this dog model of transplantation 6 days following the transplantation. The darkened color results from the ischemic changes that accompany acute rejection and secondary sepsis.

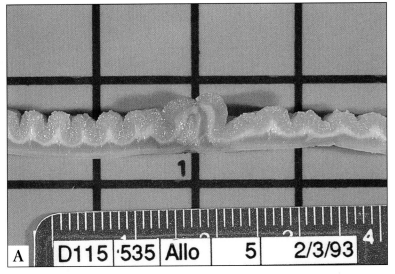 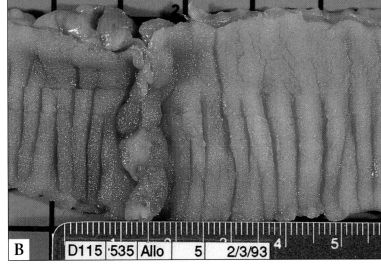

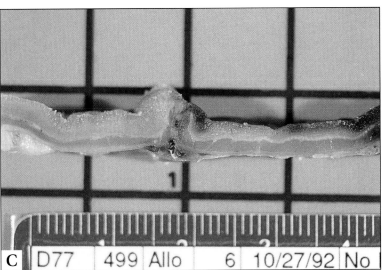 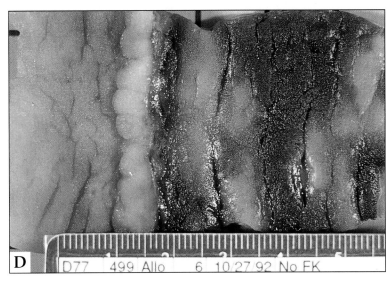

FIGURE 11-13.

Macroscopic view of acute rejection. Macroscopic views of two specimens are shown in cross-section and from the mucosal view. Each pair of specimens illustrate the anastomosis of the host jejunum on the left and the graft on the right. **A–B**, Mild thickening of the valvulae conniventes and of the submucosa. The muscularis is thickened as a result of edema and muscular hypertrophic changes. **C–D**, Characteristic changes of severe acute rejection: patchy discoloration, necrosis of the wall, and diffuse destruction of the villous architecture.

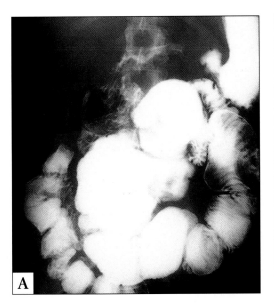 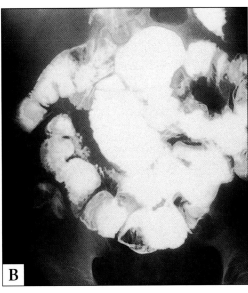

FIGURE 11-14.

Post-transplantation bowel edema and dilatation. A barium study in a recipient of combined isolated small-bowel and liver transplantation showing normal gastric emptying (**panel A**) from the host stomach and dilated loops of the small-bowel graft (**panel A** and **panel B**). The transit of contrast material through the small intestine was markedly delayed. After a transit time of several hours, the leading edge of contrast reached the ostomy, and is shown in **panel B**. The study was requested to evaluate the cause of dilated loops of small-bowel graft. Adhesions were excluded, and histologic analysis of biopsies later confirmed the presence of acute cellular rejection.

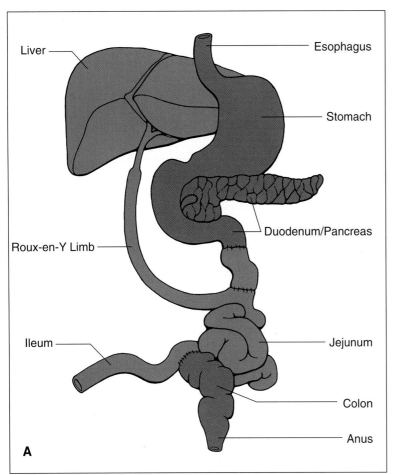

Liver

Esophagus

Stomach

Duodenum/Pancreas

Roux-en-Y Limb

Ileum

Jejunum

Colon

Anus

A

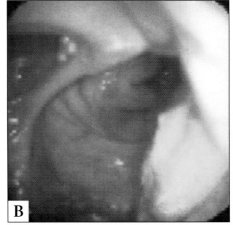

B

FIGURE 11-15.

Post-transplantation anatomy. **A,** Schematic representation of the intestinal anatomy of a patient, showing the native (green) and grafted (red) organs. **B,** Anastomosis as it is seen during endoscopy.

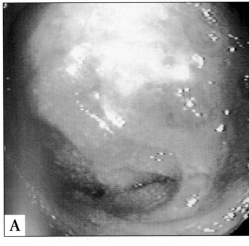

A

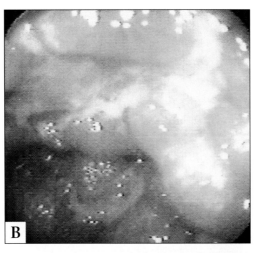

B

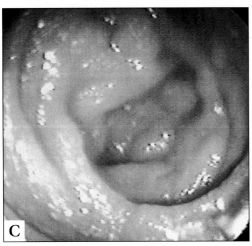

C

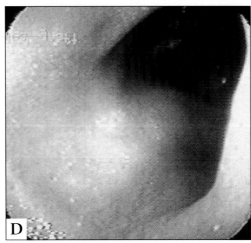

D

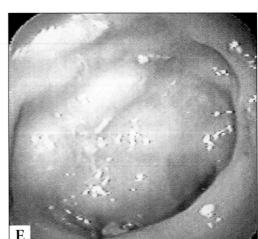

E

FIGURE 11-16.

Sequence of endoscopic findings in a patient with acute cellular rejection in the graft ileum. In clinical practice, the observation of patients with small-bowel transplantation is achieved by periodic endoscopic surveillance of the allografts that provide histologic sampling and allows the visual inspection of the intestine. This surveillance is illustrated in the series of endoscopic photographs (**A–E**) with their histologic correlates

(*continued on next page*)

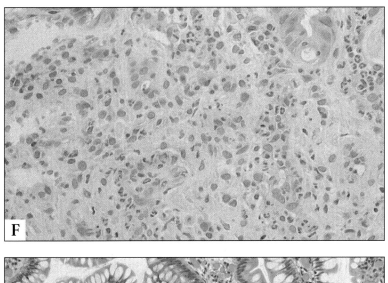

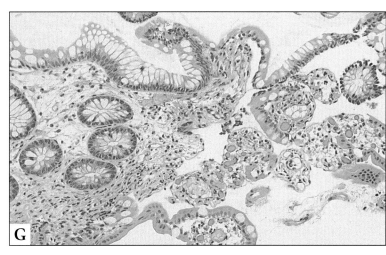

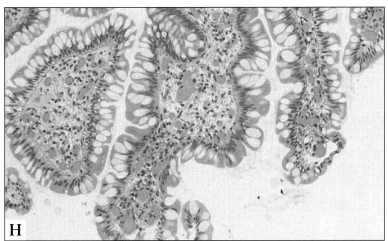

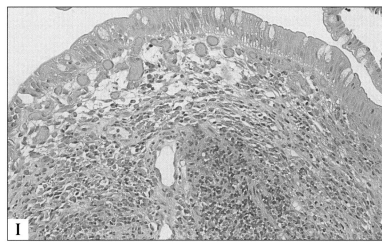

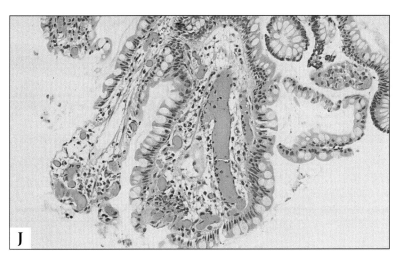

FIGURE 11-16. (*CONTINUED*)

(**F–J**) from a patient who had undergone small-bowel transplantation. The patient was a 41-year-old woman transplanted for Gardner's syndrome who presented several months following an uneventful transplantation with diarrhea, abdominal pain, and abdominal distention. **A–B**, The initial studies showed acute cellular rejection, and she was treated with an increase in the tacrolimus (FK506) dose. She had some improvement in her symptoms. **C–D**, Follow-up endoscopy, however, showed persistent ulcerations. **E–F**, A week later she developed abdominal pain and was treated with bolus steroids. **G–H**, Despite her therapy, her symptoms persisted, thus necessitating increased tacrolimus (FK506) doses. **I–J**, Finally, her clinical and laboratory parameters improved and she was discharged from the hospital.

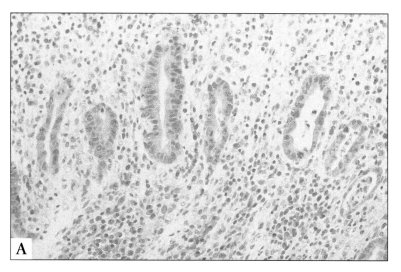

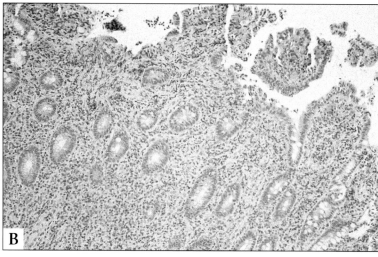

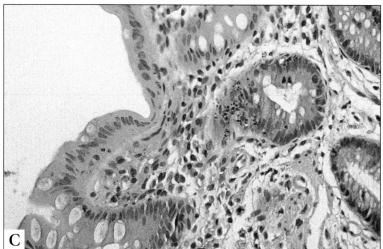

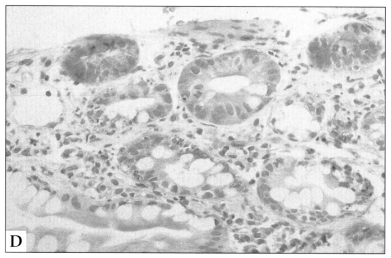

FIGURE 11-17.

Characteristic histologic features of acute cellular rejection. During acute cellular rejection there are a variety of histologic abnormalities. There is damage to the mucosa with crypt loss and regeneration (**panel A**) and loss of mucosal integrity (**panel B**). There is also crypt cell damage and drop-out (apoptosis) (**panels C and D**), which can be sequentially monitored for diagnosis and response to therapy.

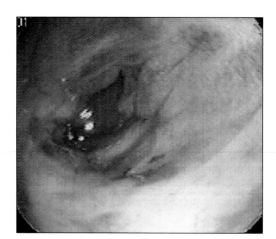

FIGURE 11-18.

Endoscopic photograph of severe acute cellular reaction during the first postoperative month, with pneumatosis cystoides and graft failure. This severe case required removal of the graft. The intensity of the resulting ischemia can be appreciated by the pallor in the mucosa.

TABLE 11-4. PARAMETERS OF INTESTINAL MUCOSAL BLOOD FLOW (IMBF) IN THE GRAFT ILEUM OF A PATIENT WITH ACUTE CELLULAR REJECTION

SEQUENTIAL IMBF IN THE REJECTING ILEUM

CORRESPONDING FIGURE	FLOW, *PERFUSION UNITS*	INTERPRETATION AND TREATMENT
11–16 a, f	50 ± 0.7	Increased FK506
11–16 b, g	161 ± 0.7	Resolving ACR
11–16 c, h	73 ± 0.8	Steroid Bolus
11–16 d, i	93 ± 1.0	Increased FK506
11–16 e, j	134 ± 1.0	Resolving ACR

Values are expressed as mean ± standard error.

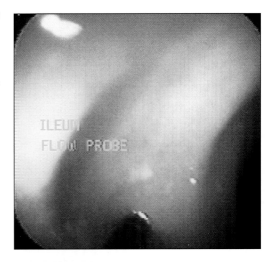

FIGURE 11-19.

Blood flow probe assesses rejection. Endoscopic photograph of the placement of a mucosal blood flow probe directly onto the mucosa of this graft ileum. Specific regions of the graft can be evaluated and compared with areas that are normal in appearance.

TABLE 11-4.

Parameters of intestinal mucosal blood flow (IMBF) in the graft ileum of a patient with acute cellular rejection. Laser Doppler flowmetry provides a mechanism to evaluate intestinal allograft mucosal blood flow in patients during rejection and after treatment. The laser Doppler apparatus calculates the flow based on measurement of velocity and of the number of erythrocytes. Recordings over time can be compared to determine the effects of treatment. The data shown here were recorded using this technique in the patient whose endoscopic and biopsy findings for similar time points are shown in Figure 11-16. In this case, sequential monitoring of her intestinal mucosal blood flow was helpful in detecting a very low flow despite improving endoscopic findings (*see* Figure 11-16, **panel C** and **panel H**). ACR—Acute cellular rejection; FK506—tacrolimus.

Chronic rejection

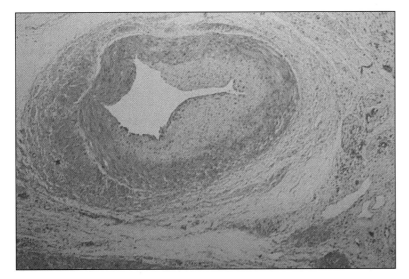

FIGURE 11-20.

Obliterative arteriopathy in chronic rejection. A photomicrograph of a medium-sized mesenteric artery. As with other organs, the hallmark of chronic rejection is obliterative arteriopathy. The specimen was obtained at autopsy of an allograft with obliterative arteriopathy that was lost to chronic rejection.

Cytomegalovirus enteritis

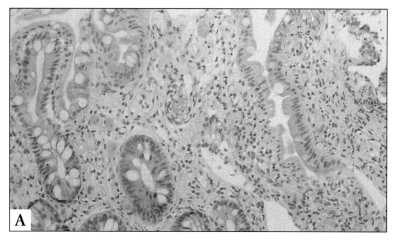

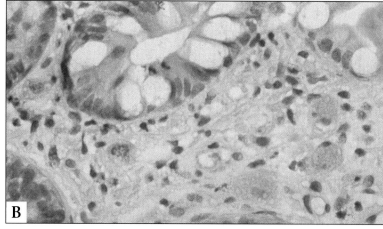

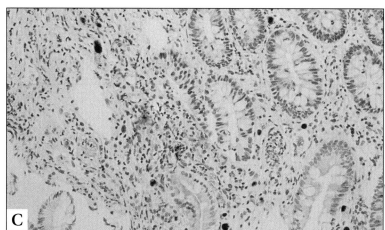

FIGURE 11-21.

Histologic characteristics of cytomegalovirus (CMV) enteritis. Histologic correlation of the endoscopic findings in Figure 11-24. **A,** CMV infection of the small-bowel graft. **B,** A magnified view of the biopsy specimen shows intracytoplasmic inclusion bodies. **C,** Specimen that tested positive (brown) with a specific immunoperoxidase staining.

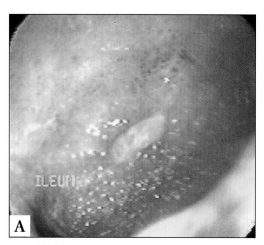

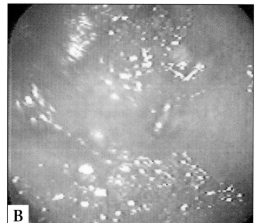

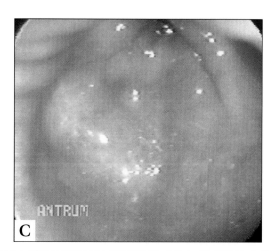

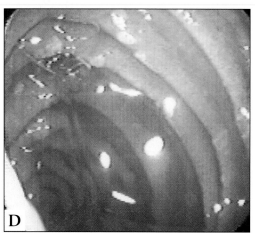

FIGURE 11-22.

Characteristic endoscopic appearance of cytomegalovirus (CMV) infection of the graft. **A–B,** CMV infection of the graft ileum with erythema and ulcerations. **C,** The infection did not affect the native stomach. **D,** No effect in the graft jejunum.

Lymphoproliferative disorder

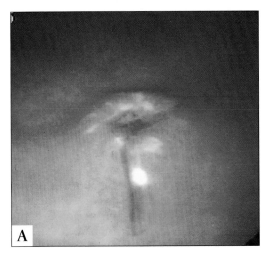 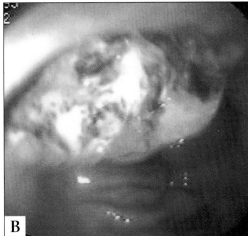 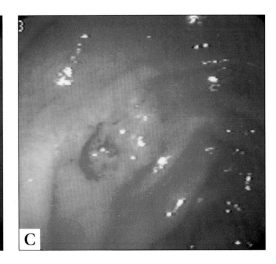

FIGURE 11-23.

Endoscopic photographs of lymphoproliferative disorder after transplantation showing several nodules with evidence of necrosis. This widespread gastrointestinal involvement with post-transplant lymphoproliferative disorder occurred in an adult patient who had undergone isolated small bowel transplantation 5 years previously. The patient did well for many months after the operation, until presenting with crampy abdominal pain and weight loss. Upper endoscopy revealed a normal esophagus and several gastric ulcers. Both the small (**panel A**) and large (**panel B**) gastric ulcers developed in the native stomach. Several ulcers were also seen endoscopically in the native jejunum (**panel C**). At histology, all of the ulcers showed a monomorphic infiltrate consistent with post-transplant lymphoproliferative disorder.

Other complications

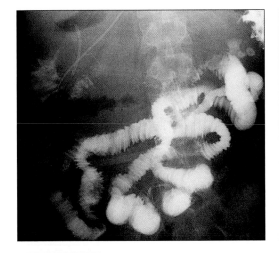

FIGURE 11-24.

Preservation injury and abnormal motility following small-bowel transplantation. This barium study shows changes consistent with preservation injury and abnormal motility following small-bowel transplantation. This patient underwent small-bowel and liver transplantation 3 weeks previously. Barium instilled into the gastrostomy tube reveals an atonic stomach with markedly enlarged folds thought to be secondary to occlusion of venous drainage through the portal system. Barium instilled through a jejunostomy tube shows thickened folds in the jejunum, consistent with the presence of submucosal edema. The caliber of the donor small-bowel graft is also variably narrowed. These nonspecific findings with a predominance of edema and no ulcerations are consistent with changes in the small intestine secondary to preservation injury.

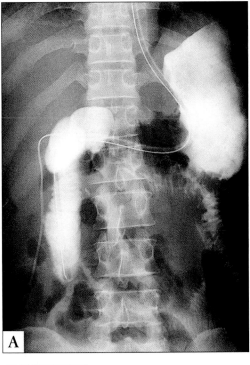 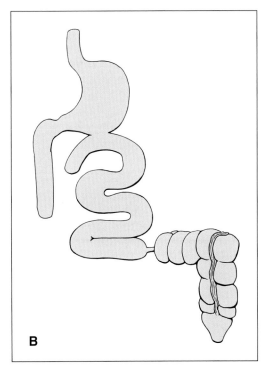

FIGURE 11-25.

A–B, Postoperative isolated small-bowel transplantation. This patient with short-bowel syndrome underwent isolated small-bowel transplantation with construction of a gastrojejunostomy caused by technical difficulties. The native duodenum ends blindly. The study shows significantly delayed gastric emptying of barium at 1 hour. Note the distal tip of the nasogastric tube positioned in the retained portion of the native duodenum.

FOLLOW-UP AND FUTURE DIRECTIONS

TABLE 11-5. FEATURES TESTED IN SMALL-BOWEL ALLOGRAFTS DURING ENDOSCOPY

MUCOSA	PERISTALSIS	LUMINAL CONTENTS
Erythema (focal, diffuse)	Absent	Absent
Erosions	Present (normal, increased, decreased)	Present (solid, semisolid, liquid)
Ulcers (single, multiple, local, diffuse)		
Edema (focal, diffuse)		
Friability		
Granularity (fine, coarse, diffuse)		
Pseudomembranes		
Exudates		
Vascular pattern		

TABLE 11-5.

The endoscopic features assessed during the surveillance of patients with small-bowel transplantation are divided into three categories: mucosal abnormalities, character of peristalsis, and character of luminal contents. Improvements in the training and agreement about these criteria among the gastroenterologists performing these procedures are likely to decrease the intra- and interobserver variations of the endoscopic interpretation.

TABLE 11-6. FUTURE DIRECTIONS FOR RESEARCH IN SMALL-BOWEL TRANSPLANTATION

Candidate and recipient selection
    Cytomegalovirus match
    Isolated small bowel with or without
        colonic transplantation
    Psychosocial evaluation
Improvement in immunosuppression and
        graft tolerance
    New immunosuppressants
    Enhancement of tolerance (chimerism?)
        Simultaneous bone marrow transplantation
        Infusion of donor-derived bone marrow cells
    Prevention of post-transplantation
        lymphoproliferative disorder
Development of early markers of rejection
    Serum markers (*eg*, IL-5, IL-10)
    In situ markers (d interferon, etc.)
    Changes in allograft perfusion
        (spectroscopy, laser Doppler)
    Changes in intestinal wall thickness
        (endoscopic ultrasound)

Improvements in the management of
        infectious complications
    New antiviral (*Cytomegalovirus*)
        and antifungal (*Aspergillus*,
        Candida) agents
    Management of bacterial translocation
    New strategies (prophylaxis,
        preemptive therapy)
Improvement of allograft motility
    Prokinetic agents
    Electrical pacing
Improvements on nutritional status after
        small-bowel transplantation
    Glutamine, new enteral formulations

TABLE 11-6.

Future directions for research in small-bowel transplantation.

ACKNOWLEDGMENTS

The authors wish to acknowledge the contributions of Randall G. Lee and A. Tsamandas in the presentation of pathologic correlates to our endoscopic data, and to T. Starzl, Satoru Todo, Hirojuki Furukawa, and Kareem Abu-Elmagd for their collegiality and visionary leadership in the efforts to develop small-bowel transplantation as a therapeutic option for patients with intestinal failure.

REFERENCE

1. Messing B: Prognosis of patients with nonmalignant chronic intestinal failure receiving long-term home parenteral nutrition. *Gastroenterology* 1995, 108:1005–1010.

Chapter 12

Infections of the Intestine

RALPH A. GIANNELLA

Infections of the intestine are common throughout the world. Agents that infect the intestine include a very large number of bacteria, viruses, protozoan parasites, and fungi. Of these, bacteria, viruses, and protozoan agents are the most common pathogens, important both in terms of frequency and in causing diarrheal disease. An estimated 750 million episodes of acute diarrheal disease occur throughout the world each year and result in approximately 5 million deaths per year. These deaths occur primarily in underdeveloped countries where coexisting malnutrition is common.

The prevalence of particular pathogenic agents as causes of diarrhea varies with the country of origin, the state of public health measures and hygiene throughout that particular community, the overall nutritional status of the host, and whether the host is healthy or immunocompromised.

In this chapter, a wide spectrum of etiopathologic agents is discussed. I have chosen to start with an overview of the general pathophysiology of diarrheal disease and then focus on the common infections. The specific agents discussed were chosen on the basis of their frequency and importance, a certain minimum base of knowledge, and the availability of some form of treatment. I have summarized the pathophysiology for each, when possible, and attempted to illustrate typical morphologic lesions when appropriate.

In addition to specific pathogenic agents, certain specific syndromes or epidemiologic classes of diarrhea are also discussed. Some of these include traveler's diarrhea, food poisoning syndromes, sexually transmitted enteric infections, and common pathogens found in patients with AIDS. Typical presentations and manifestations are emphasized throughout the chapter.

The references chosen are general in nature, provide overviews of clinical features and pathophysiology, and are excellent starting places for more in-depth reading.

GENERAL ASPECTS OF INFECTIOUS DIARRHEA

TABLE 12-1. ACUTE INFECTIOUS DIARRHEAS IN HUMANS

Bacteria

Viruses

Children—*Rotavirus, Adenovirus*

Adults—*Parvoviruses*

Astroviruses

Adenoviruses

Protozoa

Giardia lamblia

Entamoeba histolytica

Cryptosporidium

Isospora

Microsporidium

TABLE 12-1.

Acute infectious diarrheas in humans. A large number of pathogenic agents are capable of causing acute diarrhea in humans, including bacteria, viruses, and protozoan agents. The likelihood of occurence varies with the age of the individual, the country of origin, and whether the host is immunocompromised or immunocompetent. In the United States and other well-developed countries, viruses are the most common causes of acute diarrhea. Specific bacteria capable of causing diarrheal disease are listed in Table 12-8 [1–3].

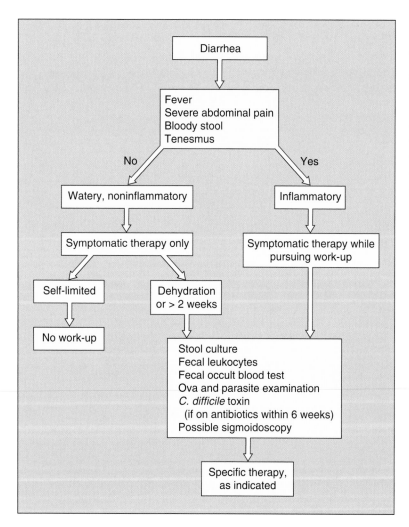

FIGURE 12-1.

Approach to the patient with acute diarrhea. Most cases of acute diarrhea are self-limited and require neither specific diagnosis nor therapy. In the absence of fever, severe abdominal pain, bloody stools, or tenesmus, watchful waiting and symptomatic therapy should be given. If either fever, severe abdominal pain, bloody stools, or tenesmus is present, this finding suggests inflammatory diarrhea and increases the likelihood of a specific, treatable enteropathogen. In such cases, symptomatic therapy can be applied while a diagnostic evaluation is pursued. (*Adapted from* Saxe and Giannella [4]; with permission.)

TABLE 12-2. MECHANISMS OF BACTERIAL ENTERIC INFECTIONS

Enterotoxins
Vibrio cholerae, Escherichia coli, Staphylococcus aureus

Invasion
Shigella, Salmonella, Campylobacter

Enteroadhesion
E. coli (EPEC)

Cytotoxins
Clostridium difficile, E. coli, Shigella

TABLE 12-2.

Mechanisms of bacterial enteric infections. Bacteria cause diarrheal disease by four major mechanisms, including the elaboration of enterotoxins, invasion of the intestinal mucosa, adhering to and obliterating the microvillous membrane (enteroadhesion), and elaborating substances cytotoxic to intestinal epithelial cells. Typical examples of each are listed [1–3].

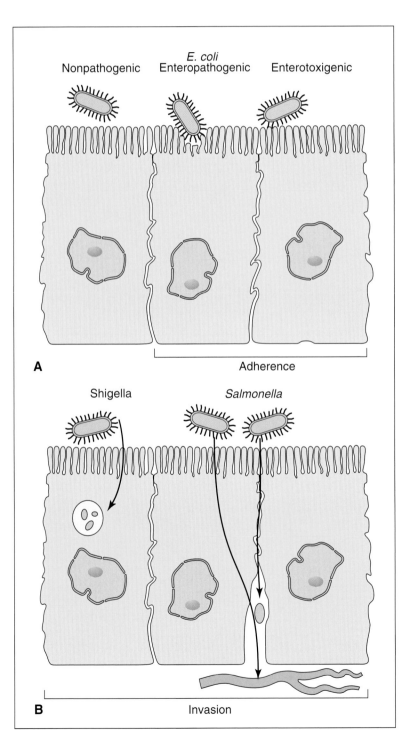

A   Adherence

B   Invasion

FIGURE 12-2.

Interaction of pathogens with enterocytes. **A,** All pathogenic bacteria must first adhere to the surface of the epithelial cell before causing disease. Various adherence mechanisms have been described. Enterotoxigenic *Escherichia coli* adheres to specific receptors on the surface of the epithelial cell through the bacterial pili. Enteropathogenic *E. coli* adheres by a poorly understood mechanism, which obliterates the microvillous membrane. **B,** Invasive organisms, such as *Shigella* and *Salmonella*, actually penetrate the intestinal mucosa. *Shigella* penetrate the brush-border membrane to enter the cell interior by an endocytotic mechanism. There the organism escapes the endocytotic vesicle and spreads laterally, causing cell damage and cell death. The organisms rarely penetrate beyond the intestinal mucosa. *Salmonella*, on the other hand, penetrates both the brush-border membrane and the tight junctions between cells. These organisms frequently penetrate the epithelial layer and enter the blood stream to disseminate widely. (*Adapted from* Banwell and Lake [5].)

TABLE 12-3. INFECTIOUS LEVELS OF ENTERIC PATHOGENS

Campylobacter jejuni	10^{2-6}
Entamoeba histolytica	10^{1-2} (cysts)
Escherichia coli	10^8
Giardia lamblia	10^{1-2} (cysts)
Salmonella	10^5
Shigella	10^{1-2}
Vibrio cholerae	10^8

TABLE 12-3.

Infectious doses of enteric pathogens. The number of organisms that must be ingested to cause disease varies greatly among enteropathogens. With *Shigella*, as few as 10 or 100 organisms can cause disease in a normal adult host. *Salmonella, Escherichia coli,* and *Vibrio cholerae* require much higher numbers. Thus, the small inoculum size accounts for the frequent person-to-person spread seen in shigellosis; the large inoculum required accounts for water-borne or food-borne transmission of *Campylobacter, Salmonella, E. coli,* or *V. cholerae*. Ingestion of only a few cysts of either *Giardia lamblia* or *Entamoeba histolytica* can initiate infection. (*Adapted from* Guerrant [6].)

TABLE 12-4. HOST FACTORS PREVENTING ENTERIC INFECTION

Nonspecific
Gastric acidity
Small intestinal motility
Normal intestinal microflora
Specific
Mucosal immune systems
Presence or absence of receptors for bacteria and toxins

TABLE 12-4.

Host factors preventing enteric infection. Various host factors act to resist the implantation of foreign organisms and the establishment of an enteric infection. Some are nonspecific mechanisms, such as gastric acidity, small intestinal motility, and the normal intestinal flora. Specific mechanisms resisting infection include the mucosal immune systems and the presence or absence of specific receptors for particular bacteria or toxins [1–3].

TABLE 12-5. BACTERIAL "VIRULENCE" FACTORS PROMOTING INFECTION

Enterotoxin elaboration
Adherence factors
Ability to invade
Chemotaxis
Motility
Mucolytic enzymes

TABLE 12-5.

Bacterial virulence factors promoting infection. Bacteria have evolved diverse virulence attributes that function to overcome host defense mechanisms and thereby establish infection. These include the abilities to elaborate enterotoxin, to adhere to the surface epithelium, to invade the mucosa, to move, to elaborate mucolytic enzymes to penetrate the mucous layer, and to respond to chemotactic signals released by the epithelium [1–3,7].

TABLE 12-6. INFLAMMATORY VERSUS NONINFLAMMATORY DIARRHEA

CHARACTERISTIC	INFLAMMATORY DIARRHEA	NONINFLAMMATORY DIARRHEA
Fecal leukocytes	Positive	Negative
Clinical presentation	Bloody, small-volume diarrhea; lower left quadrant abdominal cramps; may be febrile and toxic	Large-volume, watery diarrhea; may have nausea, vomiting, cramps
Causes	*Shigella, Salmonella,* amebic colitis, *Campylobacter, Yersinia,* invasive *Escherichia coli, Yersinia, Clostridium difficile*	Viruses, *Vibrio, Giardia,* Enterotoxigenic *E. coli,* enterotoxin-producing bacteria, food-borne gastroenteritis
Site of involvement	Colon	Small intestine
Diagnostic evaluation	Indicated	If severely volume-depleted or toxic

TABLE 12-6.

Features of inflammatory and noninflammatory diarrhea. Acute diarrhea can be divided into inflammatory or noninflammatory types. Inflammatory diarrhea is characterized by the presence of fecal leukocytes, by bloody or small-volume bowel movements, by tenesmus, and frequently by fever. Invasive or cytotoxin-producing bacteria characteristically cause this syndrome. The primary target organ is the colon. Noninflammatory diarrhea, however, is characterized by the absence of fecal leukocytes, large-volume, watery diarrhea, and lack of fever. Organisms causing noninflammatory diarrhea are enterotoxin-elaborating bacteria and certain minimally destructive viruses. The primary target organ is the small intestine [1,3]. (*Adapted from* Park and Giannella [3]; with permission.)

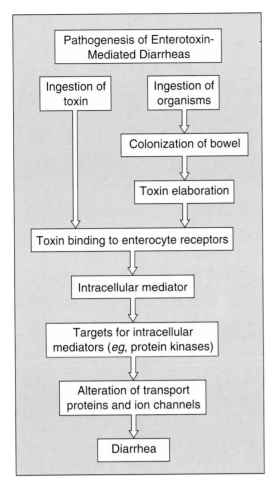

FIGURE 12-3.

Pathogenesis of enterotoxin-mediated diarrheas. This figure illustrates the general scheme whereby enterotoxin-elaborating bacteria cause diarrheal disease. Organisms are ingested, colonize the bowel, and elaborate toxin, or preformed toxin is ingested in food. The toxin binds to specific enterotoxin receptors, thereby stimulating an intracellular mediator system. Such mediators by that means activate various proteins, most commonly protein kinases, which subsequently alter transport proteins or ion channels resulting in fluid secretion and diarrhea [1–3,7,8].

TABLE 12-7. INTRACELLULAR MEDIATORS OF ENTEROTOXIN EFFECTS

Cyclic adenosine monophosphate
Cyclic guanosine monophosphate
Calcium

TABLE 12-7.

Intracellular mediators of enterotoxin effects. Three intracellular mediator systems are known to cause intestinal secretion, including cyclic adenosine monophosphate, cyclic guanosine monophosphate, and increased intracellular calcium concentrations [1–3,7,8].

CHOLERA

TABLE 12-8. TOXINS ELABORATED BY V. CHOLERAE-01

Toxin	Mechanism
Cholera toxin	↑ Adenylyl cyclase
ACE	? ATPase-like
ZOT	Zona occludens and ↑ PKC
STa (Rare)	↑ Guanylyl cyclase

TABLE 12-8.

Toxins elaborated by *Vibrio cholerae-01*. *Vibrio cholerae* can elaborate four separate enterotoxins. The first, and probably the most significant, is classic cholera toxin. This is a large protein that stimulates the adenylate cyclase system. Additional toxins include accessory cholera toxin (ACE), the mechanism of action of which is unclear, but may have activity like that of adenosine triphosphatase, and a zona occludens toxin (ZOT), which alters the zona occludens between cells and increases protein kinase c (PKC). Rare strains of *V. cholerae* elaborate a small-heat stable-like enterotoxin, which stimulates guanylate cyclase and cyclic guanosine monophosphate.

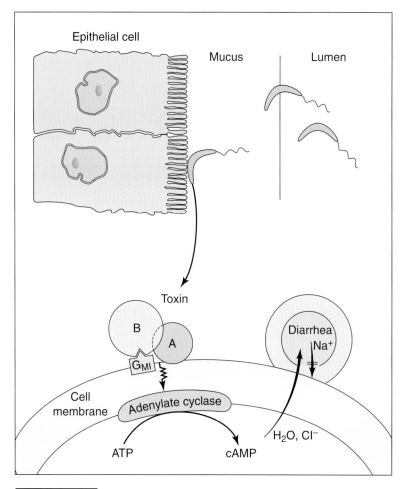

FIGURE 12-4.

The overall mechanism of diarrhea caused by cholera. After ingestion, the cholera organisms colonize the mucosal surface by penetrating the mucous layer overlying the epithelium by secreting mucolytic enzymes. The organisms adhere to the brush-border membrane and elaborate cholera enterotoxin. The toxins bind to a specific receptor, GM-1 ganglioside. The toxin receptor interaction results in the activation of adenylate cyclase and the production of cyclic adenosine monophosphate, which then results in diarrhea. This diarrhea results from the inhibition of sodium absorption and stimulation of chloride secretion. G_{M_1}—GM1 ganglioside; A—cholera Toxin A subunits; B—cholera Toxin B subunits. (*Adapted from* Holmgren and Svennerholm [9]; with permission.)

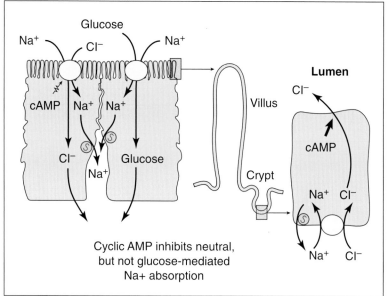

FIGURE 12-5.

Cholera toxin activation of ion transport. Cholera toxin has several actions on villus and crypt enterocytes. In villous enterocytes, cyclic adenosine monophosphate (AMP) inhibits the neutral coupled absorption of sodium and chloride. The glucose or substrate-stimulated sodium transport mechanism is unaffected. In crypt enterocytes, however, cyclic AMP activates protein kinase A to open chloride channels, resulting in chloride and water secretion. The chloride channel has been demonstrated to be the cystic fibrosis transmembrane regulator (CFTR), which is phosphorylated and activated by protein kinase A. Cholera toxin may also influence mucosal transport by effects on enteric nerves and paracrine cells. (*Adapted from* Banwell and Lake [5]; with permission.)

ESCHERICHIA COLI

TABLE 12-9. CLASSES OF DIARRHEAGENIC ESCHERICHIA COLI

Enterotoxigenic (ETEC)

Enteropathogenic (EPEC)

Enteroinvasive (EIEC)

Enterohemorrhagic (EHEC)

Enteroadherent (EAEC)

TABLE 12-9.

Classes of diarrheagenic *Escherichia coli*. At present, five classes of *E. coli* are known to cause diarrheal disease. Their popular acronyms are shown in parentheses [2,10,11].

TABLE 12-10. *ESCHERICHIA COLI* ENTEROTOXINS AND CYTOTOXINS

Toxin	Mechanism
LT-1 and LT-2	Adenylyl cyclase
STa-EAST	Guanylyl cyclase
STb	↑ Ca+ influx
SLT:(VT)	Inhibits protein synthesis
EIET	Unknown
CNF-1, CNF-2	Alters cytoskeleton

TABLE 12-10.

Escherichia coli enterotoxins and cytotoxins. *E. coli* strains can produce a variety of enterotoxic and cytotoxic substances. Their mechanism of action are also shown. CNF—cytotoxic necrotizing factor; EAST—enteroaggregative *E. coli* heat-stable enterotoxin; EIET—enteroinvasive enterotoxin; LT—*E. coli* heat-labile enterotoxin; SLT—shiga-like toxins; STa and STb—*E. coli* heat-stable enterotoxins.

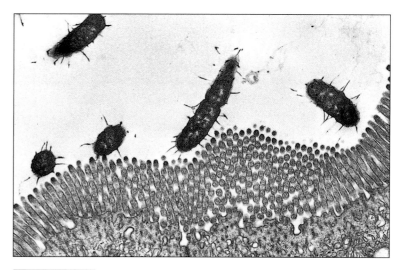

FIGURE 12-6.

Electron micrograph demonstrating adherence of enterotoxic *Escherichia coli* (ETEC) to the brush-border membrane of small-bowel enterocytes. Pili radiating from the *E. coli* are seen attaching the *E. coli* to the microvilli. Specific glycoproteins in the microvillous membrane are the specific binding sites. (*From* Cohen and Giannella [2]; *courtesy of* Dr. H. Moon, DVM, Ames, IA.)

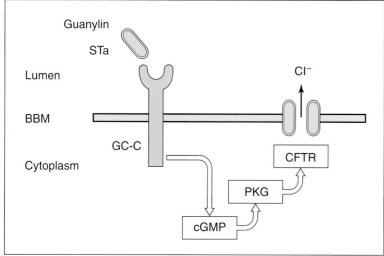

FIGURE 12-7.

Mechanism of action of *Escherichia coli* STa and guanylin-induced secretion. Guanylin and STa share the same receptor, guanylate cyclase C, which is located in the brush-border membrane of small-bowel enterocytes and colonocytes. Binding of the ligands to the binding site of guanylate cyclase activates guanylate cyclase to produce cyclic GMP. Cyclic GMP activates protein kinase G, which phosphorylates CFTR, thus resulting in chloride secretion. BBM—brush border membrane; CFTR—cystic fibrosis transmembrane regulator; cGMP—cyclic guanosine monophosphate; GC-C—guanylate cyclase C; PKG—cGMP activated protein kinase.

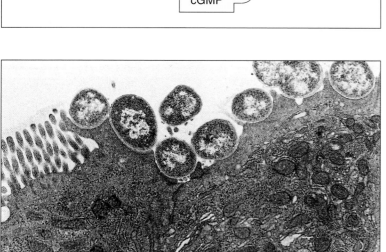

FIGURE 12-8.

Electron micrograph showing adherence of enteropathogenic *Escherichia coli* (EPEC) to brush-border membrane of enterocytes. This figure illustrates two enterocytes—one colonized by a micro-colony of EPEC and the other uncolonized. The EPEC organisms are tightly adherent to the microvillous membrane and have obliterated it, thus causing the typical indentations referred to as "pedestal" formation. (*From* Rothbaum *et al.* [12]; with permission.)

TABLE 12-11. ILLNESSES RESULTING FROM ENTEROHEMORRHAGIC *ESCHERICHIA COLI*

Hemorrhagic colitis
Nonbloody diarrhea
Asymptomatic infection
Hemolytic-uremic syndrome
Thrombotic thrombocytopenic purpura

TABLE 12-11.

Illnesses caused by enterohemorrhagic *Escherichia coli* (EHEC). The most characteristic illness caused by EHEC organisms is hemorrhagic colitis. Nonbloody diarrhea or asymptomatic infection can also occur, however. Potentially devastating complications include the hemolytic uremic syndrome and thrombotic thrombocytopenic purpura. These latter conditions occur primarily in children, but can also occur in the elderly [13,14]. (*Adapted from* Cohen and Giannella [13].)

TABLE 12-12. CLINICAL OVERVIEW OF *ESHERICHIA COLI* 0157:H7

May account for 10% of all cases of acute diarrhea
30%–95% of patients have bloody diarrhea (may account for approximately 35% of cases of acute bloody diarrhea)
2%–7% develop the hemolytic-uremic syndrome (10% mortality rate)
Overall mortality rates < 1%–35%

TABLE 12-12.

Clinical overview of infection with *Escherichia coli* 0157:H7. In the United States and Canada, infections with enterohemorrhagic *E. coli* (EHEC) organisms, predominantly *E. coli* 0157:H7, are not unusual. They may, in fact, account for approximately 10% of all cases of acute diarrhea. Many patients have bloody diarrhea; EHEC may account for approximately 35% of cases of acute bloody diarrhea.

TABLE 12-13. TRANSMISSION OF *ESCHERICHIA COLI* 0157:H7

Epidemic
Sporadic
Food: hamburger, meat, other foodstuffs
Bovine reservoir
Person to person: Family members
Daycare centers
Nursing homes

TABLE 12-13.

Transmission of *Escherichia coli* 0157:H7. Disease caused by *E. coli* 0157:H7 occurs in both epidemic and sporadic forms. The most common vehicle of transmission is hamburger, but it can be transmitted in other meat products, milk, or water. A bovine reservoir is known to exist. The organism can also be transmitted among family members, as the inoculum size required to cause disease is very low. Outbreaks occur in daycare centers and nursing homes where hygiene is suboptimal.

TABLE 12-14. *ESCHERICHIA COLI* HEMORRHAGIC COLITIS: SUMMARY

Cause: *E. coli* 0157:H7 and other serotypes
Produces a cytotoxin that inhibits protein synthesis ("Shiga" or Vero cell toxin)
Abdominal cramps, diarrhea, bloody diarrhea
Adults and children; sporadic and epidemic
Hamburger a common vehicle
Hemorrhagic colitis lasting 1 to 2 weeks (organisms shed for up to 1 month)

TABLE 12-14.

Escherichia coli hemorrhagic colitis: summary. *E. coli* hemorrhagic colitis is caused by infection with *E. coli* 0157:H7 and a variety of other serotypes. Disease is caused by the elaboration of a cytotoxin, which inhibits protein synthesis. The characteristic evolution of symptoms is a finding of abdominal cramps and diarrhea, followed 1 to 3 days later by bloody diarrhea. The disease occurs most commonly in children, but also can appear in adults. Hamburger is the most commonly ingested vehicle of transmission. The hemorrhagic colitis lasts 1 to 2 weeks whereas the organisms can be shed for up to 1 month.

TABLE 12-15. *SALMONELLA:* CLINICAL SYNDROMES

Gastroenteritis	Focal lesions
Enteric fever	Chronic carrier

TABLE 12-15.

Salmonella: clinical syndromes. The most common clinical syndromes resulting from *Salmonella* infection are uncomplicated gastroenteritis, enteric fever syndrome, focal infective lesions, or an asymptomatic carrier state [15].

TABLE 12-16. FACTORS INCREASING SUSCEPTIBILITY TO SALMONELLOSIS

LOCATION OR FACTOR	SPECIFIC CONDITION
Stomach	Achlorhydria
	Gastric surgery
Intestine	Antibiotic administration
	Gastrointestinal surgery
	(?) Idiopathic inflammatory bowel disease
Hemolytic anemia	Particularly sickle cell anemia and other hemoglobinopathies
Impaired systemic immunity	Carcinomatosis, leukemias, lymphomas
	Immunosuppressive drugs and other causes

TABLE 12-16.

Factors increasing the susceptibility to salmonellosis. Various conditions increase the susceptibility to *Salmonella* infection, including reduced gastric secretion, earlier antibiotic administration, possibly idiopathic inflammatory bowel disease, sickle cell anemia and other hemoglobinopathies, and other conditions resulting in impaired systemic immunity. (*Adapted from* Giannella [15].)

TABLE 12-17. COMPLICATIONS OF SALMONELLOSIS

Cholecystitis and cholangitis	Aortitis, endocarditis
Cholera-like syndrome	Focal infections
Ileal perforation and hemorrhage	Chronic carrier state
Osteomyelitis	Chronic colitis

TABLE 12-17.

Complications of salmonellosis. Although most cases of salmonellosis are restricted to a self-limited gastroenteritis, various complications can occur. The finding of chronic colitis is poorly understood and poorly defined. Likely, this is an ulcerative colitis-like illness that seems to have been initiated by an episode of *Salmonella* infection.

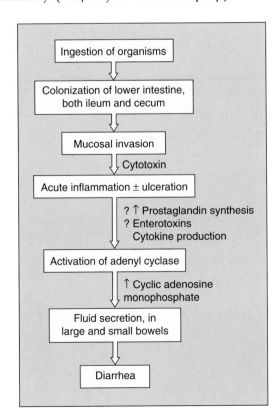

FIGURE 12-9.

Pathogenesis of *Salmonella* enteritis and diarrhea. After ingestion, the organisms pass through the acid barrier of the stomach to colonize the lower intestine, primarily the ileum and cecum. The organisms invade the intestinal mucosa and elaborate cytotoxins. The invasion and cytotoxic elaboration results in an acute inflammatory reaction within the mucosa that sometimes leads to ulceration. The acute inflammatory reaction causes an increase in prostaglandin synthesis as well as the release of various cytokines that result in intestinal secretion and diarrhea. They do so by activating adenylate cyclase and cyclic adenosine monophosphate and by neurogenic and other mechanisms. (*Adapted from* Giannella [15]; with permission.)

TABLE 12-18. SOURCES AND RESERVOIRS OF SALMONELLOSIS

Animals—poultry, cattle, pigs, domestic animals
Bone meals and animal feeds
Animal products, especially chicken, turkey, and eggs
Chronic carrier—human and animal

TABLE 12-18.

Sources and reservoirs of salmonellosis. The primary reservoirs for *Salmonella* organisms are poultry, cattle, and other domesticated animals. Thus, animal products, such as chicken, turkey, and eggs, can become contaminated and be sources of salmonella infection. A chronic carrier state, both human and animal, exists and is an important source of infection.

■ SHIGELLA

TABLE 12-19. SHIGELLOSIS: SUMMARY

Fever, cramps, diarrhea, and possible dysentery (one third have diarrhea only; one third have diarrhea preceding dysentery)
In the United States, primarily children are involved, although adult cases do occur.
Minimal inoculum required, therefore secondary cases common
Usually self-limited
Intravenous fluids not usually required
Antibiotics can shorten course of illness

TABLE 12-19.

Shigellosis: summary. The typical clinical features and clinical course are listed. It should be noted that one third of the cases of shigellosis present with only diarrhea (without obvious blood) and another one third have diarrhea that precedes frank dysentery. Fortunately, most cases are self-limited, and intravenous fluids are not usually required. Antibiotics do shorten the course of the illness, and are recommended.

TABLE 12-20. SYSTEMIC MANIFESTATIONS AND COMPLICATIONS OF SHIGELLOSIS

Bacteremia rare
Febrile convulsions
Disseminated intravascular coagulation (DIC)
Leukemoid reactions
Hemolytic uremic syndrome
Postdysenteric arthritis
Postdysenteric colitis

TABLE 12-20.

Systemic manifestations and complications of shigellosis. Although most cases of shigellosis are self-limited and uncomplicated, complications occasionally do occur. Fortunately, bacteremia is rare, but in children, febrile convulsions and hemolytic uremic syndrome may result. In adults, and particularly those with infections with *Shigella dysenteriae*, disseminated intravascular coagulation and profound leukemoid reactions may also ensue.

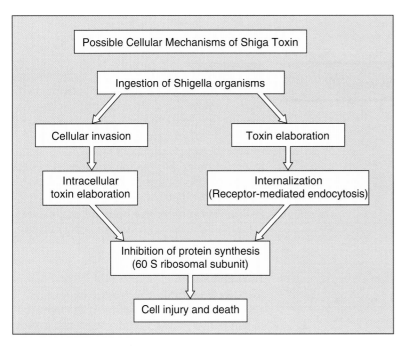

FIGURE 12-10.

Possible cellular mechanisms of *Shiga* toxin. *Shiga* toxin, elaborated by many strains of *Shigella*, contribute to the pathogenesis of the enteric infection. The mechanisms by which the toxins cause cell injury and death are not clearly understood. Toxin may be elaborated intraluminally or intracellularly after cellular invasion has occurred. The toxin inhibits protein synthesis by inhibiting the 60S ribosomal subunit. If sufficient protein synthesis is inhibited, the cell is not only injured, but killed.

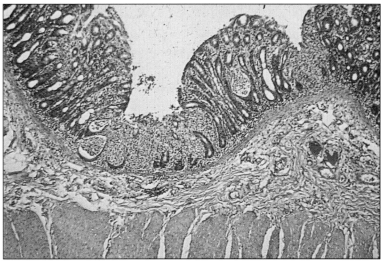

FIGURE 12-11.

Photomicrograph of *Shigella* infection of the colon. The typical appearance of shigella colitis with gross ulceration is illustrated. In addition to the obvious mucosal ulcerations, note the profound crypt abscesses. (*Courtesy of* Sam Formal, PhD, University of Maryland.)

CAMPYLOBACTER

TABLE 12-21. *CAMPYLOBACTER* DIARRHEA SUMMARY

Characteristics

Prodrome (fever, malaise, myalgias)

Colicky pain, watery diarrhea, and ± dysentery

Mimics salmonellosis, shigellosis, yersinosis, and antibiotic-associated diarrhea

Enteritis with or without colitis

Causes 5%–10% of cases of acute diarrhea

Positive stool culture for 2–5 weeks

Diagnosis

Fecal leukocytes, positive stool culture (on selective media grown at 42°C, in a CO_2-enriched environment)

Treatment

Erythromycin, tetracycline, chloramphenicol, gentamicin

Complications

Acute abdomen

Chronic diarrhea

Septicemia

Mimics idiopathic inflammatory bowel disease

TABLE 12-21.

Campylobacter diarrhea: summary. The usual clinical manifestations and course are described. The clinical syndrome mimics those of shigellosis, salmonellosis, and other enteric infections, and therefore cannot be reliably distinguished on clinical grounds alone. *Campylobacter* infection is extremely widespread and, in many surveys, is the most common definable cause of acute intestinal infection.

Most cases of *Campylobacter* infection are self-limited, resolve before a specific diagnosis is made, and do not require specific treatment. In severe cases, however, and in cases with prolonged diarrhea, antibiotic administration is required. Erythromycin is the preferred therapeutic agent. Various complications of *Campylobacter* diarrhea should be noted; they include abdominal pain so severe as to mimic an acute abdomen, occasional septicemia, and a chronic illness that mimics idiopathic inflammatory bowel disease.

YERSINIA ENTEROCOLITICA

TABLE 12-22. *YERSINIA ENTEROCOLITICA* INFECTION: SUMMARY

Fever, vomiting, abdominal pain

Enteritis with or without colitis, especially involvement of the distal ileum

Two diarrheal syndromes—watery diarrhea or dysentery

Lasts up to 2–3 weeks

Can mimic Crohn's disease—both clinically and pathologically

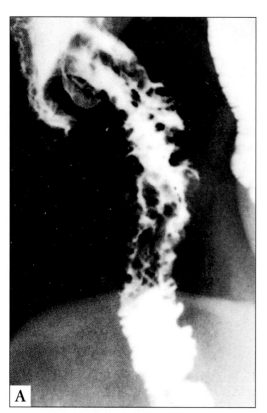 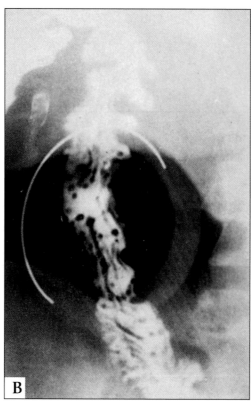

TABLE 12-22.

Yersinia enterocolitica infection: summary. *Yersinia enterocolitica* can cause both acute and chronic diarrheal syndromes. These organisms can infect both the small bowel and colon. The typical location is the distal ileum. Two clinical syndromes are possible: a watery diarrheal syndrome or a typical dysenteric syndrome. Although the typical case lasts only 2 to 3 weeks, illness *can* be prolonged for many weeks, and thus the illness can mimic Crohn's disease.

FIGURE 12-12.

A–B, Radiographic appearance of *Yersinia enterocolitica* ileitis. Spot films of the terminal ileum reveal markedly thickened folds with a nodular pattern. This can mimic Crohn's disease, lymphoma, or lymphoid hyperplasia. (*From* Vantrappen *et al.* [16]; with permission.)

CLOSTRIDIUM DIFFICILE

TABLE 12-23. *CLOSTRIDIUM DIFFICILE* COLITIS: SUMMARY

Occurs during antibiotic treatment or up to 6 weeks after cessation

Can occur with almost any antibiotic

Commonest single cause of hospital-acquired diarrhea

Spectrum of mild diarrhea to fulminant colitis

Can mimic ulcerative colitis or cause exacerbations of inflammatory bowel disease

Caused by toxin(s) elaborated by *C. difficile*

Diagnosis

Usually a colitis on signoidoscopy

Frequently with pseudomembranes

Stool assay for cytotoxin

Therapy

Discontinue antibiotics, if possible

Metronidazole

Vancomycin

TABLE 12-23.

Clostridium difficile colitis: summary. The epidemiologic and clinical features of the illness are listed. The illness is caused by one or more toxins elaborated by *C. difficile*. It should be remembered that *C. difficile* colitis can mimic ulcerative colitis or can cause exacerbations in a patient with inflammatory bowel disease.

The diagnosis of *C. difficile* colitis should be suspected when a colitis is seen on sigmoidoscopy, especially with characteristic pseudomembranes. The diagnosis is confirmed by demonstrating the presence of specific *C. difficile* cytotoxins in the stool. Treatment consists of discontinuing the antibiotic, if possible, with or without therapy with metronidazole or vancomycin [17].

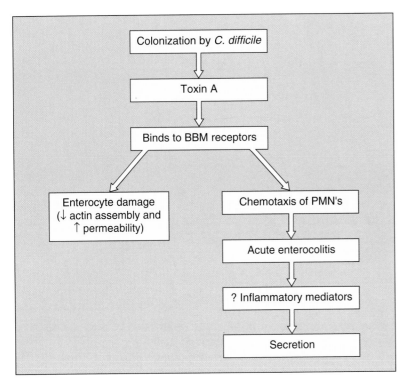

FIGURE 12-13

Pathogenesis of *Clostridium difficile* colitis. The organisms colonize the colonic mucosa and elaborate toxins. Toxin A is the major pathogenic principle. Toxin A binds to specific receptors on the brush-border membrane (BBM) and causes enterocyte damage by decreasing actin assembly and increasing mucosal permeability. In addition, toxin A results in the chemotaxis of polymorphonuclear leukocytes (PMNs) and an acute enterocolitis. The leukocytes release various inflammatory mediators that result in intestinal secretion and diarrhea. The toxin may also cause inflammation and diarrhea via the enteric nervous system.

TABLE 12-24. TESTS FOR DETECTION OF *CLOSTRIDIUM DIFFICILE* TOXINS

TEST	ANTIGEN-DETECTED	COMMENTS
Tissue culture assay	Toxin B	Most sensitive ("gold standard")
ELISA	Toxin A	Sensitive and specific
Latex agglutination test	"Latex antigen" Not specific	Nonspecific, should be confirmed with tissue culture assay or ELISA

TABLE 12-24.

Tests for the detection of *Clostridium difficile* toxins. The three most commonly used assays are listed. The gold standard is the tissue culture assay (*ie*, cytopathic changes in tissue cultures), which are blocked by specific *C. difficile* antitoxin; this assay detects toxin B. Sensitive and specific enzyme-linked immunosorbent assays (ELISA) are available to detect toxin A; they are reliable and sensitive. A rapid latex agglutination test is available; however, this test detects a "latex antigen," which is not specific. Positive results on the latex agglutination should be confirmed either by a tissue culture assay or by ELISA.

TABLE 12-25. FREQUENCY OF *CLOSTRIDIUM DIFFICILE* AND *C. DIFFICILE* CYTOTOXIN IN STOOLS FROM VARIOUS PATIENT POPULATIONS

	C. DIFFICILE, %	*C. DIFFICILE* TOXIN, %
Healthy adult	3	0
Healthy neonates	30–70	25–60
Hospitalized adults	10–20	0–1
Recent antibiotic exposure	10–20	0–1
Antibiotic-associated PMC	80–100	90–95
AAC diarrhea without PMC	20–40	15–25
Other diarrheal diseases	3	2

TABLE 12-25.

Clostridium difficile and *C. difficile* cytotoxin in the stool of various patient populations. *C. difficile* organisms can be cultured from 10% to 25% of asymptomatic hospitalized adults, as well as adults recently exposed to antibiotics. Thus, isolation of the organism by itself is not a reliable means of diagnosing *C. difficile* colitis. Detection of *C. difficile* toxin by one of the aforementioned tests is the most reliable means of making a specific diagnosis. *C. difficile* toxin is rarely found in hospitalized adults or in adults with other diarrheal diseases. It should be noted, however, that healthy neonates frequently excrete *C. difficile* cytotoxin. AAC—Antibiotic-associated pseudomembranous colitis; PMC—pseudomembranous colitis.

FOOD POISONING

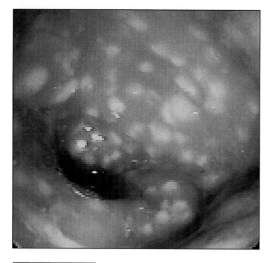

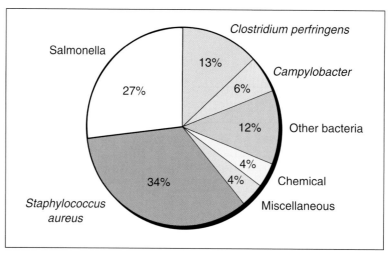

FIGURE 12-14.

Sigmoidoscopic appearance of pseudomembranous colitis. The typical appearance of *Clostridium difficile* colitis is illustrated. The mucosa is red and edematous and covered with yellow-white plaques.

FIGURE 12-15.

Causes of food poisoning. Food poisoning is a common entity resulting from either ingestion of preformed toxins or enteric bacteria, usually in food. The three most common pathogenic causes of food poisoning in the United States are *Staphylococcus aureus*, *Salmonella* spp, and *Clostridium perfringens* [5,18]. (*Adapted from* Banwell and Lake [5].)

TABLE 12-26. DIFFERENTIAL DIAGNOSIS OF FOOD POISONING SYNDROMES

SYMPTOMS	INCUBATION PERIOD, *HR*	POSSIBLE AGENTS
Acute upper gastrointestinal symptoms, nausea, vomiting	6	Preformed heat-stable toxins of *Staphylococcus aureus*, *Bacillus cereus*; also *D. latum*, anisakis, heavy metals
Upper small-bowel symptoms; watery noninflammatory diarrhea	6–72	*Clostridium perfringens* type A, *B. cereus*, enterotoxigenic *E. coli*, *Vibrio cholerae*, *Giardia lamblia*
Inflammatory ileocolitis	16–72	Salmonella, shigella, *Campylobacter jejuni*, *V. parahaemolyticus*, enteroinvasive *E. coli*, Yersinia, Aeromonas
Sensory or motor neurologic symptoms with or without gastrointestinal symptoms, suggesting botulism, fish, shellfish, or chemical poisoning	—	Histamine-like scombrotoxin, dinoflagellate neurotoxins, monosodium glutamate, mushrooms, solanine, pesticides

TABLE 12-26.

Differential diagnosis of food poisoning syndromes. Food poisoning syndromes can present in various ways. An acute syndrome characterized by upper gastrointestinal symptoms, nausea, and vomiting is one of the more common. Nausea and vomiting accompanied by watery diarrheal syndrome or inflammatory diarrhea also occurs. The least common is a syndrome characterized by sensory and motor neurologic symptoms with or without accompanying gastrointestinal symptoms. The organisms causing each of these syndromes are shown in this table. (*Adapted from* Guerrant and Bobak [7]; with permission.)

TRAVELER'S DIARRHEA

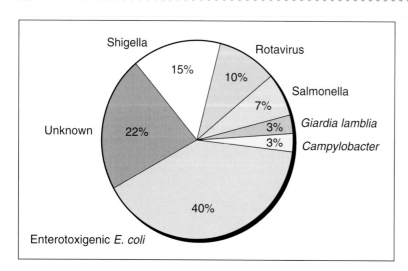

FIGURE 12-16.

Causes of traveler's diarrhea. Traveler's diarrhea is a syndrome occurring during or shortly after travel. A large array of enteropathogenic agents can cause the syndrome; however, the most common single cause is enterotoxigenic *Escherichia coli*. Other organisms causing this syndrome are shown. In all studies, 20% to 35% of patients elude specific diagnosis, thus suggesting the existence of other undefined infectious agents [5]. ETEC—Enterotoxigenic *Escherichia coli*. (*Adapted from* Banwell and Lake [5].)

TABLE 12-27. PROPHYLAXIS FOR TRAVELER'S DIARRHEA AND TARGET GROUPS

Effective Prophylaxis

Antibiotics (ciprofloxacin, TMP-Sulfa)

Bismuth subsalicylate

Groups Recommended for Prophylaxis

Patients with gastrectomy

Patients with inflammatory bowel disease

Those susceptible to dehydration (*ie*, patients with ileostomy or short-bowel syndrome)

Those with severe systemic illnesses

Immunosuppressed patients

TABLE 12-27.

Effective prophylaxis of traveler's diarrhea and specific groups recommended. Two means are effective in preventing traveler's diarrhea: antibiotics and bismuth subsalicylate; they appear to be equally effective. The preferred antibiotics in adults are ciprofloxacin or trimethoprim-sulfa.

Most authorities do not recommend routine prophylaxis for all Americans traveling to other countries. However, certain high-risk groups, as shown, should receive prophylaxis.

TABLE 12-28. DIFFERENTIAL DIAGNOSIS OF CHRONIC DIARRHEA ASSOCIATED WITH TRAVEL

Persistent infection
   Giardiasis, amebiasis, salmonellosis/*Campylobacter* infection, yersiniosis
Antibiotic-associated colitis
Lactose intolerance (transient)
Tropical sprue
Small-intestinal bacterial overgrowth
Unmasked celiac sprue
Unmasked ulcerative colitis and regional enteritis
Postdysenteric colitis
Postdysenteric irritable bowel syndrome

TABLE 12-28.

Differential diagnosis of chronic diarrhea associated with travel. One distressing syndrome is chronic diarrhea, which begins with an episode of typical traveler's diarrhea. Although the frequency of this disorder is unknown, it is not rare. Physicians caring for such patients should first exclude persistent infection with various pathogens, and then assess patients for the other entities listed in this table.

■ SEXUALLY TRANSMITTED ENTERIC INFECTIONS

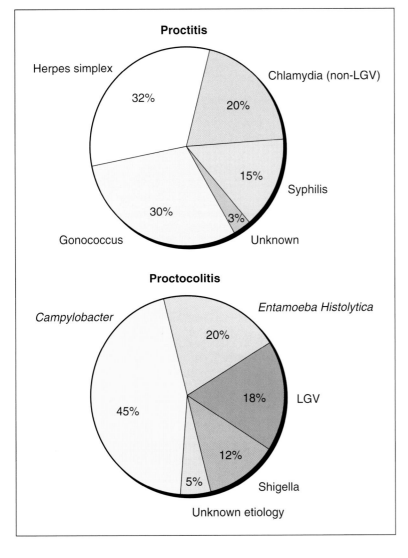

FIGURE 12-17.

Multiple causes of enteric pathogens in homosexual men. Homosexual men are susceptible to a wide range of enteropathogens, including various bacteria, protozoa, and viruses. Risk factors for such infections include sexual promiscuity, sexual practices allowing fecal-oral transmission, and the carriage of enteric pathogens by asymptomatic homosexual men. Clinical syndromes include watery diarrhea, proctitis, proctocolitis, or asymptomatic infection. In such men with proctitis, the likely pathogens include gonococcus, herpes simplex, or chlamydia. In individuals with colitis, the most common single etiologic agent is *Campylobacter*. LGV—Lymphogranuloma venereum. (*Adapted from* Banwell and Lake [5].)

GIARDIASIS

TABLE 12-29. GIARDIASIS: HIGH-RISK GROUPS

Children in daycare centers
Travelers
Homosexual males
Nursing home residents
Individuals with immunodeficiency states (AIDS, IgA deficiency)

TABLE 12-29.

Giardiasis: high-risk groups. *Giardia* causes a common enteric infection occurring particularly in children in daycare centers, travelers, homosexual men, nursing home residents, and those in various states of immunodeficiency. In individuals in all these groups, an asymptomatic infection may occur.

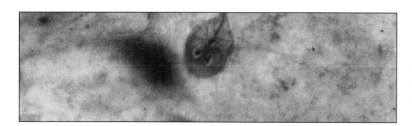

FIGURE 12-18.

Light photomicrograph of *Giardia* trophozoites from duodenal aspirate. Duodenal aspiration for *Giardia* trophozoites is frequently used to document infection with *Giardia*. Staining such aspirates with methylene blue or another stain can reveal the typical *Giardia* trophozoite as illustrated in this figure.

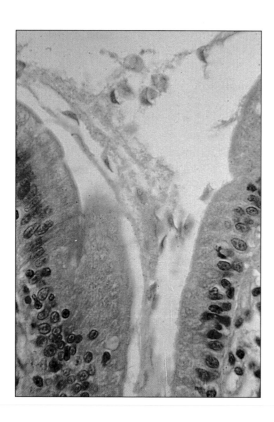

FIGURE 12-19.

Light microscopic photomicrograph of duodenal biopsy showing *Giardia* trophozoites in adherent mucus. Small-bowel biopsy is probably the most reliable way to diagnose *Giardia* infection. The trophozoites should be sought in the mucus adherent to the mucosa. The findings can be subtle, and must be sought diligently.

TABLE 12-30. GIARDIASIS: CLINICAL SYNDROMES

Asymptomatic
Acute diarrhea, self-limited
Chronic, intermittent diarrhea
Malabsorption syndrome

TABLE 12-30.

Giardiasis: clinical syndromes. These clinical syndromes of giardiasis include acute self-limited diarrhea, chronic intermittent diarrhea, a full-blown malabsorption syndrome, or an asymptomatic infection [22].

ENTAMOEBA HISTOLYTICA

TABLE 12-31. AMEBIASIS

Summary
Endemic in the United States
Transmitted by oral-fecal contamination
(Carriage in U.S. general population ± 5%;
    among homosexuals ± 30%)
Spectrum (asymptomatic to fulminant
    colitis)
Pain, diarrhea, dysentery (intermittent, wax
    and wane, weeks to months)

Complications
Fulminant colitis, toxic megacolon,
    bleeding, perforation,
    postdysenteric colitis
Liver, brain, and lung abscesses

Pathogenesis
Elaborate cytotoxins
Serotonin-like peptides
Other peptides

Diagnosis
Stool examination (3–6 specimens)
Avoid barium enema and antibiotics
Indirect hemagglutination test (especially in
    diagnosis of colitis and hepatic mass)

Differential Diagnosis
Ulcerative colitis
Bacillary dysentery

Treatment
Invasive disease: metronidazole and
    diiodohydroxyquin
Liver disease: chloroquine

TABLE 12-31.

Amebiasis: summary. Various clinical and epidemiologic features of amebiasis are listed. Amebiasis is endemic in the United States, transmitted by oral-fecal contamination, and is especially common in homosexual men. The spectrum of illness can vary from an asymptomatic carrier state to fulminant colitis. Systemic manifestations can also occur [7].

Entamoeba histolytica can cause colitis and diarrhea by several mechanisms, including the elaboration of cytotoxic substances and secretogogues, such as serotonin-like peptides. The diagnosis is usually made by examination of the stool for trophozoites or cysts, and may require as many as three to six individual specimens. The most important disorders to consider in the differential diagnosis of amebiasis include ulcerative colitis, shigellosis, and *Escherichia coli* hemorrhagic colitis. Treatment is as shown.

CRYPTOSPORIDIUM

TABLE 12-32. CRYPTOSPORIDIOSIS: SUMMARY

Features
Diarrhea, cramps, nausea, vomiting, weight loss
An enteritis or enterocolitis
Common in normal host (self-limited)
Occurs in clusters (*ie*, families and day-care centers)
Common among AIDS patients (chronic and devastating)
One third of cases have an associated second pathogen, especially giardia

Diagnosis
Acid-fast stain—oocysts in stool
Small-intestinal biopsy
Colonic biopsy

Therapy
Not required in normal host
Only partially successful in immunocompromised patients

TABLE 12-32.

Cryptosporidiosis: summary. Cryptosporidiosis is an illness characterized by diarrhea, abdominal cramps, nausea, vomiting, and weight loss. It can cause either an enteritis or an enterocolitis. It is common both in the normal immunocompetent host and especially in the immunodeficient host, such as patients with AIDS. In such patients, the diarrhea is frequently chronic and devastating, and may be associated with nutrient malabsorption.

Diagnosis of cryptosporidiosis is made by demonstration of oocysts in stool, which are most easily appreciated when stool is stained with an acid-fast stain. Small intestinal biopsy and colonic biopsy are other methods of making this diagnosis. Treatment usually is not required in the normal host and is only partially effective in the immunosuppressed host [20,21,23].

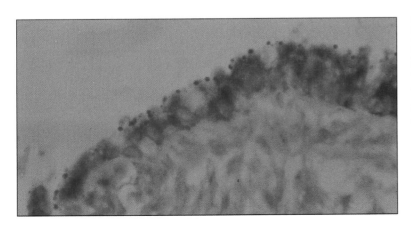

FIGURE 12-20.

Photomicrograph of intestinal biopsy—cryptosporidiosis. A small intestinal biopsy reveals cryptosporidia adherent to the surface of the enterocytes. The organism does not invade and is confined to the surface of the epithelial cell [5]. A similar appearance can be seen in the colon. (*From* Banwell and Lake [5]; *courtesy of* R.L. Owen, MD, Cell Biology Section, VA Hospital, San Francisco, CA.)

■ MICROSPORIDIA

TABLE 12-33. MICROSPORIDIOSIS: SUMMARY

Features
Profuse watery diarrhea
Abdominal pain, weight loss, no fever

Diagnosis
Endoscopic biopsy of small bowel or colon

Therapy
Albendazole

TABLE 12-33.

Microsporidiosis: summary. Infection caused by microsporidia is characterized by profuse watery diarrhea associated with abdominal pain and weight loss, but usually no fever. Diagnosis is difficult and usually made by endoscopic biopsy of the small bowel or colon.

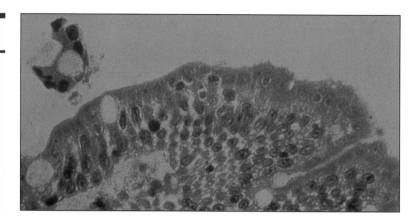

FIGURE 12-21.

Small intestinal biopsy: microsporidiosis [19]. Microsporidia invade and are seen within vacuoles in the cytoplasm of epithelial cells. Organisms are difficult to detect by light microscopy, and are best appreciated by electron microscopy. Treatment is with albendazole [19–21].

■ CYTOMEGALOVIRUS

TABLE 12-34. AIDS-RELATED PATHOGENS: PROTOZOA

PROTOZOA	SPECIFIC THERAPIES
Giardia lamblia	Metronidazole, 250 mg t.i.d.
Entamoeba histolytica	Metronidazole, 750 mg t.i.d.
Cryptosporidium sp.*	Spiramycin, azithromycin, clarithromycin, letrazuril, diclazuril, paromomycin, bovine colostrum
Isospora belli*	Trimethoprin 160 mg/sulfa 800 mg (DS) QID 10 d
Microsporidial sp.	Albendazole

*Therapies for these pathogens still in experimental stages

TABLE 12-34.

AIDS-related pathogens: protozoa—specific therapies. Protozoan enteropathogens are difficult to treat, particularly in the patient with AIDS. Although metronidazole is quite effective in patients with giardia and entamoeba infections, treatment for *Cryptosporidium*, *Isospora*, and *Microsporidia* are only partially effective at present [19–21]. (*Adapted from* Cello [19].)

TABLE 12-35. CYTOMEGALOVIRUS: SUMMARY

Features
Can infect any part of the gastrointestinal tract
Can occur in normal host, usually self-limited
Cytomegalovirus colitis common in patients with AIDS and those who have had organ transplants

Intestinal symptoms
Diarrhea, abdominal pain, bleeding perforation

Diagnosis
Typical finding is a deep, "punched-out" ulcer
Typical viral inclusion bodies on light microscopy

Treatment
Ganciclovir, foscarnet, cytomegalovirus immunoglobin

TABLE 12-35.

Cytomegalovirus: summary. *Cytomegalovirus* can infect any portion of the gastrointestinal tract in both the normal and in the immunocompromised host. Cytomegalovirus colitis is extremely common in patients with AIDS, and presents with nausea and vomiting, diarrhea, abdominal pain, and occasionally bleeding and perforation.

Diagnosis is most easily made with endoscopy and biopsy of either the upper or lower gastrointestinal tract. The typical finding is a deep, "punched-out" ulcer. Typical viral inclusion bodies are seen on light microscopy. Various treatments are available, but the agent of choice is ganciclovir [24].

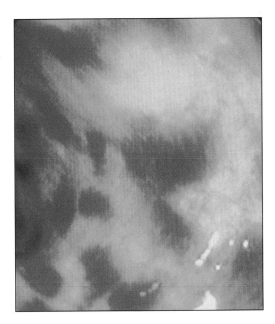

FIGURE 12-22.

Colonoscopic appearance of cytomegalovirus colitis. Typical appearance of cytomegalovirus colitis has scattered lesions throughout the colon, which in their earliest stage appear as a vasculitis or large angiodysplasia-like lesions evolving to deep "punched-out" ulcers. The intravening mucosa is frequently normal in appearance [19].

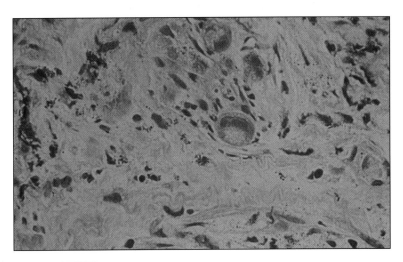

FIGURE 12-23.

Histopathology of cytomegalovirus colitis. The typical viral inclusion bodies are illustrated in this figure [19].

REFERENCES

1. Giannella RA: Gastrointestinal infections. In *Textbook of Internal Medicine.* Edited by Kelley WN. Philadelphia: JB Lippincott; 1989:554–562.

2. Cohen MB, Giannella RA: Bacterial infections of the colon: Pathophysiology, clinical features, and treatment. In *The Large Intestine: Physiology, Pathophysiology and Diseases.* New York: Raven Press; 1991:395–428.

3. Park SI, Giannella RA: Approach to the adult patient with diarrhea. *Gastroenterol Clin North Am* 1993, 22:483–497.

4. Saxe J, Giannella RA: Bacterial and traveler's diarrhea: Diagnosis and management. *Pract Gastroent* 1988, 12:20–28.

5. Banwell JG, Lake AM: *Undergraduate Teaching Project. Unit 17. Gut Immunology and Ecology.* Bethesda, MD: American Gastroenterological Association.

6. Guerrant RL: Principles and syndromes of enteric infection. In *Principles and Practice of Infectious Diseases.* Edited by Mandell GL, Bennett JE, Dolin R. New York: Churchill Livingstone; 1995:945–962.

7. Guerrant RL, Bobak DA: Bacterial and protozoal gastroenteritis. *N Engl J Med* 1991, 325:327–340.

8. Field M, Rao MC, Chang EB: Intestinal electrolyte transport and diarrheal disease. *N Engl J Med* 1989, 321:800–806.

9. Holmgren J, Svennerholm AM: Mechanisms of disease and immunity in cholera. *J Infec Dis* 1977, 136:S106–S112.

10. Cohen MB, Giannella RA: Enterotoxigenic *E. coli.* In *Infections of the Gastrointestinal Tract.* Edited by Blaser MJ, Smith PD, Ravdin JI, *et al.* New York: Raven Press; 1995:691–707.

11. Cantey JR: *Escherichia coli. Gastroenterol Clin North Am* 1993, 22:609–622.

12. Rothbaum R, McAdams AJ, Giannella RA, Partin JC: A clinicopathologic study of enterocyte-adherent *E. coli*: A cause of protracted diarrhea in infants. *Gastroenterology* 1982, 83:441–454.

13. Cohen MB, Giannella RA: Hemorrhagic colitis associated with *Escherichia coli* O157:H7. *Adv Intern Med* 1992, 37:173–195.

14. Griffin PM: *Escherichia coli* O157: H7 and other enterohemorrhagic *E. coli*. In *Infections of the Gastrointestinal Tract.* Edited by Blaser MJ, Smith PD, Ravdin JI, *et al.* New York: Raven Press; 1995:739–761.

15. Giannella RA: Salmonella. In *Medical Microbiology.* Edited by Baron S. New York: Churchill Livingstone; 1991:317–325.

16. Vantrappen G, Geboes K, Ponette E: *Yersinia enteritis. Med Clin North Am* 1982, 66:639–653.

17. Kelly CP, Pothoulakis C, LaMont JT: *Clostridium difficile* colitis. *N Engl J Med* 1994, 330:257–262.

18. Bishai WR, Sears CL: Food poisoning syndromes. *Gastroenterol Clin North Am* 1993, 22:579–608.

19. Cello JP: Diagnosis and management of AIDS-related diarrhea: A teleconference presented by California Pacific Medical Center, 1993.

20. Smith PD, Quinn TC, Strober W, *et al.*: Gastrointestinal infections in AIDS. *Ann Intern Med* 1992, 116:63–77.

21. Smith PD: Infectious diarrheas in patients with AIDS. *Gastroenterol Clin North Am* 1993, 22:549–561.

22. Farthing MJG: Giardia infections. In *Enteric Infection.* Edited by Farthing MJG, Keusch GT. New York: Raven Press; 1989.

23. Adal KA, Sterling CR, Guerrant RL: *Cryptosporidium* and related species. In *Infections of the Gastrointestinal Tract.* Edited by Blaser MJ, Smith PD, Ravdin JI, *et al.* New York: Raven Press; 1995:1107–1128.

24. Goodgame RW: Gastrointestinal cytomegalovirus disease. *Ann Intern Med* 1993, 119:924–935.

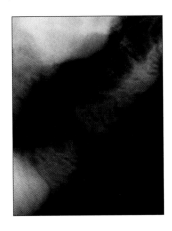

Index

Page numbers followed by *t* or *f* indicate tables or figures, respectively.

A

Abdominal pain
  with acute mesenteric ischemia, 10.2,
      10.6*f*
  with small-bowel tumors, 8.3*t*
Absorptive cells, 1.3*f*
Accessory cholera toxin, 1.14*f*
  mechanism of action, 12.5*t*
ACE. *See* Accessory cholera toxin
Acetylcholine
  in digestive function, 2.4*f*, 2.13*f*
  in vagal stimulation, 3.7*f*
Actin, 3.4*f*
  and myosin, interaction, 3.5*f*
Action potentials, 3.7*f*
Active transport, 1.5*f*, 2.2
  secondary, 1.6*f*
Activity front, 3.15*f*
Adenocarcinoma, of small intestine, 8.1
  bleeding from, endoscopic findings with,
      9.13*f*
  in Crohn's disease, 8.6*f*
  enteroclysis with, 8.5*f*
  histology, 8.5*f*
  napkin-ring lesion, 8.5*f*
  radiographic findings with, 8.5*f*
  relative frequency of distribution, 8.4*f*
  risk factors for, 8.3*t*
  signs and symptoms, 8.3*t*
Adenoma(s), of small intestine, 8.4*f*, 8.5*f*
  bleeding from, endoscopic findings with,
      9.13*f*
Adenylate cyclase, 1.13*f*
Amebiasis. *See also Entamoeba histolytica*
  summary, 12.17*t*
Amino acid(s), 2.12*f*
  acidic, 2.12*f*
  basic, 2.12*f*
  essential, 2.2*f*, 2.12*f*
  metabolism, gastric, 2.13*f*
  neutral, 2.12*f*
    aliphatic, 2.12*f*
    aromatic, 2.12*f*
    hydroxylated, 2.12*f*

    imino, 2.12*f*
    sulfur-containing, 2.12*f*
  transport, in enterocytes, 2.14*f*, 2.15*t*
5-Aminosalicylic acid prodrugs, for Crohn's
      disease of small intestine, 7.15*f*
Ampullary carcinoma, 8.6*f*, 8.7*f*
Ampullary tumors, 8.6*f*
Amylase
  activity, 2.4*f*
  pancreatic, activity, 2.11*f*
  salivary, activity, 2.11*f*
Amyloid, in small intestine, 7.13*f*
Amylopectin, 2.11*f*
Amylose, 2.11*f*
Angiodysplasia, 9.10*t*
  endoscopic treatment, 9.14*f*
  hormonal treatment, 9.15*t*
Angiography
  indications for, 9.2
  mesenteric, 10.2
Anoikis, 1.4*f*
Antiport, 1.6*f*
Aortoenteric fistula, bleeding caused by, 9.2,
      9.2*f*, 9.9*f*
Apical membrane
  lipid composition, 1.4*f*
  structure, 1.4*f*
Apoproteins, 2.10*f*
Apoptosis, 1.4*f*
Appendiceal abscess, 7.12*f*
Appendicolith, 7.12*f*
Arc of Riolan, 10.4*f*
Arteriography, with small-bowel bleeding,
      9.3*t*, 9.5*t*, 9.6*t*
Arteriovenous malformations
  classification, 9.10*t*
  distribution in gastrointestinal tract, 9.10*f*
  small-bowel
    anatomic locations, 9.11*f*, 9.12*f*
    distribution, 9.11*f*, 9.12*f*
    endoscopic findings in, 9.11*f*, 9.12*f*
    endoscopic treatment, 9.14*f*
    hemorrhage with, 9.2, 9.2*f*, 9.9*f*
    patient characteristics, 9.11*t*
    surgical treatment, 9.12*f*

  treatment, 9.13*t*
Asacol. *See* Mesalamine
Auerbach's plexus. *See* Myenteric plexus
Autonomic nervous system, in intestinal
      function, 1.11*f*
Autoregulation, 10.5*t*
Axons, in enteric nervous system, 3.9*f*
Azathioprine, for Crohn's disease of small
      intestine, 7.17*f*

B

Bacteria
  colonic, 2.6*f*
  cytotoxic, 12.3*t*
  diarrhea caused by, pathogenesis, 12.3-
      12.5
  enteric pathogens
    host defenses against, 12.4*t*
    infectious levels, 12.4*t*
    virulence factors, 12.4*t*
  enteroadhesive, 12.3*f*, 12.3*t*
  enterotoxigenic, 12.3*f*, 12.3*t*
  interactions with enterocytes, 12.3*f*
  invasive, 12.3*f*, 12.3*t*
Bacterial overgrowth
  malabsorption with, 5.5*f*
  pathophysiology, 5.5*f*
Barber-pole sign, 10.13*f*, 10.14*t*
Barium studies, with small-bowel bleeding,
      9.3*t*
Barostat system, 6.6*f*
Barrier function, of intestine, 1.2*f*, 1.3*f*
Basic electrical rhythm, 3.6*f*
Basolateral membrane, 1.4*f*
Bentiromide, oral administration, in evalua-
      tion of pancreatic exocrine func-
      tion, 5.18*f*
Bethanechol, prokinetic effects, 6.16*t*, 6.17*f*
Bicarbonate
  absorption, 1.7*f*, 1.9*f*
  secretion, 1.9*f*, 2.5*f*
  transport, 1.9*f*
Bile acid pool, 2.7*f*

Bile acids
  absorption, 2.2, 2.6f, 2.7f, 2.9f
  amphipathic properties, 2.9f
  conjugated, 2.7f
  enterohepatic circulation, 4.10f
  malabsorption
    after ileal resection, 5.12f
    causes, 4.10f
    and diarrhea, 4.10f
  micelles, 2.8f, 2.9f
  primary, 2.7f
  secondary, 2.7f
  synthesis, 2.7f
Biliary cirrhosis, primary, malabsorption
    with, 5.4f
Biotin, deficiency, signs and symptoms, 5.16t
Bisacodyl, detection, 4.11t
Bladder fistula, with Crohn's disease of small
    intestine, 7.10t
Bleeding
  acute, treatment algorithm, 9.15f
  chronic, of obscure origin, evaluation,
    9.16f
  gastrointestinal, with small-bowel tumors,
    8.3t
  small-bowel, 9.1-9.18
    arteriography with, 9.3t, 9.5t, 9.6t
    barium studies with, 9.3t
    causes, 9.2, 9.2f
    clinical presentation, 9.1-9.2
    diagnosis, 9.3t
    enteroclysis with, 9.3t
    enteroscopy with, 9.3t, 9.6t, 9.7f, 9.7t,
      9.8f, 9.8t, 9.9f, 9.9t
    evaluation, 9.1-9.2, 9.3t
    exploratory laparotomy with, 9.3t
    frequency, 9.1
    management, 9.2
    Meckel's scan with, 9.5t
    nuclear medicine studies with, 9.3t,
      9.4t
    of obscure origin, 9.1, 9.2f, 9.9f, 9.12f
    treatment, 9.13t, 9.14t
Blue rubber bleb nevus syndrome, 9.10t
Brain tumor, gastroparesis with, 6.12f
Breath hydrogen test, for transit, 3.12f, 6.6f,
    6.6t
Brunner's gland, hyperplasia, 8.13f
Brush-border membrane, amino acid trans-
    port in, 2.14f, 2.15t
Budesonide, for Crohn's disease of small
    intestine, 7.16f

C

Calcinosis cutis, 9.10t
Calcium
  absorption, 2.2, 2.16f
  content, of calcium salts, 5.13t
  daily intake, 2.16f
  deficiency, signs and symptoms, 5.16t
  intracellular

  in muscle contraction, 3.4f, 3.5f
  as second messenger, 1.13f
  supplementation, in short-bowel
    syndrome, 5.13t
Calcium-calmodulin kinase, activation, 1.13f
Calcium channels, 1.13f
Calmodulin, 1.13f, 3.4f
Calories. See Energy
cAMP. See Cyclic adenosine monophosphate
Campylobacter jejuni
  diarrhea caused by, 12.11t
  infection, summary, 12.11t
  infectious levels, 12.4t
Carbohydrate
  absorption, 2.11-2.12
    in large intestine, 2.6f
    in short-bowel syndrome, 5.9t
  dietary, 2.1, 2.2f
    average intake, 2.11f
    sources, 2.11f
  digestion, 2.11-2.12
    in large intestine, 2.6f
  malabsorption, 2.6f, 5.7f
Carboxypeptidase A, 2.14f
Carboxypeptidase B, 2.14f
Carcinoid
  diarrhea with, 4.11t, 4.16f
  in distal ileum, 7.12f
  of small intestine, 8.1, 8.7-8.8
    histology, 8.7f
    pedunculated duodenal, 8.8f
    radiographic appearance, 8.7f
    relative frequency of distribution, 8.4f
    risk factors for, 8.3t
    signs and symptoms, 8.3t
    small-bowel hemorrhage with, 9.2, 9.2f
  treatment, 4.17f
Carcinoma
  ampullary, 8.6f, 8.7f
  cecal, 7.12f
  in Crohn's disease, 7.7f, 8.6f
  gastrointestinal
    epidemiology, 8.2t
    incidence, 8.2f
Carriers, 1.6f
Catenins, 1.5f
CCK. See Cholecystokinin
Cecum, carcinoma, 7.12f
Celiac arteries, anatomy, 10.2f
Celiac artery
  compression, 10.11f
  stenosis, Doppler duplex scanning in,
    10.19t
Celiac sprue, 5.7f
Cell-cell communication, in small intestine,
    3.3f
Cell-cell interactions, 1.5f
Cell polarity, 1.4f
Cells, intestinal. See also Apical membrane;
    Basolateral membrane
  types, 1.3f
CFTR. See Cystic fibrosis transmembrane
    conductance regulator

cGMP. See Cyclic guanosine monophosphate
Chemical gradients, across intestinal epithe-
    lium, 1.5f, 1.6f
Chenic acid, 2.7f
Chloride, secretion, 1.6f, 1.8f
Chloride-bicarbonate exchanger, 1.7f, 1.9f
Chloride channels, 1.8f
Chloridorrhea, congenital, 4.9f
Cholecystokinin, 2.1
  in regulation of digestive function, 2.5f
  release, 2.5f
Cholera, 12.5-12.6
  pathophysiology, 1.14f
Cholera toxin, 1.14f
  activation of ion transport, 12.6f
  mechanism of action, 12.5t
Cholesterol, average intake, 2.8f
Cholesterol esterase, 2.8f
Cholesterol esters
  average intake, 2.8f
  synthesis, in endoplasmic reticulum of
    enterocytes, 2.10f
Cholic acid, 2.7f
  structure, 2.9f
Cholinergic agonists, 6.16t, 6.17f
Chylomicrons, 2.10f
Chyme, 2.1-2.2, 2.5f, 2.6f, 3.1
Chymotrypsin, 2.14f
Chymotrypsinogen, 2.13f
Cinitapride, 6.17t
Circular muscle, intestinal, 3.3f
Cisapride, 6.17t
  prokinetic effects, 6.16t, 6.17f, 6.18f
Clebopride, 6.17t
Clonidine, antidiarrheal activity, 4.23f
Clostridium difficile
  colitis
    pathogenesis, 12.13f
    summary, 12.12t
  cytotoxins, in stool, frequency in various
    populations, 12.13t
  infection, 12.12-12.13
  in stool, frequency in various populations,
    12.13t
  toxins, detection, 12.13t
Cobalamin. See Vitamin B$_{12}$
Coffee-grounds emesis, 9.2
Colipase, 2.8f
Colon
  vascular dysplasia, 9.10t
  vascular ectasia, 9.10t
Colonoscopy, indications for, 9.2
Copper
  absorption, 2.17t
  daily intake, 2.17t
Crohn's disease of small intestine, 7.1-7.21
  age of onset, 7.10f
  anatomic distribution, 7.2f
  anatomic pathology, 7.2-7.7
  aphthoid ulcers, 7.3f, 7.4f
  biliary tract complications, 7.10t
  bleeding in, 9.9f
  carcinoma in, 7.7f, 8.6f

chronic subserositis, 7.2f
classification, 7.3-7.7
clinical course, 7.1
clinical pathophysiology related to, 7.9-7.10
clinical presentation, 7.5f
in children and adolescents, 7.10t
clinicopathology, 7.1
diagnosis, 7.11
differential diagnosis, 7.11-7.13
endoscopic findings in, 7.4f
enterocutaneous fistula in, 7.6f
enteroenteric fistulas in, 7.5f, 7.8f
enterovesical fistulas in, 7.5f, 7.9f
epidemiology, 7.10f, 7.14
etiology, 7.14
fecal stream in, 7.21f
fistulizing pattern, 5f, 7, 7.1, 7.3f, 7.6f
clinical presentation, 7.7-7.8
granulomas, 7.2f, 7.4f
history in, 7.11t
immune dysregulation in, 7.14f
inflammatory pattern, 7.1, 7.3f, 7.4f
clinical-pathologic correlation in, 7.7
clinical presentation, 7.7
laboratory findings in, 7.11t
malabsorption with, 7.9t
natural history, 7.10
outcome, 7.1
pathologic distribution, 7.2f
perianal fistula in, 7.6f
physical findings in, 7.11t
postoperative recurrence, 7.19-7.21
prevalence, 7.14f
pseudodiverticulae in, 7.5f
radiographic appearance, 7.3f, 7.5f
radiographic findings in, 7.11f, 7.11t
renal complications, 7.10t
retroperitoneal fistula in, 7.6f, 7.9f, 7.10t
risk factors for, 7.14
staging enteric pathology, 7.3f
stenosing pattern, 7.1, 7.3f, 7.5f
clinical-pathologic correlation in, 7.8
string sign in, 7.5f
treatment, 7.15-7.21
surgical, 7.19-7.21
Crohn's ileitis, 7.1, 7.2f
Crohn's ileocolitis, 7.1, 7.2f
Cross-bridge cycling, 3.4f
Crypt cells, 1.3f
proliferative, 1.4f
Cryptosporidiosis. See Cryptosporidium
Cryptosporidium
in HIV-infected (AIDS) patients, therapy for, 12.18t
infection
intestinal biopsy in, 12.17f
summary, 12.17t
Crypts
cells in, 1.3f
dynamics, 1.4f
Crypt-villus axis

dynamics, 1.4f
heterogeneity along, 1.10f
sodium/hydrogen exchangers along, 1.9f, 1.10f
Cyclic adenosine monophosphate, as second messenger, 1.13f
Cyclic guanosine monophosphate, as second messenger, 1.13f
Cyclic nucleotides, as second messengers, 1.13f
Cyclosporin A, for Crohn's disease of small intestine, 7.17f
Cystic fibrosis transmembrane conductance regulator, 1.6f, 1.8f, 1.10f
Cytomegalovirus
gastrointestinal infection
histopathology, 12.19f
microscopic findings in, 12.19f
summary, 12.18t
infection, gastroparesis with, 6.12t
Cytomegalovirus enteritis, after small-bowel transplantation, 11.12f
Cytotoxin, of Escherichia coli, 12.7t

D

DAG. See Diacylglycerol
Deconvolution, for computation of gastrointestinal transit, 3.13f
Deoxycholic acid, 2.7f
Desmin, 3.4f
Desmosomes, 1.5f
Diabetes mellitus
gastric emptying in, 6.9f
secretory diarrhea in, 4.19f
small-bowel transit in, measurement, 6.6f
Diabetic gastroparesis, 6.1, 6.2
clinical features, 6.8t
motor activity in, 6.9f
pathophysiology, 6.9t
Diacylglycerol, 1.13f
Diarrhea
bacterial
Campylobacter, 12.11
in cholera, 1.14f, 12.5-12.6
Clostridium difficile, 12.12-12.13
enterotoxin-mediated
intracellular mediators, 12.5t
pathogenesis, 12.5f
Escherichia coli and, 12.6-12.8
mechanisms, 12.3t
Salmonella, 12.9-12.10
Shigella, 12.10-12.11
Yersinia enterocolitica, 12.12
bile acid malabsorption and, 4.10f
carbohydrate-induced, 5.7f
chronic
approach to patient with, algorithm for, 4.20f-4.21f
associated with travel, differential diagnosis, 12.15t
plasma peptide determinations in, 4.13f

definition, 4.1
in diabetes mellitus, 4.19f
differential diagnosis, 4.1
in food poisoning, 12.14
ileostomy, causes, 4.7t
infectious (See also Food poisoning; Infection(s); Traveler's diarrhea)
approach to patient with, 12.2f
epidemiology, 12.1
etiopathologic agents, 12.1, 12.2t
inflammatory versus noninflammatory, 12.4t
pathogenesis, 12.3-12.5
sexually transmitted, 12.15f
osmotic, 4.1
pathophysiology, 1.11f
protozoan
AIDS-related, therapy for, 12.18t
Cryptosporidium, 12.17
Entamoeba histolytica, 12.17
etiopathologic agents, 12.1, 12.2t
Giardia, 12.16
Microsporidium, 12.18
secretory, 1.8f, 4.1-4.24
with carcinoid syndrome, 4.11t, 4.16f
causes, 4.4t
circulating secretagogues and, 4.11-4.18
clinical features, 4.2-4.4, 4.4t
definition, 4.1
differential diagnosis, 4.4t
drug- and toxin-induced, 4.18t
in enteritis, mechanisms, 4.8t
evaluation of patient with, 4.1
with glucagonoma, 4.11t, 4.18f
idiopathic, 4.20f
with loss of electrolyte transport function, 4.9f
luminal secretagogues and, 4.10-4.11
mechanisms, 4.4t
with medullary thyroid carcinoma, 4.11t, 4.16f
with mucosal inflammation, 4.8f
nonspecific treatment, 4.22f
oral rehydration therapy for, 4.22f
pathogenesis, 4.1
postresection, 4.5f-4.7f
with somatostatinoma, 4.11t, 4.17f
specific syndromes, 4.5-4.21
with systemic mastocytosis, 4.18f
treatment, 4.2
tumor-induced, 4.12f
in Verner-Morrison syndrome, 4.11t, 4.15f
in Zollinger-Ellison syndrome, 4.11t, 4.13f
steatorrhea with, 5.18f
treatment
clonidine for, 4.23f
octreotide for, 4.23f
opiates for, 4.23f
viral
cytomegalovirus, 12.18-12.19
etiopathologic agents, 12.1, 12.2t

I.3

Diet, composition, 2.2
Dieulafoy's syndrome, 9.10t
Digestion, 2.1-2.18, 5.1
  cephalic phase, 2.1, 2.2-2.3
  gastric phase, 2.1, 2.4-2.5
  intestinal phase, 2.1, 2.5-2.15
  in oral cavity, 2.3t
Diglycerides, 2.8f, 2.10f
Dipeptides, transport, 2.14f
Disaccharidases, 2.11f
Disaccharides, intake, 2.11f
Diverticula, small-bowel
  bleeding caused by, 9.2, 9.2f
  bleeding with, 9.9f
Domperidone, prokinetic effects, 6.16t, 6.17t
Dopamine antagonists, 6.16t, 6.17f, 6.17t
Doppler duplex scanning, for intestinal
  ischemia, 10.18f, 10.19t
Drugs, secretory diarrhea caused by, 4.18t
Dumping syndrome, 6.1, 6.7t
Duodenum
  anatomy, 3.2f
  length, 3.2f
Dyspepsia
  dysmotility and, 6.11f
  etiology, 6.10t
  and motility, 6.10f, 6.10t, 6.11f
  nonulcer, antral hypomotility in, 6.10f

E

E-cadherins, 1.5f
Elastase, 2.14f
Electrical control activity, 3.6f
Electrical gradients, across intestinal epithe-
  lium, 1.5f, 1.6f
Electrical response activity, 3.6f
Electrochemical gradient
  across intestinal epithelium, 1.5f, 1.6f
  for sodium, 1.7f, 1.8f
Electrogastrography, 6.2, 6.3f, 6.4t
Electromyography, in small intestine, 6.6t
Electrophysiology, 1.6f
Endometrioma, small-bowel involvement,
  bleeding with, 9.2, 9.2f
Endopeptidase, 2.13f, 2.14f, 2.14t
Endoscopy, upper gastrointestinal, 9.1, 9.2
Energy
  absorption, in short-bowel syndrome,
    5.10f
  deficiency, signs and symptoms, 5.16t
  intake, and energy requirements, in short-
    bowel syndrome, 5.10f
  requirements, in malnourished patient,
    5.19t
  sources, 2.1, 2.2f
Entamoeba histolytica
  colitis, summary, 12.17t
  diarrhea caused by, summary, 12.17t
  in HIV-infected (AIDS) patients, therapy
    for, 12.18t
  infectious levels, 12.4t

Enteric nervous system, 1.11f, 3.9f
  and mucosal transport function, 4.8f
  stimulation by cholera toxin, 1.14f
Enteritis, diarrhea in, mechanisms, 4.8t
Enteroclysis
  with adenocarcinoma, 8.5f
  indications for, 8.1, 9.2
  with small-bowel bleeding, 9.3t, 9.12t
Enterocytes
  cholera toxin and, 1.14f
  interaction of bacterial pathogens with,
    12.3f
  villus tip, effect of ischemia on, 10.5f
Enteropathy, malabsorption caused by, 5.7-
  5.8
Enteropeptidase, 2.13f, 2.14t
Enteroscopy
  indications for, 9.1, 9.2
  with small-bowel bleeding, 9.3t, 9.6t, 9.7f,
    9.7t, 9.8f, 9.8t
  intraoperative, 9.9f, 9.9t
Enterotoxin
  diarrhea caused by
    intracellular mediators, 12.5t
    pathogenesis, 12.5f
  of Escherichia coli, 12.7t
  of Vibrio cholerae, 12.5t
Eosinophilic gastroenteritis, malabsorption
  with, 5.8f
Epithelial cells. See also Apical membrane;
  Basolateral membrane
  apical membrane, barrier function, 1.2f
  interaction with cholera toxin, 1.14f
  turnover, 1.4f
Epstein-Barr virus, infection, gastroparesis
  with, 6.12t
Erosions, small-bowel, bleeding caused by,
  9.2, 9.2f
Erythromycin, prokinetic effects, 6.16t, 6.19f
Escherichia coli
  cytotoxins, 12.7t
  diarrhea caused by, 12.6-12.8
  diarrheogenic, 12.6t
  enterohemorrhagic, illnesses caused by,
    12.8t
  enteropathogenic, 12.3f
    adherence, 12.7f
  enterotoxigenic, 12.3f
    adherence, 12.7f
  enterotoxins, 12.7t
    mechanism of action, 12.7f
  0157:H7
    infection
      clinical overview, 12.8t
      summary, 12.8t
      transmission, 12.8t
    hemorrhagic colitis, 12.8t
  infectious levels, 12.4t
Exfoliation, 1.4f
Exopeptidase, 2.13f, 2.14f, 2.14t

F

Familial adenomatous polyposis, 8.4f
Fat
  dietary (See Lipids)
  fecal, 5.2f
    analysis, 5.17f
    and fecal weight, relationship between,
      5.18f
    with primary biliary cirrhosis, 5.4f
    and stimulated pancreatic lipase
      output, 5.3f
Fatty acids
  essential, 2.1, 2.2f, 2.8f
    deficiency, signs and symptoms, 5.16t
  hydrolysis, 2.8f
  saturated, 2.8f
  short-chain, metabolism, 2.6f
  unsaturated, 2.8f
Fiber, digestion, 2.2
Fistula(s)
  aortoenteric, bleeding caused by, 9.2, 9.2f,
    9.9f
  in Crohn's disease
    bladder, 7.10t
    enterocutaneous, 7.6f
    enteroenteric, 7.5f, 7.8f
    enterovesical, 7.5f, 7.9f
    perianal, 7.6f
    retroperitoneal, 7.6f, 7.9f, 7.10t
Fluid flow, intestinal, radioscintigraphic
  assessment, 3.13f
Fluid secretion, intestinal, 1.8f
Folate
  absorption, 2.16f
  deficiency, signs and symptoms, 5.16t
Folate conjugase, 2.16f
Food poisoning, 12.14
  causes, 12.14f
  differential diagnosis, 12.14t
Fructose, digestion and absorption, 2.11f,
  2.12f

G

Galactose, digestion and absorption, 2.11f,
  2.12f
Gallstones, in Crohn's disease, 7.10t
Gap junctions, 1.5f, 3.3f
Gastrectomy, malabsorption after, 5.5f
Gastric acid, secretion, 2.3f, 2.3t, 2.4f, 2.13f
Gastric emptying, 2.4f, 2.5f
  in diabetes, 6.9f
  measurement, 6.2f, 6.3f, 6.3t
Gastric secretion, 2.2f
Gastrin, in digestive function, 2.4f, 2.13f
Gastroduodenostomy, gastric resection with,
  malabsorption with, 5.5f
Gastroesophageal reflux disease, gastroduo-
  denal motor function and, 6.11t
Gastrojejunostomy
  gastric dysmotility after, 6.7t, 6.8f

gastric resection with, malabsorption with, 5.5*f*

Gastroparesis, 6.1, 6.7*t*
  in acid-peptic disease, 6.7*t*
  in anorexia nervosa, 6.7*t*
  with brain tumor, 6.12*f*
  causes, 6.2
  in collagen vascular disease, 6.7*t*
  in endocrine disorders, 6.7*t* (*See also* Diabetic gastroparesis)
  etiology, 6.7*t*
  in gastric mucosal disease, 6.7*t*
  idiopathic, 6.7*t*
  management, 6.16*t*
  in metabolic disorders, 6.7*t*
  in neuromuscular disorders, 6.11*t*
  postsurgical syndromes, 6.7*t*, 6.8*t*
  postviral, 6.12*t*
  prokinetic drugs in, 6.16*t*
  with pseudo-obstruction, 6.7*t*
  psychiatric causes, 6.7*t*
  in scleroderma, 6.7*t*
  viral, 6.12*t*

Gastroschisis, small-bowel transplantation for, 11.3*f*

Gastrostomy, in gastric dysmotility, 6.16*t*

Giardia lamblia
  in HIV-infected (AIDS) patients, therapy for, 12.18*t*
  infection, 12.16
    clinical syndromes, 12.16*t*
    high-risk groups, 12.16*t*
    infectious levels, 12.4*t*
    trophozoites, 12.16*f*

Giardiasis. *See Giardia lamblia*

Glucagonoma, diarrhea with, 4.11*t*, 4.18*f*

Glucocorticoid(s), for Crohn's disease of small intestine, 7.16*f*

Glucose, digestion and absorption, 2.11*f*, 2.12*f*

Glucose transporters
  GLUT-2, 1.7*f*, 2.12*f*
  GLUT-5, 2.12*f*

Glycerol-3-phosphate, 2.10*f*

Goblet cells, in small intestine, 1.3*f*

G-proteins, 1.13*f*

Gut brain, 3.9*f*

H

Haptocorrin, 2.15*f*

HCO₃. *See* Bicarbonate

Hemangioma, of small intestine, 8.14*f*, 8.15*f*

Hematemesis, 9.2

Hematochezia, 9.2

Hemorrhage. *See* Bleeding

Henoch-Schönlein purpura, mesenteric vascular insufficiency in, 10.12*f*

Hereditary hemorrhagic telangiectasia, 9.10*t*

Hernia, strangulated, intestinal ischemia with, 10.15*f*

Herpes simplex virus, infection, gastroparesis with, 6.12*t*

Histamine, in digestive function, 2.4*f*, 2.13*f*

HIV-infected (AIDS) patients, protozoa in, therapy for, 12.18*t*

Homosexual males, enteric pathogens in, 12.15*f*

Hyperthyroidism, diarrhea with, 4.11*t*

I

Ileocolonic resection, diarrhea after, 4.7*f*

Ileostomy
  diarrhea due to, causes, 4.7*t*
  stoma fluid, characteristics, 4.7*f*

Ileum
  anatomy, 3.2*f*
  jejunization, 7.13*f*
  length, 3.2*f*
  lymphoma in, 7.12*f*
  nutrient absorption in, 2.6*f*
  resection
    bile acid malabsorption and, 4.10*f*
    diarrhea after, 4.6*f*
    malabsorption after, 5.8*t*
  vasculitis and edema, 7.13*f*

Ileus, acute, radiographic findings in, 6.12*f*

Immune cells, intestinal, 1.12*f*

Immunoglobulin A, secreted, 1.2*f*

Immunomodulators, for Crohn's disease of small intestine, 7.17*f*

Indium-111 amberlite resin pellets, in measurement of small-bowel transit, 6.6*f*

Infection(s), 12.1-12.19. *See also* Diarrhea
  causes, 12.1
  enteric
    host defenses against, 12.4*t*
    sexually transmitted, 12.15

Inositol trisphosphate, 1.13*f*

Intermediate filaments, 3.4*f*

Intermediate junctions, 1.5*f*, 3.3*f*

Interstitial cells of Cajal, 3.5*f*, 3.6*f*, 3.9*f*

Intestinal angina, 10.2

Intestinal failure
  costs, 11.2*f*
  morbidity and mortality, 11.2*f*

Intestinal resection, predicted nutritional outcome in, 5.8*t*

Intestinal wall, layers, 3.3*f*

Intestinocolonic inhibitory reflex, 3.8*f*

Intestinointestinal reflex, 3.8*f*

Intrinsic factor, 2.6*f*, 2.15*f*
  secretion, 2.4*f*

Intussusception
  causes, 10.14*f*
  clinical presentation, 10.14*f*
  diagnosis, 10.14*f*-10.15*f*
  mesenteric vascular insufficiency with, 10.13-10.14
  pathophysiology, 10.14*f*

Ion-specific channels, 1.6*f*

Ion transport
  across intestinal epithelium, 1.6*f*
  electrogenic, 1.6*f*
  electroneutral, 1.6*f*

Ipecac, detection, 4.11*t*

Iron
  absorption, 1.10*f*, 2.16*f*
  daily intake, 2.16*f*
  deficiency, signs and symptoms, 5.16*t*
  supplementation, in short-bowel syndrome, 5.14*t*

Irritable bowel syndrome
  manometric features, 6.16*f*
  motility disorder in, 3.15*f*

Ischemia
  intestinal (*See also* Mesenteric vascular insufficiency)
    associated conditions, 10.8*t*
    chronic, 10.9*f*
    classification, 10.7*f*, 10.7*t*
    clinical presentation, 10.6*f*
    clinical syndromes, 10.7*t*, 10.7-10.20
    conditions contributing to, 10.8*t*
    evaluation, 10.18*f*, 10.18*t*, 10.19*t*
    stages, 10.6*f*
    traumatic, 10.17*f*
  small-bowel
    classification, 10.7*t*
    histopathology, 10.10*f*
  of small intestine, 10.1 (*See also* Mesenteric vascular insufficiency)

Ischemia-reperfusion injury, gastrointestinal, 10.1

Ischemic hypoxia, of gut, cytototoxicity, 10.5*f*, 10.6*f*

Isospora belli, in HIV-infected (AIDS) patients, therapy for, 12.18*t*

J

Jaundice, with small-bowel tumors, 8.3*t*

Jejunoscopy, with small-bowel bleeding, 9.6*t*, 9.7*f*, 9.7*t*, 9.8*f*

Jejunostomy
  in dysmotility, 6.16*t*
  short bowel with
    magnesium balance with, 5.13*t*
    and sodium-water absorption, 5.11*f*
  sodium balance after, 5.11*f*
  stoma fluid, characteristics, 4.7*f*

Jejunum
  anatomy, 3.2*f*
  length, 3.2*f*
  macronutrient digestion and absorption in, 2.6*f*
  manometry, clinical use, 3.17*t*
  resection
    diarrhea after, 4.5*f*
    malabsorption after, 5.8*t*

Junctional complexes, of paracellular pathway, 1.5*f*

Juvenile polyps, 8.13*f*

K

Kaposi's sarcoma, of small intestine, 8.11*f*
Kidney stones, with Crohn's disease of small intestine, 7.10*t*

L

Lactase, 2.11*f*
    deficiency
        malabsorption with, 5.6*f*
        pathophysiology, 5.6*f*
Lactose, intake, 2.11*f*
Laparotomy, indications for, 9.2
Large intestine, in carbohydrate absorption and digestion, 2.6*f*
Latch state, 3.5*f*
Law of the intestine, 3.10*f*
Laxatives
    abuse, 4.11*t*
    detection, 4.11*t*
Lecithin, 2.10*f*
Leiomyoma
    bleeding from, endoscopic findings with, 9.13*f*
    of small intestine, 8.9*f*, 8.11*f*
Leiomyosarcoma, of small intestine, 8.1, 8.9*f*, 8.10*f*, 8.11*f*
    relative frequency of distribution, 8.4*f*
    signs and symptoms, 8.3*t*
Leukemia, small-bowel involvement, bleeding with, 9.2, 9.2*f*
α-Limit dextrin, digestion, 2.11*f*
Linoleic acid, 2.8*f*
Linolenic acid, 2.8*f*
Lipase
    gastric, 2.8*f*
        activity, 2.4*f*, 2.8*f*
        secretion, 2.4*f*
    intraluminal activity, with pancreatic enzyme replacement, 5.3*f*
    output, in duodenum and ileum
        in normal subjects, 5.4*f*
        with pancreatic insufficiency, 5.4*f*
    pancreatic, stimulated output, and fecal fat excretion, 5.3*f*
Lipid emulsion droplets, 2.8*f*
Lipids
    absorption, 2.8-2.10
        in short-bowel syndrome, 5.9*t*, 5.10*f*
    average intake, 2.8*f*
    dietary, 2.1, 2.2*f*
    digestion, 2.8-2.10
    energy content, 2.8*f*
    malabsorption, after ileal resection, 5.12*f*
Lipid vesicles, in endoplasmic reticulum of enterocytes, 2.10*f*
Lipolysis, 2.1
    gastric, 2.8*f*
Lipoma, of small intestine, 8.14*f*
Lithocholic acid, 2.7*f*

Liver, injury, from total parenteral nutrition, 11.1, 11.4*f*
Lung cancer, metastatic, small-bowel involvement, 8.12*f*
Lymphangiectasia, malabsorption with, 5.15*f*
Lymphangioma, of small intestine, 8.15*f*
Lymphoma
    intestinal involvement, 7.12*f*
    of small intestine, 8.1, 8.8-8.9
        clinical presentation, 8.9*f*
        clinical staging, 8.8*f*
        polypoid, 8.9*f*
        primary, 8.8*f*, 8.8*t*, 8.9*f*
        prognosis for, 8.8*t*
        relative frequency of distribution, 8.4*f*
        risk factors for, 8.3*t*
        signs and symptoms, 8.3*t*
        small-bowel hemorrhage with, 9.2, 9.2*f*
Lymphoproliferative disorder, after small-bowel transplantation, 11.13*f*
Lysolecithin, 2.9*f*, 2.10*f*

M

Macronutrients, 2.1, 2.2*f*
    absorption, 2.1-2.2, 2.2
        in jejunum, 2.6*f*
        in short-bowel syndrome, 5.9*t*
    digestion, 2.1-2.2
        intestinal phase, 2.6*f*
    enzymatic breakdown, in stomach, 2.4*f*
Magnesium
    compounds, magnesium content, 5.13*t*
    daily intake, 2.16*f*
    deficiency
        in short-bowel syndrome, 5.13*t*
        signs and symptoms, 5.16*t*
    as laxative, detection, 4.11*t*
    supplementation
        in malnourished patient, 5.19*t*
        in short-bowel syndrome, 5.13*t*
Malabsorption, 5.1-5.19
    after gastrectomy, 5.5*f*
    with bacterial overgrowth, 5.5*f*
    carbohydrate, 5.6*f*
    causes, 5.1, 5.2*t*
    with celiac sprue, 5.7*f*
    classification, 5.2*t*
    enteropathies producing, 5.7-5.8
    with eosinophilic gastroenteritis, 5.8*f*
    with lactase deficiency, 5.6*f*
    with lymphangiectasia, 5.15*f*
    mucosal, 5.6-5.14
        causes, 5.2*t*
    nutritional therapy in, complications, 5.19*f*
    with pancreatic exocrine insufficiency, 5.2-5.4
    postmucosal, 5.15
        causes, 5.2*t*
    premucosal, 5.2-5.5
        causes, 5.2*t*

    with primary biliary cirrhosis, 5.4*f*
    with short-bowel syndrome, 5.8-5.14
    signs and symptoms, 5.16*t*
    suspected
        evaluation for, 5.15-5.18
            algorithm for, 5.16*f*
            initial evaluation of patient, 5.15*t*
    with Whipple's disease, 5.8*f*
Malignancy, of small intestine, 8.1
Malrotation, radiologic abnormalities in, 10.13*f*, 10.14*t*
Maltase-glucoamylase, 2.11*f*
Maltose, 2.11*f*
Maltotriose, 2.11*f*
Manganese
    absorption, 2.17*t*
    daily intake, 2.17*t*
Manometry
    antroduodenal, 6.4*f*-6.5*f*
    intestinal, 3.15-3.17, 6.7*f*
        perfusion system, 6.4*f*, 6.4*t*
        solid-state system, 6.4*t*, 6.5*f*
    of intestinal neuropathy, 6.15*f*
    of intestinal obstruction, 6.12*f*
    of intestinal pseudo-obstruction, 6.13*f*
    of irritable bowel syndrome, 6.16*f*
    jejunal, clinical use, 3.17*t*
    small-bowel, 6.6*t*
Marginal artery of Drummond, 10.4*f*
Mass, with small-bowel tumors, 8.3*t*
Mastocytosis
    diarrhea with, 4.11*t*
    systemic, 4.18*f*
M cells, 1.3*f*
Meandering mesenteric artery, 10.4*f*
Meckel's diverticulum, bleeding caused by, 9.2, 9.2*f*, 9.13*t*
Meckel's scan, with small-bowel bleeding, 9.5*t*
Meissner's plexus internus. *See* Submucosal plexus
Melanoma, metastatic, small-bowel involvement, 8.11*f*, 8.12*f*
Melena, 9.2
6-Mercaptopurine, for Crohn's disease of small intestine, 7.17*f*, 7.18*f*
Mesalamine
    for Crohn's disease of small intestine, 7.15*f*, 7.16*t*
    and Crohn's disease recurrence, 7.20*f*
    pharmacology, 7.16*t*
Mesenteric ischemia
    acute
        clinical presentation, 10.2
        treatment, 10.2
    chronic
        clinical presentation, 10.2
        treatment, 10.2
Mesenteric vascular anatomy, 10.2-10.4
    arterial, 10.2*f*, 10.3*f*
    collateral channels, 10.2*f*, 10.4*f*
    intramural, 10.4*f*
    venous, 10.2*f*

Mesenteric vascular insufficiency, 10.1-10.20
  associated conditions, 10.8t
  causes, 10.5t
  with celiac artery compression syndrome, 10.11f
  classification, 10.7f, 10.7t
  clinical features, 10.2
  clinical syndromes, 10.7t, 10.7-10.20
  conditions contributing to, 10.8t
  with embolism, 10.8f
  evaluation, 10.18f, 10.18t, 10.19t
  in Henoch-Schönlein purpura, 10.12f
  with intussusception, 10.13-10.14
  management, 10.19f-10.20f
  with mesenteric venous thrombosis, 10.10f
  morbidity and mortality, 10.1
  pathophysiology, 10.1-10.2, 10.5-10.6
  with pneumatosis intestinalis, 10.9f
  with polyarteritis nodosa, 10.11f
  presentation, 10.2
  in sickle-cell disease, 10.16f
  stages, 10.6f
  with strangulated hernia, 10.15f
  in superior mesenteric artery syndrome, 10.17f
  in systemic lupus erythematosus, 10.12f
  trauma-related, 10.17f
  treatment, 10.2
  with vasculitis, 10.11-10.12
  with volvulus, 10.13-10.14
Mesenteric venous thrombosis, 10.10f
  clinical presentation, 10.2
Metastases, small-bowel involvement, 8.12f, 9.13t
Methotrexate, for Crohn's disease of small intestine, 7.17f, 7.18f
Metoclopramide, prokinetic effects, 6.16t, 6.17f, 6.17t
Metronidazole, for prevention of Crohn's disease recurrence, 7.20f
Micelles, 2.8f, 2.9f
Micronutrients, 2.1, 2.2f
  absorption, 2.2, 2.15-2.17
Microsporidium
  in HIV-infected (AIDS) patients, therapy for, 12.18t
  infection
    small intestinal biopsy in, 12.18f
    summary, 12.18t
Microvilli, 1.3f
Microvillus membrane, surface area, 1.2f
Migrating motor complex, 3.15f, 6.4f-6.5f
Minerals, 2.1, 2.2f
  absorption, 2.16f
  daily intake, 2.16f
Monoglycerides, 2.8f, 2.9f
Motility
  disorders, 3.15f, 6.1-6.20
  dyspepsia and, 6.10f, 6.10t, 6.11f
  foregut, disorders
    assessment for, 6.1-6.2
    causes, 6.2

    management, 6.2
    signs and symptoms, 6.1
  gastric
    antroduodenal, evaluation, 6.4f-6.5f
    assessment, 6.2-6.4
    disorders, 6.1-6.20
      clinical syndromes, 6.7t
      management, 6.16-6.20
      postsurgical syndromes, 6.7t, 6.8t
      signs and symptoms, 6.1
      surgery for, 6.20t
    in fundus and corpus, evaluation, 6.6f
  gastroduodenal, disorders, in diffuse motility disorders, 6.10t
  intestinal
    assessment, 6.1-6.2, 6.4-6.7
      contrast radiographs in, 3.11f
      plain radiographs in, 3.11f
      radioscintigraphy in, 3.13f, 6.2
    chemical regulation, 3.10f
    disorders
      management, 6.16-6.20
      surgery for, 6.20t
    endocrine regulation, 3.10f
    neural modulation, 3.6f, 3.8f
    normal fasting and fed patterns, 3.15-3.16
    paracrine regulation, 3.10f
    slow waves in, 3.6f
    study, historical perspective on, 3.2t
  small-bowel, 3.1-3.18
    anatomical considerations, 3.2-3.7
    assessment, 6.1-6.2, 6.4-6.7
    disorders, 6.1-6.20
      clinical features, 6.12-6.16
      management, 6.16-6.20
      signs and symptoms, 6.1
      surgery for, 6.20t
Mucosa
  intestinal, 3.3f
  small-bowel, inflammation, diarrhea with, 4.8f, 12.4t
Mucosal immune system, 4.8f
Mucosal transport
  abnormalities, in cholera, 1.14f
  heterogeneity, 1.10
  principles, 1.5-1.9
  regulation, 1.11-1.13
    immune, 1.11f, 1.12f
    intracellular, 1.13f
    neural, 1.11f
    paracrine, 1.11f
Mucus, intestinal
  barrier function, 1.2f
  secretion, 1.3f
Multilamellar vesicles, 2.8f
Multiple endocrine neoplasia, 4.12t
Muscularis mucosae, 3.3f
Myenteric plexus, 3.5f, 3.9f
Myofilaments, in small intestine, 3.4-3.7
Myopathy, intestinal, 6.14f
Myosin, 3.4f
  cross-bridges, 3.4f, 3.5f

    interaction with actin, 3.5f
Myosin light chain kinase, activation, 3.4f
Myosin phosphatase, 3.5f

N

Neoplastic diseases, of small intestine, 8.1-8.16
  benign vs. malignant, frequency, 8.2f
  bleeding with, 9.12f, 9.12t, 9.13t
  clinical presentation, 8.1
  diagnosis, 8.1
  endoscopic findings with, 9.13f
  epidemiology, 8.2t
  imaging, 8.1
  incidence, 8.2f
  low frequency of, proposed pathogenetic mechanisms, 8.3t
  malignant (See Adenocarcinoma; Carcinoid; Lymphoma)
  signs and symptoms, 8.3t
  small-bowel hemorrhage with, 9.2, 9.2f
Neurofibroma, of small intestine, 8.14f
Neuromodulators, in enteric nervous system, 3.9f
Neuromuscular disorders, gastroparesis in, 6.11t
Neuropathy, intestinal, manometric features, 6.15f
Neurotransmitters, 1.13f
  in enteric nervous system, 3.9f
NHEs. See Sodium/hydrogen exchangers
Niacin, deficiency, signs and symptoms, 5.16t
Nitric oxide
  in digestive function, 2.4f
  in vagal inhibition, 3.7f
Nitrogen, absorption
  with pancreatic insufficiency, 5.4f
  in short-bowel syndrome, 5.10f
Nonsteroidal anti-inflammatory drugs, bleeding caused by, 9.2, 9.2f
Nuclear medicine studies, with small-bowel bleeding, 9.3t, 9.4t
Nucleus of solitary tract, 3.8f, 3.9f
Nutrients
  absorption, 2.1-2.18
  dietary, 2.2f
  digestion, 2.1-2.18
  malabsorption (See Malabsorption)
  types, 2.1
Nutrition, in motility disorders, 6.16t
Nutritional support, 5.1-5.2
Nutritional therapy, complications, 5.19f

O

Obstruction
  intestinal, manometric features, 6.12f
  with small-bowel tumors, 8.3t

Octreotide
    for diarrhea, 4.23*f*
    prokinetic effects, 6.19*f*-6.20*f*
    for VIPoma, 4.15*f*
Oligopeptides, hydrolysis, 2.14*f*
    in brush border, 2.14*t*
Oligosaccharides, digestion, 2.11*f*
Opiates, for diarrhea, 4.23*f*
Oral cavity, in digestive process, 2.3*t*
Oral rehydration therapy
    mechanism of action, 4.22*f*
    and ostomy output, 5.12*f*
    for secretory diarrhea, 4.22*f*
    in short-bowel syndrome, 5.11*f*
Osler-Weber-Rendu syndrome, 9.10*t*
Osmotic gap, calculation, 4.3*f*
Ostomy. *See also* Ileostomy; Jejunostomy
    output
        oral rehydration therapy and, 5.12*f*
        zinc loss in, 5.14*f*

P

Pacemaker potentials, 3.6*f*
Pancreas, heterotopic, 8.12*f*
Pancreatic enzyme replacement, and intraluminal lipase activity, 5.3*f*
Pancreatic enzymes, proteolytic, 2.13*f*, 2.14*f*
Pancreatic exocrine function, evaluation, 5.18*f*
Pancreatic exocrine insufficiency, malabsorption with, 5.2-5.4
Pancreaticoduodenal arcade, 10.4*f*
Pancreatic secretion, 2.2*f*, 2.5*f*
Paneth cells, 1.3*f*
Paracellular pathway, 1.2*f*, 1.5*f*
Paracellular transport, 1.5*f*
Parasympathetic nervous system, 1.11*f*
Passive transport, 1.5*f*, 2.2
Pentasa. *See* Mesalamine
Pepsin
    activity, 2.4*f*, 2.13*f*
    formation, 2.13*f*
Pepsinogen I, secretion, 2.4*f*, 2.13*f*
Pepsinogen II, secretion, 2.4*f*, 2.13*f*
Peptidases, 2.14*f*
Peptide YY, release, 2.5*f*
Perforation, with small-bowel tumors, 8.3*t*
Periampullary tumors, 8.6*f*
Peristalsis, gastric, 2.4*f*
Peristaltic reflex, 3.10*f*
Peutz-Jeghers polyp, 8.13*f*
Phenolphthalein, detection, 4.11*t*
Pheochromocytoma, diarrhea with, 4.11*t*
Phlegmon, in fistulizing Crohn's disease of small intestine, 7.7*f*
Phosphate, as laxative, detection, 4.11*t*
Phosphatidic acid, 2.10*f*
Phosphoinositol, 1.13*f*
Phospholipase A$_2$, 2.8*f*
Phospholipase C, 1.13*f*

Phospholipid, average intake, 2.8*f*
Phospholipids, synthesis, in endoplasmic reticulum of enterocytes, 2.10*f*
Phosphorus, supplementation, in malnourished patient, 5.19*t*
PI. *See* Phosphoinositol
PINES (acronym), 1.11*f*, 1.14*f*
Plexuses, 3.5*f*, 3.9*f*
Pneumatosis intestinalis, 10.9*f*
    causes, 10.9*t*
Polyarteritis nodosa
    mesenteric vascular insufficiency with, 10.11*f*
    small-bowel bleeding with, 9.9*f*
Polyp(s)
    adenomatous, 8.4*f*, 8.5*f*
    bleeding with, 9.2, 9.2*f*
    juvenile, 8.13*f*
    lipomatous, 8.14*f*
    lymphomatous, 8.9*f*
    Peutz-Jeghers, 8.13*f*
Polysaccharides, intake, 2.11*f*
Potassium, supplementation, in malnourished patient, 5.19*t*
Potassium channels, 1.8*f*
Primary biliary cirrhosis, malabsorption with, 5.4*f*
Procarboxypeptidase, 2.13*f*
Proelastase, 2.13*f*
Prokinetic drugs, 6.16*t*, 6.17*f*, 6.17*t*, 6.18*f*, 6.19*f*-6.20*f*
Protein
    absorption, 2.12-2.15
        in short-bowel syndrome, 5.9*t*, 5.10*f*
    average intake, 2.12*f*
    deficiency, signs and symptoms, 5.16*t*
    dietary, 2.1, 2.2*f*
    digestion, 2.12-2.15
    recommended dietary allowance, 2.12*f*
    sorting, in intestinal cells, 1.4*f*
    structure, 2.12*f*
    synthesis, 2.1
    transport, in intestinal cells, 1.4*f*
Protein kinase C, 1.13*f*
Protein kinases, 1.13*f*
Proteolysis
    gastric, 2.13*f*
    in proximal small intestine, 2.14*f*
Protozoa, in HIV-infected (AIDS) patients, therapy for, 12.18*t*
Psammoma bodies, 7.12*f*
Pseudomembranous colitis, 12.14*f*
Pseudo-obstruction
    gastroparesis with, 6.7*t*
    intestinal
        acute, radiographic findings in, 6.12*f*
        chronic, 11.4*f*
            clinical features, 6.15*t*
            evaluation, 6.15*t*
            manometric features, 6.13*f*
            radiographic features, 6.13*f*
        classification, 6.13*f*
        etiology, 6.13*f*

    management, 6.16*t*
    motility disorder in, 3.15*f*
Pumps, 1.6*f*
Push enteroscopy, with small-bowel bleeding, 9.6*t*, 9.7*f*, 9.7*t*, 9.8*f*
Pyloric gland, hyperplasia, 8.12*f*
Pyridoxine, deficiency, signs and symptoms, 5.16*t*

R

Radiation enteritis, 7.13*f*
Radiation injury, to small intestine, 10.16*f*
Raynaud's phenomenon, 9.10*t*
Regional enteritis. *See* Crohn's disease of small intestine
Renzapride, 6.17*f*
R factors, 2.15*f*
Riboflavin, deficiency, signs and symptoms, 5.16*t*
Roux-en-Y anastomosis, gastric dysmotility after, 6.7*t*, 6.8*f*

S

Salivary secretion, 2.2*f*, 2.3*t*
Salmonella
    clinical syndromes caused by, 12.9*t*
    diarrhea caused by, 12.9-12.10
        pathogenesis, 12.3*f*
    infection
        complications, 12.9*t*
        pathogenesis, 12.9*f*
        reservoirs, 12.10*t*
        sources, 12.10*t*
    infectious levels, 12.4*t*
    susceptibility to, factors affecting, 12.9*t*
Salmonellosis. *See Salmonella*
Schabadasch's plexus externus. *See* Submucosal plexus
Scintigraphy
    indications for, 9.2
    in measurement of gastric emptying, 6.1-6.2, 6.2*f*, 6.3*f*
    in measurement of small-bowel transit, 6.6*f*, 6.6*t*
    with small-bowel bleeding, 9.4*t*
Sclerodactyly, 9.10*t*
Scleroderma
    gastroparesis in, 6.7*t*
    small-bowel transit in, measurement, 6.6*f*
Second messengers, 1.8*f*, 1.13*f*
Secretin, 2.1
    in regulation of digestive function, 2.5*f*
    release, 2.5*f*
Secretory vesicles, 2.10*f*
Segmenting waves, 3.1
Selenium
    absorption, 2.17*t*
    daily intake, 2.17*t*
Senna, detection, 4.11*t*

Serosa, 3.3f
Sham feeding response, 2.3f, 2.3t
Shiga toxin, cellular mechanisms, 12.11f
Shigella
    diarrhea caused by, 12.10-12.11
        pathogenesis, 12.3f
    infection
        complications, 12.10t
        microscopic findings in, 12.11f
        summary, 12.10t
        systemic manifestations, 12.10t
    infectious levels, 12.4t
Shigellosis. *See Shigella*
Short-bowel syndrome, 5.8-5.14
    calcium supplementation in, 5.13t
    calorie absorption in, 5.10f
    carbohydrate absorption in, 5.9t
    endoscopic findings in, 11.4f
    energy intake and energy requirements in,
        5.10f
    fat absorption in, 5.9t, 5.10f
    macronutrient absorption in, 5.9t
    magnesium deficiency in, 5.13t
    magnesium supplementation in, 5.13t
    nitrogen absorption in, 5.10f
    nutritional outcome in, 5.8t
    oral rehydration therapy in, 5.11f
    protein absorption in, 5.9t, 5.10f
    small-bowel transplantation for, 11.3f
    sodium balance in, 5.11f
    sodium-water absorption in, 5.11f
    therapeutic goals in, 5.9t
    trace mineral supplementation in, 5.14t
    vitamin supplementation in, 5.14t
    zinc losses in, 5.14f
Sickle-cell disease, intestinal ischemia in,
    10.16f
Signal transduction, 1.13f
Slow waves, 3.6f
Small-bowel transplantation, 11.1-11.14
    candidates for, 11.1
    complications, 11.6t, 11.6-11.13
    contraindications to, 11.1, 11.2t
    cytomegalovirus enteritis after, 11.12f
    endoscopic features assessed during
        surveillance after, 11.14t
    follow-up, 11.14t
    future directions, 11.2, 11.14t
    for gastroschisis, 11.3f
    indications for, 11.1, 11.2t
    lymphoproliferative disorder after, 11.13f
    operative procedure, 11.4f
    postoperative isolated, 11.13f
    post-transplantation anatomy, 11.8f
    post-transplantation bowel edema and
        dilatation, 11.7f
    preservation injury and abnormal motility
        after, 11.13f
    rejection
        acute
            endoscopic findings in, 11.8f, 11.10f
            histology, 11.9f, 11.10f
            intestinal mucosal blood flow with,

11.11f, 11.11t
        intraoperative view, 11.6f
        macroscopic view, 11.7f
    chronic, 11.11f
    for short-bowel syndrome, 11.3f
Small intestine
    anatomy, 3.2-3.7
    axial heterogeneity, 1.1
    bleeding (*See* Bleeding)
    cell types in, 1.3f
    contractile activity, measurement, trans-
        ducers for, 3.14f
    Crohn's disease (*See* Crohn's disease)
    electromyography, 6.6t
    epithelium, 1.1
    fluid and electrolyte absorption in, 1.1-
        1.14
    functional anatomy, 1.1-1.14, 1.2f
    innervation, 3.7-3.10
        extrinsic, 3.7-3.8
        intrinsic, 3.9
        parasympathetic pathways, 3.7f
        sensory pathways, 3.7f, 3.8f
        sympathetic pathways, 3.7f, 3.8f
    ischemic injury, 10.1 (*See also* Mesenteric
        vascular insufficiency)
    length, 3.2f
    local reflexes, 3.10f
    motility (*See* Motility, small-bowel)
    motor activity (*See also* Motility)
        assessment, 6.6t
    mucosal inflammation, diarrhea with,
        4.8f, 12.4t
    neoplastic diseases, 8.1-8.16
    radiation injury, 10.16f
    surface area, 1.2f
    transit, assessment, 6.6f, 6.6t
    transplantation (*See* Small-bowel trans-
        plantation)
    transport function
        factors affecting, 4.8f
        heterogeneity, 1.10f
    vertical heterogeneity, 1.1
Smooth muscle, intestinal, 3.3f
    contractile activity, 3.3f, 3.4f
    myofilaments, 3.4-3.7
Sodium
    absorption, 1.6f
        electrogenic, 1.8f
        glucose-stimulated, and oral rehydra-
            tion therapy, 4.22f
        nutrient-coupled, 1.7f
        in short-bowel syndrome, 5.11f
    balance, in short-bowel syndrome, 5.11f
    intake, in malnourished patient, 5.19t
Sodium-bicarbonate symport, 1.9f
Sodium channels, 1.6f, 1.8f
Sodium-chloride absorption, 1.7f
Sodium-glucose cotransport, and oral rehy-
    dration therapy, 4.22f
Sodium-glucose transporter, SGLT-1, 1.7f,
    2.12f
Sodium-hydrogen antiporter, 1.7f

Sodium-hydrogen exchange, 1.7f
Sodium-hydrogen exchangers, 1.9f
Sodium-potassium ATPase. *See* Sodium
    pump
Sodium-potassium-two chloride carrier, 1.8f
Sodium pump, 1.6f, 1.7f, 1.8f
Solute transport, 1.6f
Somatostatinoma, diarrhea with, 4.11t, 4.17f
Sonde enteroscopy, with small-bowel
    bleeding, 9.6t, 9.7f, 9.8t, 9.9f
Spike bursts, 3.7f
Splanchnic nerves, 3.8f
Stack of coins appearance, 7.13f
Starch
    components, 2.11f
    digestion, 2.11f
STa toxin, of *Vibrio cholerae*, 12.5t
Steatorrhea, 5.2f
    detection, 5.17f
    with diarrhea, 5.18f
    with primary biliary cirrhosis, 5.4f
Stem cells, 1.4f
Steroids, for Crohn's disease of small intes-
    tine, 7.16f
Stomach
    functions, 2.1
    protein digestion in, 2.13f
Stool
    fat (*See* Fat, fecal; Steatorrhea)
    fat concentrations, in steatorrhea, 5.2f
    osmolality, 4.3f
Stromal cell tumor, of small intestine, 8.1,
    8.9-8.11. *See also* Leiomyoma;
    Leiomyosarcoma
Submucosa, intestinal, 3.3f
Submucosal plexus, 3.5f, 3.9f
Sucrase-isomaltase, 2.11f
Sucrose, intake, 2.11f
Sulfasalazine, for Crohn's disease of small
    intestine, 7.15f
Sulfate, as laxative, detection, 4.11t
Superior mesenteric artery
    anatomy, 10.2f, 10.3f
    arteriography, 10.3f
    embolic occlusion, 10.8f
    stenosis, Doppler duplex scanning in,
        10.19t
Superior mesenteric artery syndrome, 10.17f
Surgery, for gastrointestinal dysmotility, 6.20t
Symport, 1.6f
Systemic lupus erythematosus, mesenteric
    vascular insufficiency in, 10.12f

T

Technetium 99m-labeled RBC, with small-
    bowel bleeding, 9.4t
Technetium 99m-labeled sulfur colloid, in
    assessment of intestinal fluid
    flow, 3.13f
Technetium 99m-sodium pertechnetate scan,
    with small-bowel bleeding, 9.5t

Technetium 99m-sulfur colloid scan, with small-bowel bleeding, 9.4*t*

Telangiectasia, 9.10*t*

Thiamine, deficiency, signs and symptoms, 5.16*t*

Thyroid carcinoma, medullary, diarrhea with, 4.11*t*, 4.16*f*

Tight junctions, 1.5*f*

Total parenteral nutrition
costs, 11.2*f*
liver injury from, 11.1, 11.4*f*
prolonged, 11.1
survival, 11.2*f*

Trace elements, 2.1, 2.2*f*
absorption, 2.17*t*
daily intake, 2.17*t*
supplementation, in short-bowel syndrome, 5.14*t*

Transcellular transport, 1.5*f*

Transducers, for measurement of contractile activity, 3.14*f*

Transit, gastrointestinal
breath hydrogen test for, 3.12*f*
definition, 3.12*f*

Transplantation, of small intestine. *See* Small-bowel transplantation

Trauma, intestinal ischemia related to, 10.17*f*

Traveler's diarrhea
causes, 12.14*f*
differential diagnosis, 12.15*t*
prophylaxis, 12.15*t*

Triglycerides
average intake, 2.8*f*
digestion, 2.8*f*
structure, 2.8*f*
synthesis, in endoplasmic reticulum of enterocytes, 2.10*f*

Tripeptides, transport, 2.14*f*

Trypsin, 2.13*f*, 2.14*f*

Trypsinogen, 2.13*f*

Tuberculosis, intestinal involvement, 7.13*f*

Tumors. *See* Neoplastic diseases

U

Ulcers, bleeding caused by, 9.2, 9.2*f*, 9.9*f*, 9.13*t*

Unstirred layer, 1.2*f*

V

Vagus nerve, 3.7*f*, 3.8*f*
dorsal motor nucleus, 3.7*f*, 3.9*f*

Valvulae conniventes, 3.2*f*

Varices, small-bowel, bleeding caused by, 9.2, 9.2*f*

Vascular anomalies
with associated skin lesions, 9.10*t*
classification, 9.10*t*
not associated with skin lesions, 9.10*t*
small-bowel hemorrhage with, 9.2, 9.2*f*, 9.9*f*

Vascular ectasia, 9.10*t*

Vascular resistance, 10.5*t*

Vasculitis, mesenteric vascular insufficiency with, 10.11-10.12

Vasoactive intestinal polypeptide, 2.4*f*

Verner-Morrison syndrome, 4.12*t*
diarrhea in, 4.11*t*, 4.15*f*

Very low density lipoproteins, 2.10*f*

Vibrio cholerae
infectious levels, 12.4*t*
toxins elaborated by, 12.5*t*

Villus, ischemic, 10.5*f*

VIPoma, diarrhea with, 4.12*f*, 4.14*f*

Vitamin A, deficiency, signs and symptoms, 5.16*t*

Vitamin B$_{12}$
absorption, 1.10*f*, 2.2, 2.6*f*, 2.15*f*
daily requirement, 2.15*f*
deficiency, signs and symptoms, 5.16*t*

Vitamin C, deficiency, signs and symptoms, 5.16*t*

Vitamin E, deficiency, signs and symptoms, 5.16*t*

Vitamin K, deficiency, signs and symptoms, 5.16*t*

Vitamins, 2.1, 2.2*f*
fat-soluble, absorption, 2.16*f*
supplementation, in short-bowel syndrome, 5.14*t*
water-soluble
absorption, 2.15*f*, 2.16*f*
transport, in enterocytes, 2.16*f*

VLDL. *See* Very low density lipoproteins

Volvulus
mesenteric vascular insufficiency with, 10.13-10.14
midgut
ischemia secondary to, 10.13*f*
radiographic findings in, 10.13*f*, 10.14*t*

W

Water
absorption
intestinal, 4.2*f*
in short-bowel syndrome, 5.11*f*
fluxes, intestinal, 4.2*f*
as laxative, detection, 4.11*t*
transport, during steady-state total gut perfusion, 4.3*f*

Watershed regions, 10.4*f*

Whipple's disease, malabsorption with, 5.8*f*

X

d-Xylose, in evaluation of small-bowel absorptive function, 5.17*f*

Y

Yersinia enterocolitica
diarrhea caused by, 12.12
ileitis, radiographic appearance, 12.12*f*
infection, 12.12*t*

Z

Zacopride, 6.17*f*

Zinc
absorption, 2.17*t*
daily intake, 2.17*t*
deficiency, signs and symptoms, 5.16*t*
excretion, 5.14*f*
loss, and stool output, 5.14*f*
supplementation, in short-bowel syndrome, 5.14*t*

Zollinger-Ellison syndrome, 4.12*t*, 7.13*f*
diarrhea in, 4.11*t*, 4.13*f*
pathogenesis, 4.13*f*
treatment, 4.14*f*

Zona adherens, 1.5*f*

Zona occludens, 1.5*f*

Zona occludens toxin, 1.14*f*
mechanism of action, 12.5*t*

ZOT. *See* Zona occludens toxin